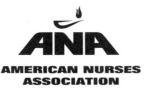

AMERICAN NURSES
ASSOCIATION

D0127275

Nursing and Health Care Ethics
A Legacy and A Vision

Winifred J. Ellenchild Pinch, RN, EdD, FAAN
Amy M. Haddad, BSN, MSN, PhD
EDITORS

American Nurses Association
Silver Spring, MD • 2008

Library of Congress Cataloging-in-Publication data

Nursing and healthcare ethics : a legacy and a vision / editors, Winifred J. Ellenchild Pinch, Amy M. Haddad.
    p. ; cm.
  Includes bibliographical references and index.
   ISBN-13: 978-1-55810-261-3 (soft cover)
   ISBN-10: 1-55810-261-2 (soft cover)
  1. Nursing ethics. 2. Medical ethics. I. Pinch, Winifred. II. Haddad, Amy Marie.
  III. American Nurses Association.
  [DNLM: 1. Ethics, Nursing. 2. Nursing Research--ethics. 3. Nursing Theory.
  WY 85 N9742 2008]
  RT85.N877 2008
  174.2'9073--dc22

                                                              2008037136

The opinions in this book reflect those of the authors and do not necessarily reflect positions or policies of the American Nurses Association. Furthermore, the information in this book should not be construed as legal or other professional advice.

Published by Nursesbooks.org
The Publishing Program of ANA

American Nurses Association
8515 Georgia Avenue, Suite 400
Silver Spring, MD 20910-3492
1-800-274-4ANA
http://www.nursesbooks.org/

ANA is the only full-service professional organization representing the nation's 2.9 million Registered Nurses through its 54 constituent member associations. ANA advances the nursing profession by fostering high standards of nursing practice, promoting the economic and general welfare of nurses in the workplace, projecting a positive and realistic view of nursing, and lobbying the Congress and regulatory agencies on healthcare issues affecting nurses and the public.

Page and cover design: Laura C. Johnson, Grammarians, Inc., Alexandria, VA
Development editing: Rosanne O'Connor Roe ⌒ *Production editing:* Eric Wurzbacher
Copyediting: Steven A. Jent, Denton, TX ⌒ *Proofreading:* Ashley Mason, Atlanta, GA
Indexing: Estalita Slivoskey, Ellendale, ND
Composition: Laura C. Johnson, Grammarians, Inc.
Printing: McArdle Printing, Upper Marlboro, MD

ISBN-13: 978-1-55810-261-3   SAN: 851-3481   3.5   5M   09/08

First printing September 2008.

Acknowledgments

As co-editors of this book, we are most grateful for the opportunities afforded us through our work at the Center for Health Policy and Ethics (CHPE) at Creighton University. We are especially indebted to the University and the Vice President for Health Sciences and Dean of the School of Medicine, Cam Enarson, MD, for supporting the project through his affirmation of directing CHPE resources to it when external funding sources were not possible. In addition, we thank the School of Nursing and its Dean, Eleanor Howell, PhD, RN, who offered to support an event at the seminar when all of the participants convened at Creighton University. To her credit, the School sponsored the Dorothy Vossen Lecture and dinner as the opening event for the Legacy Seminar.

As we moved through the several years of planning and implementation of the project, beginning in the spring of 2005 with our initial musings about a focus on nursing ethics, the project would have not come to fruition unless we had the kind of staff support that exists at the Center. These individuals were priceless not only in their work as it related to the specific needs of the project, but they were also excellent prospective thinkers and problem solvers as various needs arose. The staff included Becky Crowell, Marybeth Goddard, Chris Jorgensen, Helen Shew, and Kate Tworek. We also owe our deepest appreciation to every one of the nurse scholars and other invited participants we contacted, even those who because of conflicts were unable to participate in our project. We in turn want them all to know how much they are respected and admired for their contributions to ethics and the profession of nursing above and beyond this project. As these individuals were contacted, we were met with the highest level of interest, cooperation, and praise for our endeavors which continued throughout the project.

In the early drafts of the papers, every participant in our project wanted to extend thanks to many persons, but given the space constraints we were unable to include those individual expressions of gratitude. Instead we want to emphasize here that they all mentioned a multitude of people: their families, our Center and Creighton University, mentors, teachers, colleagues, students, deans, librarians, and not least of all, patients. Finally, in the course of planning the project and recognizing the need for professional facilitators during a seminar of the caliber we anticipated, we would like to thank John Hall, Vice President, Client Services, of Right Management Consultants, who was so impressed by the plan for the seminar that he volunteered his services. As the seminar neared, Sue Twitt, also of Right Management Consultants, joined in the seminar to assist John. The seminar greatly benefited from their very active roles; their energy and enthusiasm could not have been higher. The gathering was particularly inspirational. We close with thanks for anyone we might have inadvertently missed who deserves specific recognition. There were many details involved in a project of such magnitude and we were awed by how seamlessly it finally came to completion.

Winifred J. Ellenchild Pinch
Amy M. Haddad

Permissions

"Suffering" by Cortney Davis in Section IX. First published in *The Body Flute*. Copyright © 1994 by Cortney Davis. Reprinted by permission of the author.

"There Are No Poems at Hospital Management Meetings" by Cortney Davis in Section III. Published in a special issue called *Workers Write! Tales from the Clinic* published by Blue Cubicle Press (2008). Copyright © 1994 by Cortney Davis. Reprinted by permission of the author.

"To the Mother of the Burned Children" by Cortney Davis in Section V. First published in *Kaleidoscope: International Magazine of Literature, Fine Arts and Disability*. Copyright © 1994 by Cortney Davis. Reprinted by permission of the author.

The quote on page 139 in Section IV, Chapter 12 was first published in the article "Champions of Human Rights and Social Reform" by G. Rockfield in *The College of New Rochelle Alumnae Magazine*. Copyright © 2006 by The College of New Rochelle. Reprinted by permission of the publisher.

The quote on page 48 in Section V, Chapter 15 was first published in *Nursing, Images and Ideals: Opening Dialogue with the Humanities* by S. F. Spicker and S. Gadow. Copyright © 1980 by Springer Publishing Company, Inc.

The quote on page 234 in Section VII, Chapter 21 was first published in *Essentials of Teaching and Learning in Nursing Ethics: Perspectives and Methods* by A. J. Davis, V. Tschudin, & L. de Raeve (Eds.). Copyright © 2006 by Elsevier Limited. Reprinted by permission of the publisher.

The quote on page 308 in Amy M. Haddad's essay "Endnotes: A Mix of Metaphors" was first published in *Metaphors We Live By* by G. Lakoff and M. Johnson. Copyright © 1980 by University of Chicago Press. Reprinted by permission of the publisher.

The quote on page 310 in Amy M. Haddad's essay "Endnotes: A Mix of Metaphors" was first published in *The Cancer Journals* by Audre Lorde. Copyright © 1980 by Aunt Lute Books. Reprinted by permission of the publisher.

American Nurses Association Code of Ethics for Nurses in Appendix A. Used with permission from American Nurses Association.

The Evolution of the Nursing Code of Ethics in Appendix B. Used with permission from American Nurses Association.

ANA Center for Ethics and Human Rights Mission Statement in Appendix C. Used with permission from American Nurses Association.

Contents

Appendixes

Winifred J. Ellenchild Pinch

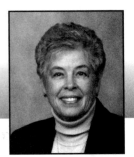

Preface: Crafting a Dream

For a nurse ethicist, gathering a group of outstanding scholars in nursing ethics in order to discuss and exchange ideas is a dream come true. Motivation to consider such an undertaking came from a belief that the dawn of the 21st century was an appropriate time to examine the unique contributions of nurses to ethics and health care. As with many health professionals, nursing has an extensive history of explicit scholarly work in ethics. Beginning with the Nursing Studies Index, a heading of "ethics" existed for organizing manuscripts covering the years 1900 to 1959 (Henderson, 1963, 1966, 1970, 1972). Of course, most of those early scholars were no longer available for ethical research, debate, or dialogue. However, more germane to the current scholarship in nursing, ethics, and health care was the specific set of circumstances which Jonsen designates as the "birth of bioethics" (1993, 1998). In his book, he sets the stage for the genesis of modern bioethics in "academic medicine, medical practice, and public policy" (Jonsen, 1998, p. xiii).

Jonsen began his chronology in the late 1960s when bioethical discourse was largely focused on the physician-patient relationship and ensuing ethical problems as they existed in the clinical and research contexts. In general, physicians did not usually seek advice or consultation from outside the profession although they eventually faced several challenges that motivated them to begin to do so. Advances in science and technology provided practitioners with a vast array of treatment options for their patients. Not all of these approaches were successful; rather many left patients without a cure—neither improved nor dead. Naturally these physicians were then confronted with the ethical responsibility to decide whether to continue aggressive treatment. Additionally, questions arose regarding options for future patients.

In the late 1950s and early 1960s, philosophers and theologians began to grapple with those ethical dilemmas as defined by physicians. There was a demand to replace abstract and analytical discussions with "practical, concrete and even political terms" in this developing discipline of bioethics (Toulmin, 1982, p. 749). Subsequently a shift occurred in the discourse from theoretical to functional. Therefore, mainstream bioethics evolved into a more narrowly defined dialogue focusing on the practice of medicine. As the decades passed, ethical debate became broader, covering the entire breadth of the health care arena. Scholars gradually became more aware of the complexity of health care delivery and the role of other health professionals.

In large part, the role of the nurse in the early bioethical dilemmas or case studies was often omitted or ignored, yet their provision of the health care services in most circumstances was integral to the problem solving or outcome. Those nurses were enmeshed in the same dilemmas addressed by the physicians, theologians, and philosophers (Jonsen, 1998). However, scholars in nursing were already addressing a wide variety of ethical issues and pursuing their own examination of problems the profession faced in numerous practice areas—often unrecognized by the field at large. The profession of nursing reached a significant crossroads whereby in this most recent, modern phase of bioethics (beginning about the late 1960s into the early 1970s), early scholars as well as newer faces and voices are contributing together to advance scholarship in nursing ethics.

At this point, several questions come to mind. How can these contributions positively affect professional practice for a variety of situations: in the individual patient-professional relationship, the professional in the service institution, or in the broader community, country, or world? Collectively, what do these voices say? How did the investigations of nurse ethicists differ from other scholarly work in bioethics? The meaning of this work for the broader field of health care ethics and for the future requires further exploration. No previous project in ethics convened a group of nurse ethics scholars in one place to examine and discuss their total contributions to health care ethics and to capture these contributions in one source for future generations of nurses.

Since this birth of bioethics, nurses continued to address ethical issues in practice like the early scholars (1900–1960) who preceded them but with some different strategies and goals. Nurses began to obtain specialized education and skills in this area to enhance the credibility of their scholarship. Opportunities included the Joseph P. Kennedy, Jr., Foundation Fellowships in Medical Ethics; the Intensive Bioethics Course offered by the Joseph and Rose Kennedy Institute of Ethics at Georgetown University; the National Endowment for the Humanities summer seminars; doctorates with a concentration in bioethics; and postdoctoral fellowships. Obviously, until formal educational opportunities expanded, these programs served a limited number of professionals. Also a number of nurses, even with these options, simply chose to emphasize bioethics in existing doctoral programs or complete clinical internships with an emphasis on ethics. Interest and preparation for work in the area by nurses intensified over the next three or more decades, and they took their scholarship in a number of different directions after completing such experiences. Over those years, membership and leadership roles that focused on bioethics were enacted in conferences, meetings, committees, institutes, and associations.

The focus of scholarly activity in ethics and nursing took various paths. Early scholars were more likely to pattern their contributions in a manner similar to the work of philosophers, theologians, and physicians who targeted general health care and the ethical problems that arose there. As the cohort of nurse ethicists grew it also carved out new areas for discussion and debate. In some cases there was a significant paradigm shift represented by the work in nursing ethics. For example, the work of nurses focused on the patient's perspective, which was minimized or omitted from the earlier discussions in medical ethics. Another characteristic of nurse scholars' contributions to bioethics included their comfort using both quantitative and qualitative approaches in their research in ethics.

A certain maturity factor operated in the discipline as well. Bioethics experienced its own growth phases. Forty-plus years of influence in health care brought bioethics to a point where the legacy of early contributors should be examined in the context of the challenging complexity of present health care delivery. Subsequently, a look into the future was warranted in order to set goals for a path other scholars could follow. Therefore, a multistage project was planned by Dr. Haddad and me to document the legacy and vision of these nurse ethicists in a book.

Utilizing the expertise of all or even a majority of nurse scholars in ethics to implement such an ethics project would have been impractical and unmanageable. To begin the search for possible participants, a list of the publications in nursing ethics cited in CINAHL was first examined. Next the authors of those publications were noted, and leading scholars who played various leadership roles in bioethics conferences, professional associations, and related ethics events were identified. Both the individuals' credentials and the content of their publications were examined. The process was necessarily selective. A list of possible nurse scholars was prepared and the themes of their work noted. The selected individuals, however, were representative of both noted scholars who have been active in the creation of scholarship in bioethics and nursing, as well as more recent contributors, building on the work of those early scholars. A balance was sought among these individuals including such factors as their interdisciplinary connections, practice settings, areas of expertise, and research contributions.

Eight themes were identified through this examination of the work of these scholars to best represent their combined work in bioethics. The themes were philosophical and theoretical issues; political, administrative, and systems aspects; perspectives on advocacy; relationship issues; concerns related to vulnerability; care and caring in nursing; diversity and disparity issues; and pain and suffering. Assignment to a theme did not imply its sole representation in any one individual's work. Rather these themes and other concepts as well appeared across a number of different publications.

The list of potential participants was developed and contact began. Scholars who agreed to participate in the project prepared essays summarizing their career and contributions to ethics (legacy) as well as their thoughts about the impact of their work and implications for the future (vision)—the first stage in the project. The second stage included a working seminar, the Legacy seminar. DeMarco, Horowitz, and McCurry (2005) lament the "valuable opportunities for professional growth" that are missed when critique and dialogue at scholarly conferences do not occur (p. 232). Although their model for "giving voice to critique" (p. 236) does not transfer directly to the present project, their observation that the profession of nursing would benefit from constructive scholarly dialogue supported the implementation of the Legacy seminar. Bringing nurse scholars in ethics together to directly share their ideas with one another, to discuss, explore, and debate these ideas, as well as forge a vision for the future in health care ethics, is based upon similar strategies and goals. Essays were submitted prior to the seminar so the joint meeting time could be devoted to an exchange of ideas related to the themes and their papers, rather than a presentation of the papers.

The exception to this strategy was the keynote address, The Institutionalization of Nursing Ethics, which was not distributed prior to the gathering but rather delivered when the participants met the evening prior to the working sessions. The seminar itself was organized around the eight major themes and the papers related to those themes (see the Table of Contents). Themes from Sections II through V were scheduled the first day and Sections VI through IX the second day. The group facilitators monitored the sessions, and although participants were provided with 30 minutes for a discussion of their papers, only 5 to 10 minutes were allowed for a brief introduction of the participants' ideas. The facilitators were diligent in keeping the group on schedule so that everyone's allotted time was respected. After attending the very exciting and meaningful two-day seminar, participants returned home to revise their papers for this publication, the final stage.

Papers varied in the degree of revision, often depending upon the stage of preparation prior to the seminar and the individual's response to her colleagues' commentary. Although participants were directed to prepare "manuscript length" papers, these were later edited to about 10 pages each for publication. Of course some details were lost, but the essence of each contribution remained and major events and ideas faithfully reflect each person's story. One of the exceptional benefits of the gathering for us, the editors, was the establishment of each participant's commitment to the Legacy project and for some, the recognition of the need to continue and expand the dialogue initiated at the seminar.

Given the historical importance of the gathering and the unique nature of the Legacy seminar itself, both a nurse historian and a medical sociologist were invited to attend. These individuals observed the dynamics of the seminar and carefully noted the content as discussion ensued over the two days. Subsequently each wrote a reflective paper related to the seminar itself based on the expertise and particular analytical skills they brought to the event. Their contributions would not have been as relevant if they had not been part of the working seminar. A humanities dimension was also planned and is represented by a poet who selected pieces of her work reflecting each of the seminar's themes.

The results of this project are now offered to the reader. Readers include not only undergraduates and graduate students in academic settings, but also those in professional development programs. Although nurses in varying types of professional practice would benefit from examining and discussing the different essays, other health professionals as well as philosophers, theologians, and anthropologists interested in health care would find the contributions enlightening. The Critical Thinking Activities provide examples of a range of possible strategies to utilize not only with the designated theme but also revised appropriately to target additional essays. After several years of work—dreaming, planning, and implementing our ideas—we can say that we have captured a unique point of view on nursing and ethics as portrayed in the contributions from this stellar group of nurse scholars and other contributors.

References

DeMarco, R. F., Horowitz, J. A., & McCurry, M. K. (2005). Effective use of critique and dialogue at scholarly conferences. *Nursing Outlook, 53*(5), 232–238.

Henderson, V. (1963). *Nursing studies index 1957–1959* (Volume IV). Philadelphia: J. B. Lippincott Company.

Henderson, V. (1966). *Nursing studies index 1950–1956* (Volume III). Philadelphia: J. B. Lippincott Company.

Henderson, V. (1970). *Nursing studies index 1930–1949* (Volume II). Philadelphia: J. B. Lippincott Company.

Henderson, V. (1972). *Nursing studies index 1900–1929* (Volume I). Philadelphia: J. B. Lippincott Company.

Jonsen, A. R. (Ed.). (1993). The birth of bioethics, Special supplement. *Hastings Center Report, 23*(6), S1–S16.

Jonsen, A. R. (1998). *The birth of bioethics.* New York: Oxford University Press.

Toulmin, S. (1982). How medicine saved the life of ethics. *Perspectives in Biology and Medicine, 25*(4), 736–750.

Warren T. Reich

Foreword: The Legacy of Nursing Ethics

It is a privilege to offer the foreword to such an important work on the legacy and vision of nursing and health care ethics.

The purpose of this book is to document the work of nurse scholars in ethics, but it effectively goes well beyond a mere documentation of what has transpired and a list of what can be done in the future. It creatively looks back to assess previous accomplishments and forward to find new directions and strengthen future scholarly contributions of scholars in nursing ethics.

This book fills a real need. Although thousands of articles and books appear annually in the field of nursing ethics, the sheer volume of scholarly publications points to the need to provide assessment and focus, and that is what this book offers.

Furthermore, publications in nursing ethics have a quality that is unique among the various components of the broader field described as bioethics. Nurse scholars, more than others, tend to describe and argue for new theories and explanations to account for their experiences, insights, and ethical analyses. Those theories and explanations have become so numerous that they require a fresh assessment so as to give intellectual guidance and scholarly direction to the field. This book, produced by what its initiators have called "The Legacy Project," is designed to offer that sort of helpful analysis.

What I find most fascinating and creative about this book is the way Winifred Pinch, Amy Haddad, and their colleagues have organized it around a rich set of major themes: philosophical and theoretical issues; political, administrative, and systems aspects; advocacy; relationship; vulnerability; caring and care; diversity and disparities; and pain and suffering. I'm convinced that only nurse scholars would have selected this range and depth of issues; no other group within the broader field of bioethics and health-related humanities would be expected to take this approach. The diversified set of themes selected for inclusion in this work provides it with depth of analysis and clarity of focus; its method of combining poetry with philosophical analysis and "critical thinking activities," and the inclusion of work by experts in historical and sociological approaches challenge the reader in a very comprehensive sort of way.

Finally, a word about the distinctiveness of the nursing ethics that is examined and proposed in this work. Some 40 years ago the field of bioethics was born; it has been a broad field of learning, with characteristics never found before in any of the humanities or life sciences. Nonetheless, as proposed by some leading scholars, bioethics quickly became rather strongly medicalized: one profession—the medical profession and its traditional medical ethics—has tended to dominate the concerns, goals, and products of bioethics. However, that emphasis does not really reflect the global, interdisciplinary, and interprofessional character of the initial ethos of bioethics.

This book provides a major argument why nursing ethics does not need to chronicle its evolution or measure its importance against a historical standard that has insinuated itself into the center stage of bioethics. The larger field of bioethics should afford equal standing to the celebrated life-and-death issues involving established centers of power and the more hidden issues of home nursing care for the unknown, neglected, and vulnerable poor. This book, which in so many ways arises from and returns to the nurse–patient relationship, nicely reaches back to a rich past and forward to an even richer future of a distinctive nursing ethics. That is as it should be.

SECTION I

Historical and Sociological Issues

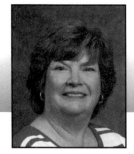

Laurie Badzek

CHAPTER 1

Legacy and Vision: The Perspective of the American Nurses Association on Nursing and Health Care Ethics

A s I ponder the legacy and vision of nursing ethics, I am overcome with an emotion best described as pride. I am proud to be a nurse and to be counted as a member of the most trusted and honorable profession. As the current Director at the Center for Ethics and Human Rights (1998–99; 2003–present), I am privileged to be both a member and a leader in the American Nurses Association (ANA). The role of the director is to ensure that considerations of ethics and human rights are integral to the association's activities and to further the guiding objectives of the Center. In my role at the ANA, I have had the opportunity to share with colleagues and the public knowledge of the organization and its objectives. I am humbled and honored to have had the privilege of meeting the editors and the authors of this book, as well as countless other nurses, who value nursing ethics and believe as I do that ethics is the foundation for nursing practice.

For over a century, nurses have identified ethical issues, shared information and knowledge related to ethics, developed strategies to address issues impacting the ethics of nursing practice, and subscribed to a code of ethical conduct. Much of the work in nursing ethics has been supported by ANA. As a full-service professional organization in existence for over 100 years, ANA represents the nation's 2.9 million registered nurses (RNs) through 54 constituent member associations. The core purpose of ANA (2006) is stated as "nurses advancing [the] profession for the health of all." This purpose is accomplished by fostering high standards of nursing practice, promoting the rights of nurses in the workplace, projecting a positive and realistic view of nursing, and lobbying the Congress and regulatory agencies on health care issues affecting nurses and the public.

In 1896, when representatives of the Nurses' Associated Alumnae of the United States and Canada, later incorporated in 1901 as the ANA, met in New York to establish a constitution and articles of incorporation, one clearly stated purpose was to establish and maintain a code of ethics. Informally since ANA's inception and formally since 1921 (ANA, 1991), there has been a specific entity or committee within ANA that addresses ethical issues and nursing practice. Members of ANA through their collective voices have identified and clarified the values and commitments of the nursing profession. These core values have withstood the test of time. Values and commitments in nursing today may be interpreted in a new or different social context; however, the essence of the values remains unchanged.

A profession by its very definition is a group defined by a code of ethics. Even though the initial members of ANA struggled to come to consensus on what should be included in the profession's ethical code, the need and desire for a formal code was present from the beginning and remains a foundation of the organization today. After rejecting two problematic proposed documents in 1926 and 1940, the ANA delegates formally and unanimously adopted the first formal *Code for Professional Nurses* in 1950 at the national business meeting (ANA, 1991).

Our current *Code of Ethics for Nurses with Interpretive Statements* (see Appendix A) reflects both the commitments and ideals of nurses from the past, in the present, and into the future. The 2001 *Code of Ethics for Nurses with Interpretive Statements* articulates enduring core values in a contemporary, useful statement of nurses' ethical obligations and duties. Many of the ethical beliefs within the current Code can be traced to similar values and commitments found in the writing of Florence Nightingale (1860/1969), contained within the Nightingale Pledge (Gretter, 1893 as cited in Roberts, 2007), and articulated in the initial 1950 *Code for Professional Nurses*. The document although grounded in history and nurses' long-held beliefs about professional duties and values provides an ethical framework for decision-making that is responsive to current nursing practice and a changing world. The *Code of Ethics for Nurses* is not negotiable and only through formal processes within the ANA can the Code be changed (ANA, 1994). The values and commitments of nurses found in the ethical code assure the public that nurses will advocate to protect the rights of patients and provide quality nursing care. This foundational document is nursing's most treasured and enduring legacy.

The authors of this book are some of the most famous and prolific nurses of our time. Most, if not all, are leaders in nursing ethics whose contributions have been instrumental in guiding the profession and the public to a better understanding of nursing ethics. These authors through their individual and collective work have contributed to ANA's legacy and current vision of nursing ethics. A majority of the book authors are among the nurses who have had a significant impact on the current or past versions of the *Code of Ethics for Nurses*. Several authors were instrumental in the formation of the ANA Center for Ethics and Human Rights. Two authors served prior to my tenure in the position of the Director of the ANA Center for Ethics and Human Rights. The first director was Gladys White, MSN, PhD (1990–92; 2000–03). Colleen Scanlon, MS, JD, served as the second director from 1992–1998. Both contributed immensely to the development of the Center and the creation of important policies and documents. The guiding objectives set for the Center when it became operational on September 4, 1990, are still in use today (see Appendix C).

A formal advisory board created in 1991 guides the work of the Center. Winifred Ellenchild Pinch, EdD, and Mila Aroskar, EdD, two noted nursing ethics leaders, an editor and author respectively for this book, served as ethics experts on the first advisory board. Dr. Aroskar, now retired, continued to serve the committee both as a member and Chair for over a decade. Issues addressed by the Center in the first decade of its existence included advance directives, assisted suicide, capital punishment, and the revision of the 1985 *Code for Nurses*. More current topics addressed by the Center relate to stem cell research, genomics competencies for nurses, and torture and abuse of prisoners. Pamela Miya, PhD, another nursing leader and author included in this book, serves as the current Chair of the Center advisory board. Dr. Miya with knowledge of the legacy and its strong foundation is responsible for leading the current advisory board in the creation of a vision for the future. The contributions of all the authors are too numerous to list.

The current vision of nursing and health care ethics at ANA revolves around addressing emerging issues that will likely have a profound impact on future health. Emerging issues include but are not limited to genetics, technology, safety, and resources. Each year new issues become known that require nurses at the forefront of patient care to reflect and draw upon the strength, knowledge, and traditions from the past. This collection of writings, along with available contributions from other nurses related to nursing and ethics, will provide further guidance and support for the cornerstone work of ANA and the Center for Ethics and Human Rights both now and in the future. The nursing ethics legacy at ANA is strong, the profession reflects a proud heritage, and the vision for the future is bright.

References

American Nurses Association. (1991). *Informational report: Progress report on integrating ethics and human rights in the American Nurses Association* introduced by L. Joel, President. (Available from the American Nurses Association, 8515 Georgia Avenue, Suite 400, Silver Spring, MD 20910-3492).

American Nurses Association. (1994). *Position statement on the non-negotiable nature of the Code of Ethics.* Available to members at http://www.nursingworld.org

American Nurses Association. (2006). *Annual report: A global enterprise...Caring for those who care.* Available to members at: http://www.nursingworld.org

Gretter, L. E. (1893). *The Florence Nightingale Pledge.* Detroit, MI: Farrand Training School for Nurses, Harper Hospital.

Nightingale, F. (1969). *Notes on nursing: What it is, and what it is not.* New York: Dover. (Original work published in 1860).

Roberts, C. (2007). Museum news. Retrieved November 24, 2007, from http://www.florence-nightingale.co.uk/collection

Laurie Badzek, RN, MS, JD, LLM, is currently Director for the American Nurses Association Center of Ethics and Human Rights, a role in which she previously served from 1998–1999. During that time, Badzek was instrumental in developing a plan that ultimately resulted in the approval of a new Code of Ethics for Nurses by the 2001 House of Delegates. Currently a tenured, full professor at the West Virginia University School of Nursing, Badzek, a nurse attorney, teaches nursing, ethics, law and health policy. Having practiced in a variety of nursing and law positions, she is an active researcher, investigating ethical and legal health care issues. Her current research interests include patient and family decision making, nutraceutical use, mature minors and professional health care ethics. Her research has been published in nursing, medical and communication studies journals including the *Journal of Nursing Law, Nephrology Nursing Journal, Annals of Internal Medicine, Journal of Palliative Care,* and *Health Communication.*

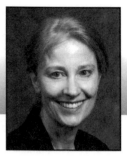

Patricia D'Antonio

CHAPTER 2

Nursing and Health Care Ethics: A Legacy

To provide the historical context for understanding the seminal contributions made by nursing's ethics scholars, one would first turn to the body of historical research on this subject, read it, and then reorganize themes and arguments in such a way as to create a sense of direction for succeeding remarks. There is, to be sure, substantive research on the history of medical ethics.[1] But to date, relatively little attention has been paid, as historian Beth Linker (2005, p. 320) points out, to the meaning of the post-World War I "ethics boom," when most self-identified American professional groups—including nursing and others both inside and outside the health care arena—began outlining, deliberating, and ultimately codifying their own standards of principled practice.[2] We do know that the American Nurses Association formally endorsed its own Code of Ethics in 1950.

But I am a historian trained to see documents not only as consensus statements of purpose and vision, but also as windows into the expression of sharp conflicts, deep divisions, and dearly held beliefs. I wonder, then, why American nurses came relatively late to the ratification of a Code of Ethics, even among predominately female professions: the Dental Hygienist Association ratified its Code in 1923, the American Physiotherapy Association in 1935, and the American Association for Social Workers in 1947. I wonder why the 1926 editors of the *American Journal of Nursing* believed they were presenting a code that, in their words, "bears the scars of past conflicts." And why they felt they were girding for battle and for the "expected avalanche of criticism..." they knew awaited (A Code of Ethics, p. 622).

Such kinds of historical questions and consciousness also pervade the chapters in this book. Contributors know of their place in the lineage of ethics thought leaders that begins with Florence Nightingale and continues through the early 20th century with Isabel Hampton Robb, Charlotte Aikens, Sara Parsons, and Annie Goodrich. In important respects, this is not surprising. Many nursing concerns are timeless. Moreover, history, as taught in early nursing schools, always provided exemplars of ethical decisions—or, in Sara T. Fry's more recent words, concrete examples of nurses making the right choices for the right reasons. History guided neophytes in the historical homes and hospitals of America's health care system. And it provided sustenance for the day-to-day conflicts inherent in nursing practice—in the past as well as in the present. If you think you have problems, to paraphrase a 1937 section in Aikens' *Studies in Ethics for Nurses,* just think of the "physical dirt and disorder, immorality, drunkenness, neglect, indifference, graft, and political corruption" your foremothers confronted to earn you your respected place in a heroic tradition of care (p. 34).

My sense of the historical consciousness in these chapters, however, also means a commitment to understanding the many different and often quite intricate ways in which patients and practitioners are deeply connected to and influence both each other and the world in which they exist. Perhaps here is where I might make some contribution. I share my ethics colleagues' interest in concepts and contextualization, but my training pulls me into the past, and my methods allow me to exploit the distance of time to offer a different perspective on what I see as a keenly felt concern running through all these chapters. In one way or another, I think these chapters wonder: Is the nursing ethic endangered? More specifically, is the discipline's sense of itself as embodying certain moral values that may be reflected in its particular code, but that is always represented in its day-to-day practice, threatened by the increasingly impersonalized and market-driven hospital and health care system in which it works? And are nurses silenced at the bedside and around the globe by assumptions about their gender, race and class, prevailing knowledge paradigms, and their own sense of distress? I think history suggests not.

Bringing Order to Chaos

Many, if not most, of the chapters in this book explore their authors' intellectual quest to understand, to explicate, and to support the ethical basis of nursing practice at a very particular place: the bedside of very sick and very vulnerable patients in hospitals. At this point, then, it may be useful to concentrate on the history of nursing in this place. And it may be even more useful to remember that the arc of nursing's history in hospitals has been one of constant struggle to bring order to chaos.

Certainly, we can see this in Florence Nightingale's exploits in the Crimea in the mid-19th century. We see this process as well in the development of training schools in hospitals across late 19th- and early 20th-century America. I have, in other places, described these students and their instructors as powerful—as less the "foot-soldiers" of health care reform, as historian Charles Rosenberg has called them, and more akin to the marines: establishing, maintaining, and to a fair degree controlling the beachhead from which science and medicine would later launch a stunning and seemingly successful assault on crippling injuries and diseases (D'Antonio, 1999). These women tamed the eternal chaos of sickrooms and wards—the stagnant air, foul smells, contaminated effusions, pitiful sufferings, and searing pain—by establishing routines, systematizing procedures, and honing disciplined and depersonalized personas. The constant emphasis on the well-made bed and well-run ward, however, was more than the installation of mindless and rote behavior. It concretely reflected nursing's ability to rescue patients whose recovery teetered on the brink of the very real disorder and disarray that always surrounds sickness and suffering.

But the most important work of these trained and student nurses lay in how they tamed the cacophony of voices—of authoritative and legitimate opinions about diagnoses and treatments freely given by 19th-century family, friends, pharmacists, physicians of widely varying backgrounds, nurses, and midwives—at the bedside of sick patients in homes or in hospitals. Historians have correctly argued that the 19th-century bedside did provide space for powerful female voices—voices that were increasingly silenced by the growing legitimacy of scientific medicine and by the work of trained nurses who actively believed in and supported its practices. But, as I have argued elsewhere, this may be too simplistic a picture. My own historical research emphasizes how American physicians, middle-class mothers, and nurses joined to reorder the chaos of voices at the patient's bedside. They established a class-based hierarchy in support of a medically structured therapeutic relationship—with the physician supervising the middle-class woman, who, in turn, would supervise the hired, and almost always working-class, nurse (D'Antonio, 1993; O'Brien, 1987). Later in the century, nursing leaders—almost always the superintendents of the training schools—drew on this particular kind of hierarchical reordering. They became managers of the domestic life on the wards, in the schools, and in the sickrooms of their patients' homes. In matters of ordering clinical care of the patient, the physician had absolute command. In matters of organizing the clinical care of patients, nurses took charge. Indeed nurses in hospitals maintained power through the skillful manipulation of these hierarchical relationships: their tight organizational structure and almost unyielding emphasis on a sacrosanct chain of command, in fact, seems to have strengthened their position in the often uncharted and treacherous waters of interprofessional bureaucracies.[3] Many nurses, in fact, may well have loathed relinquishing this very real power and control. Judith Walzer Leavitt's (1998) most recent work on obstetrical nurses, for example, suggests that they held on tenaciously to rigid routines and regimented experiences even as their leaders, their medical colleagues, and birthing women themselves pushed for a more fluid and flexible, patient-centered hospital experience in the mid-20th century.

It is again in mid-century America that we see nursing's struggle to bring order to chaos. The fault lines of a health and nursing care system that was quintessentially private and oriented toward local traditions, customs, and values had appeared first during the Great Depression of the 1930s and had hardened during the years of the Second World War. The environment nurses were to control was itself spinning out of control. The too-often prohibitive costs of private duty nursing care in one's home limited it to the very rich (who could pay) or the very poor (when subsidized by the philanthropy of the very rich or the work of students). But one's home was losing its centrality as a preferred place of care. The demand for hospital care sky-rocketed as increasingly available indemnity insurance plans covered parts of its costs for middle- and working-class Americans, and federal legislation deliberately placed this institution at the center of the American health care system.

But the wards and the semiprivate rooms in which patients awaited new, exciting, and life-saving treatments and procedures were again too often places of chaos, confusion, and instability. Very ill and injured patients arrived at all hours of the day and night, adding to a constantly changing mix of different patients with different expectations of both medical and nursing care. Moreover, there were extraordinarily high levels of turnover among staff. On the one hand, bureaucratic policies and procedures increasingly structured nursing practice. Carefully delineated rules and regulations accommodated the episodic work trajectories of registered nurses as well as the demands of providing increasingly complicated medical and surgical procedures placed upon relatively inexperienced student nurses. But on the other hand, these same pressures created spaces of opportunity for some nurses to experiment with different forms of practice.

We are only now beginning to historically analyze this postwar period. We have glimpses of how some nurses responded—how they wrung order from chaos—by manipulating their traditional control of environmental spaces and gathering their sickest and least stable patients together in what would come to be called intensive care units (Fairman & Lynaugh, 1998). Julie Fairman (2002) has explored the testing and negotiation of professional boundaries that gave rise to the nurse practitioner movement. And Wanda Hiestand (2006) has painted the indelible image of Frances Reiter, then dean of the new Graduate School of Nursing at the New York Medical College and staunch advocate of baccalaureate prepared "nurse clinicians," gathering her colleagues around the "Whiskey File" and toasting to less exhausting days nursing patients while proving that educated and expert care did make substantive differences.

The Moral Center of Nursing Practice

I am, of course, approaching that moment in time when the first generation of nurse ethicists came into nursing. Historians place this generation at the center of a "rights revolution" in American history: a time when struggles for civil rights, women's rights, and, for our purposes, patients' rights challenged an established political, social, and, to a large extent, moral consensus about what was good, right, and just in society and in health care. Nursing's leadership both affected and was affected by such changes that, in important ways, centered on individuals—and on a particular individual's particular rights in particular contexts. Certainly, our organizational leaders played important roles in the construction of such institutions as Medicare, Medicaid, and the National Institutes of Health—but these institutions, in addition to their stated missions, also signified the increasingly direct responsibility of the federal government in an individual's physical health and illness experience.[4] And, in fact, our intellectual leaders—people we sometimes group together as "the theorists"—contributed more than just their particularly grand theories of care: they also gave us what I suggest is an as yet-unacknowledged sense of scholarly self-confidence that we needed as we moved into academia in a more substantive way. Their emphasis on context continued a tradition that allowed us to understand and critique an increasingly reductionistic, fragmented, and specialized nature of both medical and nursing practice. But it was in their constant emphasis on the individual patient, I would argue, that we see their most striking impact.

I need to make an important caveat: I would never deny the persistent historical importance of nursing's concern about an individual's care and treatment. Still, I do think the 1960s and 1970s ushered in a fundamental change: the nurse-patient relationship became the moral center of nursing practice; and the felt quality of the nurse-patient relationship became the moral compass by which nurses found their way to experiences of satisfaction or distress with their work.

I will admit to being on very tentative ground. But I will temporarily stand my ground to make two points: that however important our emphasis on the nurse-patient relationship, this emphasis is itself both the product of a particular moment in historical time and that it is best understood within a history of nursing practice (or, at the very least, institutionally based practice) that involves both the care of the patient "and" the control of the environment. I use the word "control" deliberately, fully admitting its conflicted place in our postmodern, neo-Foucaultian intellectual world, but also acknowledging its equally conflicted place as an inescapable and, perhaps, even just component of a complicated matrix of social and societal relationships. In fact, I will go further. As I have argued in my work on early 19th-century psychiatric care, what becomes problematic is not the tension between care and control in our work, per se. Rather, the problem lies in the ways in which ideas and practices rarely support acknowledging, discussing, and deconstructing the duality that surrounds our day-to-day work.

I come to this argument through my own historical research on the day-to-day experiences of patients and staff inside the Friends Asylum in early 19th-century Philadelphia. The Asylum was the first private insane asylum in the United States dedicated to the implementation of a radically new model of care called moral treatment. But, as I discovered, the model's theoretical focus was on the individual and, in the crucible of the intimate and often chaotic world of day-to-day institutional life, it suggested few pragmatic strategies for the central dilemma facing staff: how did one balance the needs of an individual for kind, compassionate, and personalized care against the equally compelling needs of the larger group to which he or she belonged for stability, predictability and, in the oft-repeated words of the Asylum's staff, "peace and tranquility." This, in fact, proved to be moral treatment's fundamental flaw. It left staff floundering—without a language to discuss such a dilemma and without a framework within which to understand it. Staff ultimately abandoned moral treatment and introduced, in its place, a more medically driven and depersonalized model of care (D'Antonio, 2006). I have argued and still argue that their experiences inform 21st-century practice: they remind us that, although we ourselves bring new and different perspectives to bear on the needs of individuals in our care, we, too, can never avoid that point where their needs might collide with those of the larger group—with those of the unit, our colleagues, our administration—to whom we have similar responsibilities.

In some ways, we have certainly ranged far afield—and we seem far from the issues of the technologically oriented, bureaucratically structured, and market-driven context that creates the conundrums that 21st-century ethics and ethical nursing practice must address. But when thinking about the history that produced our current context, I wonder if, when we dip beneath the surface, the themes of similarities are not stronger than those of differences. Nursing is and always has been that discipline most responsible for determining the actual experiences of very vulnerable individuals (and families) when they need the resources, the structure, or the safety a hospitalization might bring. Nursing is and always has been that discipline that knows—whatever the rhetoric and whatever the plan—that moments of felt stability and control are illusory. And nursing is and always has been that discipline—in different ways at different times—that does bring some sense of order to the chaos and crisis that surrounds serious illness. We do need to maintain (and strengthen) both our analytic and our practice focus on the nurse-patient relationship. This relationship is the place where individual motivations, impersonal science, the forces of the market, and the ramifications of public policy all meet and mix. More importantly, this relationship is now our legitimating ideal and the fulcrum of what we expect from ourselves and what our public expects from us.

But as we move from the present to the past and back again to the present (and as we go deeper into the relationship and even deeper still—with our emphasis on genetics and molecular biology—into the patient and the patient's physical body) we might remember that we who give an institution its form have as long a history and as deep a commitment to reconciling our simultaneous, often conflicting, rarely articulated, and ever-present obligation to "both" the individual and to the institutional environment in which we meet this individual.

Still, as several contributors point out, the possibility that nurses' voices may not be heard within the ambiguous and always complicated social and intellectual world of actual clinical practice raises real concern. But as Bronwyn Rebekah McFarland-Icke's chilling examination of nurses' participation in the euthanasia policies of the German T4 program shows, the process of being silenced also depends on the collusion of those who would be silenced (McFarland-Icke, 1999). In the end, it may be here—in challenging the silences—that we might see the enduring legacy of the nurse ethicists who present their work in this book.

These scholars, charged by their training in the humanities to consider and critique the complicated nature of human experience, assume no hubris. They are well aware and, in their worry about the state of the nursing ethic in today's too-often callous medical marketplace, deeply concerned about the universal fragility of moral human relationships. Some worry about issues that my history has not directly addressed, issues such as those related to gender or those involving traditions of spirituality. But all, whatever their particular perspective, help nurses give voice to their experiences. This is why I do not think the nursing ethic is endangered. The work of nurse ethicists fills silences by creating an awareness of, a sympathy for, and a space to talk about the ambiguity, pressures, ambivalence, and uncertainties that have, do, and will still, in the future, exist within the clinical moment and that more aptly characterize nurses' experience of day-to-day clinical practice.

Endnotes

1. For an excellent collection of essays that covers the terrain of historical research, see Baker, Caplan, Emanuel, & Latham, 1999.

2. For another important pre-20th century study, see Lederer, 1977. The important work done on nursing ethics in this period includes Fowler 2000. See also Cianci, 1992; Freitas, 1990; and Sward, 1978.

3. This argument is detailed in D'Antonio,1999. See also Monteiro, 1987.

4. See, for examples, Hardy, 1988; and Woods, 1989.

References

Aikens, S. (1937). *Studies in ethics for nurses* (4th ed.). Philadelphia: W. B. Saunders Company.

A Code of Ethics [Editorial]. (1926). *The American Journal of Nursing, 26*(8), 621–625.

Baker, R. B., Caplan, A. L., Emanuel, L. L., & Latham, S. R., Jr. (Eds.). (1999). *The American medical ethics revolution: How the AMA's Code of Ethics has transformed physicians' relationships to patients, professionals, and society.* Baltimore: Johns Hopkins University Press.

Cianci, M. M. (1992). The Code of Ethics and the role of nurses: An historical perspective. *Nursing Connections, 5*(1), 37–42

D'Antonio, P. (1993). The legacy of domesticity: Nursing in early nineteenth century America. *Nursing History Review, 1*(1), 229–246.

D'Antonio, P. (1999). Revisiting and rethinking the rewriting of nursing history. *Bulletin of the History of Medicine, 73*(2), 268–290.

D'Antonio, P. (2006). *Founding friends: families, staff and patients at the Friends Asylum in early nineteenth century Philadelphia.* Bethlehem, PA: Lehigh University Press.

Fairman, J. (2002). The roots of collaborative practice: Nurse practitioners pioneers' stories. *Nursing History Review, 10*, 159–174.

Fairman, J., & Lynaugh, J. E. (1998). *Critical care nursing: A history.* Philadelphia: University of Pennsylvania Press.

Fowler, M. (2000). The evolution of the ANA Code of Ethics. *Imprint, 47*(5), 53–54.

Freitas, L. (1990). Historical roots and future perspectives related to nursing ethics. *Journal of Professional Nursing, 6*(4), 197–205

Hardy, M. A. (1988). Political savvy or lost opportunity: Evolution of the American Nurses Association Policy for Nursing Education Funding, 1952–1972. *Journal of Professional Nursing, 4*(3), 205-217

Hiestand, W. (2006). Frances U. Reiter and the Graduate School of Nursing at New York Medical College, 1960–1973. *Nursing History Review, 14*, 213–226.

Leavitt, J. W. (1998). Strange young women on errands: Obstetric nursing between two worlds. *Nursing History Review, 6*, 3–24.

Lederer, S. (1977). *Subjected to science: Human experimentation in America before the Second World War.* Baltimore: Johns Hopkins Press.

Linker, B. (2005). The business of ethics: Gender, medicine, and the professional codification of the American Physiotherapy Association, 1918–1935. *Journal of the History of Medicine and Allied Sciences, 60*(3), 320–354.

McFarland-Icke, B. R. (1999). *Nurses in Nazi Germany: Moral choice in history.* Princeton, NJ: Princeton University Press.

Monteiro, L. A. (1987). Insights from the past. *Nursing Outlook, 35*(2), 65–69.

O'Brien (D'Antonio), P. (1987). 'All a woman's life can bring:' The domestic roots of nursing in Philadelphia, 1830–1885. *Nursing Research, 36*(1), 12–17.

Sward, K. (1978). The Code for Nurses: An historical perspective, In *Perspectives on the Code for Nurse,* Kansas City, MO: American Nurses Association.

Woods, C. Q. (1989). *Evolution of the American Nurses Association's Position on Heath Insurance for the Aged: 1933–1965,* Unpublished doctoral dissertation, University of Kansas, Lawrence, KS.

Patricia D'Antonio, RN, PhD, FAAN is an Associate Professor of Nursing, the Associate Director of the Barbara Bates Center for the Study of the History of Nursing, University of Pennsylvania, and a Fellow of the American Academy of Nursing. She is also the editor of the *Nursing History Review,* the official journal of the American Association for the History of Nursing. She received her BS from Boston College, her MSN from the Catholic University of America, and her PhD from the University of Pennsylvania. Her clinical background includes specialization in psychiatric nursing; her research focuses on the history of psychiatry and psychiatric nursing, and 19th and early 20th century nursing and health care.

CRITICAL THINKING ACTIVITIES

Nursing and Health Care Ethics: A Legacy

✦ The theme of "bringing order to chaos" is an important one in the history of nursing according to D'Antonio. Think of a present-day clinical problem with an ethical dimension that requires bringing order to chaos. What routines, organizations, structures, and relationships need to be established, maintained, and controlled to address the problem you identified?

✦ How are nurses' voices being silenced today? Does drawing attention to the ethical issues in nursing (as distinct from other health professions) help in giving voice to nurses' concerns? Why or why not?

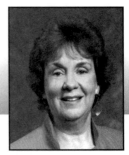

Gladys B. White

CHAPTER 3

The Dorothy Vossen Lecture: The Institutionalization of Nursing Ethics

We in nursing have something that is the envy of other professional groups, namely, a strong code of ethics. Our *Code of Ethics for Nurses with Interpretive Statements* is a succinct statement of (a) the ethical obligations and duties of every individual who enters the nursing profession, (b) the profession's nonnegotiable ethical standard, and (c) nursing's own understanding of its commitment to society. At the outset of this historic meeting of leaders in nursing and champions of its ethics, I will address the "Institutionalization of Nursing Ethics," as exemplified by the development, revision, and dissemination of our Code and the organizational infrastructure that has supported this over the years, namely the American Nurses Association (ANA). The institutionalization of nursing ethics is a given. Professionally, we are distinctive in that the ethics at our core was one of the key motivational forces in the founding of ANA in the first place. In 1896, the Nurses Associated Alumnae of the United States and Canada, which later became ANA, had as its first purpose the establishment and maintenance of a code of ethics for nurses. Other contemporary professional groups such as bioethicists are just beginning to consider the need for a code of ethics and unfortunately do not seem to be aware of the serious ethics work that exists in nursing (Baker, 2005).

Common ties bind all of the contributors to the Legacy project. The first common tie is that we are all nurses, whether we were originally educated in diploma or baccalaureate nursing programs or entered nursing from another field. Each of us, almost without exception, has been capped, pinned, graduated, and sat for state licensure exams. We have, at various times, been more or less active in our professional association, but we have generally been known as nurses throughout our professional lives.

A second tie is that we have each taken the road less traveled: that is, we have taken an unconventional route both within nursing and in health care as a whole. Each of us is unique in terms of our vantage point. Some of us are perched at the bedside casting the experienced eye of the nurse researcher on the responses of patients to illness and to death; some of us are conceptually located within the circle of the family and community, applying anthropological and sociological insights to our observations of human interactions, and responses to health and illness. Others have devoted their considerable energy and skills to the policy arena. For me, the excitement has often been at the cutting edge of science and technology, both in attempting to understand the dimensions of new scientific discoveries and then also considering the ethical features of novel questions about human birth, life, and death. Our paths have not been easy ones, but our multiplicity is stunning. If I have computed correctly, the participants in the Legacy project cumulatively represent about 850 years of effort in the fields of nursing and ethics.

A third tie is our long-standing commitment to the revision, dissemination, and maintenance of a strong Code of Ethics for the nursing profession. We have cleaved to the ethical core of the profession and, as a result, we have had longevity throughout our careers, somewhat independent of particular positions or jobs of the moment. Fourth and finally, we are all female and our personal stories and professional paths have been shaped by the politics of our time including the crosscurrents of at least radical and liberal feminism.

In the remarks that follow, I would like to accomplish a number of things. First, I want to examine the nature of the Code as normative and its place within the hierarchy of ethical reasoning. Second, I would like to describe the Code and consider its resilience with respect to current realities in clinical care. Third, I would like to consider the capacity of the Code to embrace new possibilities in science and health care, and fourth, I want to indicate how respect for the enduring value of the Code has implications for possible future revisions and continuing dissemination. I will touch on the uneasy alliance between nursing ethics and the field of bioethics as well as our need to continue to develop a robust meta-level of nursing ethics scholarship. Finally, I would like to consider how we can leverage the positive relationship that we have with the American public in order to influence the major health care debates and ethical dilemmas of our time.

Over the years, I have found it convenient and effective to think about philosophical ethics in terms of a hierarchy of ethical reasoning. This hierarchy proceeds from simple to complex, starting with ethical judgment at the first level and proceeding through ethical rules and principles, culminating at the level of ethical theory. The hierarchy proceeds from those ethical statements or claims that are least generalizable to those that are most generalizable, namely those theories that have the widest purchase with respect to encompassing the key ethical polarities or arguments across the range of ethical disputes and dilemmas. I consider an ethical dilemma to be a problem of one of two types: either a situation for which no matter what action is taken, some harm will occur, or a problem for which there are strong arguments for different courses of action. I mention these foundational points now, realizing that everyone may not share these basic assumptions. From my perspective, given these assumptions, the Code is primarily a rule-oriented ethical document, situated at the second level in the hierarchy of ethical reasoning. However, its detailed accompanying interpretive statements push the relevant analyses to the levels of ethical principles and theories. Nonetheless, first and foremost, the Code is a set of nine rules that can be conveniently quoted on a bookmark. This economy of thought in terms of the major provisions, as well as available elaboration in the longer interpretive statements, is a positive characteristic of the Code. How did we work to produce the current version of the Code?

After having had the privilege of serving as the first director of ANA's Center for Ethics and Human Rights in the early 1990s, and followed in that role by Colleen Scanlon, RN, JD, and Laurie Badzek, RN, JD, I returned to ANA in 2000 at the request of the organization. ANA had hit some snags in its work on the latest Code revision, namely an inability to win approval from the ANA House of Delegates (HOD). One of the issues was the perception on the part of the delegates that the document had not received enough input and review from staff nurses. ANA is the professional association that represents the nation's approximately 2.9 million registered nurses. Regrettably, only a small percentage of these nurses are actually ANA members at any point in time. Even though all nurses are not ANA members, the ideal is that the Code should be relevant and applicable to the professional concerns of all nurses, so making the match between what nurses care about and what the Code said was imperative. The draft Code was once again circulated for comment many times, and the thorny issue of collective bargaining versus workplace advocacy strategies was accommodated in a revised Provision 6 (ANA, 2001, p. 4). Additional changes were made, and the new Code was finally approved by the ANA HOD in July 2001 and represented the first full revision of the document to have taken place in 25 years. The current version was the result of 5 years of effort by members of the Code of Ethics Project Task Force, an advisory board of state liaisons, and ANA staff. The provisions of the new Code break down as discussed below.

In Provisions 1, 2, and 3 (see Appendix A), the Code reiterates the fundamental values and commitments of the nurse. These obligations have shaped nursing's mission to care for individuals for their own sakes and not merely as means to the objectives or ends of others. Nurses should always be concerned about the health, safety, and rights of patients. This portion of the Code emphasizes the importance of patient autonomy and also considers the idea that members of some cultures "place less weight on individualism and may choose to defer to family or community values in decision making" (ANA, 2001, p. 9).

The Code discusses conflicts of interest and personal boundaries and notes that there may be situations in which public health considerations override individual rights. The Code identifies the boundaries of duty and loyalty (see Provisions 4, 5, and 6). The management strategies and cost containment efforts that characterize inpatient facilities, as well as the variety of settings in which nurses practice, present ethical challenges for nurses who must have the ability and authority to make professional judgments, plan and prioritize the use of their time, and ensure that the work environment supports them in these efforts. Nurses need to be able to delegate tasks appropriately, continue to grow as health care professionals, and preserve personal integrity. The Code supports efforts to improve the workplace and working conditions.

There are times when nurses will become aware of impaired or inappropriate practice among colleagues. The Code supports nurses in whistle blowing or acting in response to incompetent, unethical, illegal, or impaired practice by any member of the health care team. It also supports the nurse's right (with stipulations) to refuse to participate in specific treatments, interventions, or practices that are morally objectionable to the nurse. In Provisions 7, 8, and 9, the Code describes nursing duties beyond individual patient encounters. Nurses work in many arenas, including practice, research, administration, and it is critical that nurse researchers develop new knowledge while protecting the rights and interests of their subjects and minimize the risks. Nurse administrators assume the responsibility for facilitating professional nursing practice and ensuring the delivery of high-quality care. Nurse educators are those who help ensure a steady flow of professional nurses into the future (White, 2001, pp. 73–74). It is really necessary to read the Code and its interpretive statements carefully: appreciate its breadth, utility, and sophistication. The Code is clearly normative: that is, it describes how the nurse ought to act. In addition, as a whole it stipulates some of the features of the "good nurse" as an ethical matter.

Our Code has many positive features, and in my opinion, negotiates some of the trickiest ethical issues in health care. For example, one of the current debates in medical practice has to do with how physicians handle personal religious belief and the dictates of conscience when asked to become involved in controversial clinical practices (Curlin, Lawrence, Chin, & Lantos, 2007, p. 593). As reported in the *New England Journal of Medicine* in February 2007, a random sample of 2,000 practicing physicians were asked about ethical rights and obligations when a patient requests a legal medical procedure to which the physician might object for religious or moral reasons. One of the key conclusions of this study was that many physicians do not consider themselves obligated to disclose information about or refer patients for legal but morally controversial medical procedures. Our Code advises us along another path. Nurses are not and have never been directed by our Code to simply omit telling patients about legal interventions with which we might disagree.

Another example of the virtues of our Code has to do with its resilience in coming to grips with the current realities of clinical care. By resilience, I mean the ability of the Code to endure some bending and stretching without compromising its integrity and relevance as a document. Several of the Legacy Project members and other authors have referred to the fact that nursing is a moral art. Just as Catherine Murphy (1978) noted in her seminal article, the nurse is frequently in the position of not being able to do the "right thing." I returned to the bedside two summers ago after taking a nurse refresher course. I worked as a staff nurse on a medical oncology unit at a local community hospital. It was truly an eye-opening experience. All the things that we had been saying at ANA in recent years proved to be true. The staff nurse faces a welter of pressures and conflicting demands in the process of delivering patient care. Patients in hospitals are sicker than ever, that is, patient acuity has increased in recent years and nursing work continues to be devalued, misunderstood, and often not respected. There are all kinds of impediments to nurses serving as patient advocates, and a case in point is the implementation of barcode medication administration.

Developed originally by nurses in Veterans Administration facilities, this technology is intended to address the serious and ongoing problem of medication errors (Aspden, Wolcott, Bootman, & Cronenwett, 2007; Kohn, Corrigan, & Donaldson, 2000). Nonetheless, barcode medication administration has introduced a new and troubling computer interface between nurse and patient (Patterson, Cook & Render, 2002). In many cases, the role of the nurse on acute care units has devolved into pushing heavy, ergonomically faulty carts from room to room for most of the hours of the shift. Getting the meds out, for a six-patient assignment per nurse may involve administering as many as 100 medications during an 8- (most often 9- or 10-) hour shift. Medication administration alone has become the overwhelming, and in many cases, almost infeasible priority on acute care units. Dan Dugan, a clinical ethicist, described it as follows: "Nurses already have a major challenge these days getting assignments without regard for continuity and being pressured to the max to list out and complete the task list, further diluting the nurses' attention to old-fashioned care. More and more, nurses feel that they are getting paid from the shoulders down" (Dan Dugan, personal communication, July 10, 2006).

The computer is like a seventh patient added to the assignment: it must be fed (powered up at all times, along with the barcode scanner), interacted with (prompts answered), and treated with respect (if the power goes down or the battery pack is low, the nurse can lose all of the information from the entire shift, resulting in hours of overtime to rerecord). Although the issue of barcode medication administration is not addressed in the Code, the competing commitments that this issue reveals are pertinent to Provision 1 of the Code, which discusses patient dignity and the importance of sustaining relationships with patients, and Provision 3, the obligation of the nurse to promote and protect the health, safety, and rights of the patient. Therefore, in terms of this one specific issue, the Code is resilient: that is, the provisions are pertinent, but the Code is not determinative. It cannot determine where a balance point needs to be struck in avoiding errors on the one hand, and effectively removing a significant portion of the nurse's attention from patient to machine, on the other hand. Using this topic as an example, I think that the Code comes to rest exactly where it should.

The capacity of the Code to address new realities in science and health care will continue to be tested. The issues that will demand the most of nurses ethically are those that are often unfamiliar. The map and sequence of the human genome has led to new precision in the development and use of genetic tests, but we have not yet created the necessary safeguards to guarantee genetic privacy, or protect against genetic discrimination. The genetic map and sequence will aid in the development of somatic and germ line gene transfer research, yet we have achieved no social consensus about oversight of this field, despite the fact that it has already yielded dramatic harms and benefits. It is now possible through preimplantation genetic diagnosis to ascertain the sex and other characteristics of the human embryo, well in advance of birth and even before pregnancy, yet it is undecided whether the infant has a right to genetic privacy at birth and, if so, how such privacy will be ensured. The fact that the use of embryonic stem cells holds promise for the treatment of spinal cord injuries, and Alzheimer's and Parkinson's diseases, does not resolve the question of whether it is acceptable to use such cells. And finally, we know that we have the scientific and technical ability to clone mammals, but we have not fully examined the ethical implications of human cloning (White, 2000). And beyond that, we will be forced as well to face the health and safety issues involved with nanotechnology involving small particles measuring one-billionth of a meter, as well as neuroethics or the ethical issues raised by advances in neuroscience (National Institute for Occupational Safety and Health [NIOSH], 2007; Illes, 2006).

The Code may not offer specific direction on any one of these topics, but it should be possible to obtain some general guidance as we approach these matters. However, we cannot leave this work to bioethicists alone, or the eventual insights and analyses will suffer from the lack of a nursing perspective.

The enduring value of the Code results from the fact that it occupies an important and helpful position between the specific and the abstract. This has important implications for ANA's role as keeper of the Code with its inherent responsibilities. It is a role involving stewardship rather than ownership. What are the responsibilities of stewardship with respect to the Code? First, making it widely available; second, recognizing that it is owned by the profession as a whole; third, defending and clarifying what it says and means on the occasion of disputed interpretation; and fourth, in light of the intended enduring quality of the Code, pushing for revisions only when necessary.

The major provisions of the Code are posted online, at my strong urging, at no cost so that an individual nurse who is interested and may even have a need to see the content of the Code can do so for free. But responsible stewardship of the Code does not mean moving toward a new revision before its time. One of the key characteristics of a professional code of ethics is its enduring value. If the Code is revised too often, then its value could be weakened as nurses will wonder: Should I consult the Code or is it likely that I do not have the latest edition anyway, so why bother? More about this in a moment.

Nursing and the American Public: The Untapped Potential for Communication

Today, nursing continues to rank as one of the most trusted of the health professions. The American public trusts us, and we need to leverage this trust into generating a wider awareness about what nurses think about important issues of the day. This can have educational benefits for patients, families, and communities and involve us to a greater degree in important public policy debates such as access to health care. In recent decades, ANA has endorsed one of the candidates for president during each election cycle, but there continues to be a debate about whether this is money well spent for a cash-strapped organization. I would rather see more resources and efforts expended on getting the word out about how nurses view the profession and their ethical commitments to patients and the health deficits of the American public.

We have the trust and respect of the American public, but in the terms that Marsha Fowler has used in her paper in this volume, I think that we need to strengthen the power structure in nursing, that is, all those capabilities that allow us to get things done and create what she terms "a reciprocating balance between this and our meaning and value structure," which is already strong. One way to do this is to draw on the features of the art of persuasion, as described by Aristotle in the *Rhetoric* (McKeon, 1941). The ability to be persuasive according to Aristotle consists of three powers: (a) ethos, or the speaker's power of evincing a personal character that will make his speech credible to others (nurses have this); (b) pathos, or the power of stirring the emotions of our hearers, (we have this too, i.e., empathy); and (c) logos, the power of proving a truth or apparent truth by means of persuasive arguments (we can do this) (McKeon, p. 1341). Our logical arguments, however, are not as apparent in the public domain as they should and could be.

Conclusion

The 2001 *Code of Ethics for Nurses with Interpretive Statements* (ANA) continues to serve the nursing profession well. The ANA continues to bear the responsibilities of stewardship for the Code, which involves recognizing that, in its most meaningful sense, the Code is owned by the profession as a whole. Although the document essentially offers rule-oriented ethical guidance, it offers considerably more through the elaboration and description offered in the interpretive statements.

The Code is not a new idea or an afterthought in nursing. It has been an inherent feature of our professional association from its beginning more than 100 years ago. ANA's stewardship of the Code involves a recognition of the need to make the Code fully available to all nurses, and an understanding that in order to protect the enduring value of the document, it should not be revised too often. From my perspective, I do not think the Code should be revised again until at least 2015. In the meantime, I believe that through serious investment and support of the ANA Center for Ethics and Human Rights, the organization should do all that it can to stimulate a robust meta-level of nursing ethics scholarship. This should include a focus on the cutting-edge issues in science and technology such as reprogenetics, neuroethics, and the uses and abuses of nanotechnology, to name a few. Finally, we need to recognize that our ethics and the public perception of nurses should be used to amplify and magnify our outrage regarding the American crisis of access to health care. We should address the ways in which the broader utilization of nurses can increase the availability and accessibility of health care in the United States, and the strategies for doing this should come from us.

References

American Nurses Association. (2001). *Code of ethics for nurses with interpretive statements.* Washington, DC.

Aspden, P., Wolcott, J., Bootman, J. L., & Cronenwett, R. R. (Eds.). (2007). *Preventing medication errors: Quality chasm series.* Washington, DC: National Academy Press.

Baker, R. (2005). A draft model aggregated code of ethics for bioethicists. *American Journal of Bioethics, 5*(5), 33–41.

Curlin, F. A., Lawrence, R. E., Chin, M. H., & Lantos, J. D. (2007). Religion, conscience, and controversial clinical practices. *New England Journal of Medicine, 356*(6), 593–600.

Illes, J. (Ed.). (2006). *Neuroethics, defining the issues in theory, practice and policy.* New York: Oxford University Press.

Kohn, L. T., Corrigan, J. M., & Donaldson, M. S. (Eds.). (2000). *To err is human: Building a safer health system.* Washington, DC: National Academy Press.

McKeon, R. P. (Ed.). (1941). *The basic works of Aristotle.* New York: Random House.

Murphy, C. P. (1978). The moral situation in nursing. In E. L. Bandman & B. Bandman (Eds.), *Bioethics and human rights: A reader for health professionals* (pp. 312–320). Boston: Little, Brown.

National Institute for Occupational Safety and Health. (2007). Centers for Disease Control and Prevention, Department of Health and Human Services. *Progress toward safe nanotechnology in the workplace: A report from the NIOSH Nanotechnology Research Center.* DHHS (NIOSH) Publication no. 2007-123. Retrieved November 14, 2007, from http://purl.access.gpo.gov/GPO/LPS81440

Patterson, E. S., Cook, R. I., & Render, M. L. (2002). Improving patient safety by identifying side effects from introducing bar coding in medication administration. *Journal of the American Medical Informatics Association, 9*(5), 540–553.

White, G. B. (2000). What we may expect from ethics and the law. *American Journal of Nursing, 100*(10), 114–116, 118.

White, G. B. (2001). The code of ethics for nurses. *American Journal of Nursing, 101*(10), 73–75.

Gladys B. White is an adjunct faculty member at Georgetown University, University of Maryland University College, and Montgomery College. She teaches bioethics, workplace ethics and philosophy at these three institutions. She is a graduate of Duke University (BSN), Catholic University of America (MSN), and Georgetown University (PhD in philosophy). Bioethics has been the focus of her work since 1985. Special interests include reprogenetics, access to health care, and ethical issues in the professions.

CRITICAL THINKING ACTIVITIES

The Institutionalization of Nursing Ethics

✦ White states in the opening of her address that, "We in nursing have something that is the envy of other professional groups, namely, a strong code of ethics" [*Code of Ethics for Nurses with Interpretive Statements,* 2001, American Nurses Association]. Is this a questionable claim or a fact? Compare and contrast the ANA Code of Ethics with another professional code found on the following websites: American Dental Association (http://www.ada.org), American Medical Association (http://www.ama-assn.org), American Occupational Therapy Association (http://www.aota.org), American Pharmaceutical Association (http://www.pharmacist.com) or American Physical Therapy Association (http://www.apta.org). How does the ANA Code fare? What is there for other professions to envy?

✦ Provision 6 of the ANA Code of Ethics was particularly difficult to draft according to White since it dealt with the "thorny issue of collective bargaining versus workplace advocacy strategies." Review the provision and describe the sorts of ethical issues that would be in conflict and why.

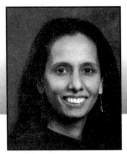

Shireen S. Rajaram

CHAPTER 4

Nursing Ethics and Sociology

After being immersed in the world of sociology and public health, it was a distinct pleasure for me to share a couple of days with prominent nurse ethicists at the Legacy Seminar. As I ponder over participants' papers and discussions at the seminar, I am left with several sociological musings which I will address: What power do nurses have to define issues as ethical? Are there issues within the profession such as inherent class, gender, and race/ethnic biases that are not necessarily defined as ethical issues, and hence receive less attention from nursing leaders and nurse ethicists? How can sociological perspectives—concepts, theories, and research methodologies—help shed light on some of these issues?

Nursing Ethics and the Nursing Profession

Nurses face many moral dilemmas in their different spheres of activities and role responsibilities—as clinicians, researchers, public health specialists, administrators, patient advocates, and health policy analysts. What then constitutes ethical issues in nursing, and within which nursing role do ethical issues arise? When one talks about "nurse" and "nursing" and "ethical dilemmas in nursing," are we referring to the bedside nurse, the nurse as an administrator, or the nurse as a leader within a professional organization? Joan Liaschenko rightly raises this issue in her essay and in a postconference e-mail discussion. She clearly articulated how some nurses do clinical ethics, while others are more academic. Some are empirical researchers, while others are not. Judith Erlen stated that nursing was both an art and a science, as well

29

as a discipline and practice, and that multiple perspectives were essential—one of them being nursing ethics—to fully understand the profession and practice of nursing. Leah Curtin eloquently responded that nurses create the profession of nursing—for better or for worse—with each action and interaction. Clearly, ethical issues are present in all spheres of the nursing profession.

Most participants' essays defined nursing ethics broadly to include issues relating to allocation of resources, adequate health care coverage, global and national health disparities, adequate education, microcredit, and gainful employment. In the discussion at the Legacy Seminar, nursing ethics appeared to be primarily focused on the role of the nurse as clinician, operating on the front line within the structure of the medical establishment. Within this role, nurses face many ethical dilemmas. Are moral dilemmas of nurses truly moral dilemmas—ones that involve not knowing what to do, or being torn between two difficult solutions? Or are they an artifact of the lack of power that nurses experience, being a female-dominated profession that occupies a lower position in the professional hierarchy of medical care? The moral dilemmas of nurses probably involve both issues. Here, the voice of the sociologist can provide a unique perspective in addressing the dilemmas that nurse ethicists face in the constantly changing health care world (Zussman, 1997). For issues to be considered as "ethical," does one need to have the autonomy and power to be able to apply moral theories to guide one's course of action? Chambliss (1996) reminds us that ethics is the privilege of powerful people such as physicians, who have the ability to choose one course of action over another. Nurses, on the other hand, often lack this power. He states, "How, a nurse may reasonably ask, should one act when one 'isn't' powerful" (p. 5). He prefers to conceptualize difficult issues that nurses face as moral issues rather than ethical ones. Even so, he states, "In a setting where one's work is governed by others, how can one person claim her own moral integrity?" (p. 3).

Sociologists and Nursing Ethics

What role can sociologists play in nursing ethics? I will focus on three broad possibilities outlined in the sociology literature and which grew out of my observations at the seminar. First, sociologists can help shed light on how social context, structures, cultures, and organizational arrangements influence the work of nurse ethicists. Second, sociological and anthropological research methodologies such as ethnography can help draw attention to the underlying social process in ethical decision-making among nurses. Third, sociologists can further sensitize nurses to social justice issues and knowledge about multiple axes of subordination that may exist "within" their profession: race/ethnicity, nationality, social class, gender and sexual orientation biases, and attributions of differential social worth.

Social Context and Moral Issues

The sociologist's approach to nursing ethics is grounded in a social context perspective which acknowledges a hierarchal organizational structure of health care. Understanding this lack of power, perhaps adopting a broader sociological perspective, might help. Sociologists can work with nurse ethicists to illustrate how social structures, culture, social settings, and social interactions influence their work on the front line (DeVries & Subedi, 1998; Zussman, 1997).

Through adopting sociological imagination, sociologists can help nurse ethicists articulate how the social context is important in defining and determining ethical issues. Sociological imagination is the ability to connect personal troubles or everyday life dilemmas to larger structural processes (Mills, 1959). Sociological imagination will allow nurse ethicists to see how the social context in which ethical issues arise is influenced by disciplinary norms, structural processes, interpersonal professional relationships, social arrangements of power and prestige, economic demands, institutional agendas, and personal conscious or unconscious biases (DeVries & Subedi, 1998; Smith, 1990).

At the Legacy Seminar, there was some discussion about the lack of power that nurses had within the organizational structure of the health care system, which made it difficult for them to bring attention to ethical issues that are relevant from a nursing perspective. However, seminar participants might benefit from further examination of the underlying social processes and structural dynamics that exist within a hierarchal organization that may result in the silencing of nurses, who are often at the periphery of the power base due to gender, race/ethnicity, social class, and social position, among other factors.

Also at the Legacy Seminar there were discussions as to which role within nursing participants were referring to when discussing nurse ethics. Clearly, issues of power within an organization are determined by one's social position within the structure. A better articulation of the role or multiple roles that nurses occupy is essential to understand nursing ethics and nurses' ability to bring attention to ethical issues. For example, an associate degree nurse will have relatively less decision-making power than a doctorally prepared nurse administrator to define an issue as an "ethical issue." Sociologists, through the use of scientific research methodologies of ethnography or survey research, can help nurses understand how these social processes are shaped by arrangements of power and privilege and are influenced by sociohistorical factors. Through systematic research that deconstructs commonly held assumptions (Berger, 1963), sociologists can help nurse ethicists ask the tough questions and take a critical analysis of their strengths and weakness.

Ethnography and Nursing Ethics

Ethnography uses rigorous scientific methods through systematic observation and data collection to understand the everyday practices of people in society. Ethnography provides insights into the social construction of meaning and the part that different actors play in the social construction of meaning. Ethnography requires the collection of qualitative data through in-depth interviews and participant observation, and focuses on the nuances of meaning, interaction, and hierarchal relationships (Atkinson, Delamont, Coffey, Lofland, & Lofland, 2007; Denzin & Lincoln, 2005; DeVries & Subedi, 1998). Several of the Legacy Seminar participants were familiar with, and conduct, qualitative research projects, but given the time constraints of the seminar, participants were not able to discuss this issue. In her essay, Catherine Murphy noted the need to further explore this research methodology in addition to philosophical and historical research approaches in defining ethical directions for the future. Anne Davis and Joan Liaschenko also mentioned the importance of using this research methodology in nursing ethics research.

Ethnographers are more concerned with how the social context—within a symbolic-cultural framework or a social-structural framework—shapes interactions and the decision-making process. Symbolic interaction, a theoretical framework in sociology, focuses on how people socially construct reality through their everyday interactions (Cooley, 1962; Mead, 1959). Within a social organization, ethical issues arise and are framed as such through the process of interaction. This interactional process is influenced by different players within the health care system that lack the same level of power and control. Although reality can be considered "soft," it is real to the people who have so created it. The W. I. Thomas theorem states that situations that are defined as real are real in their consequences (1966, p. 301). Ethnography helps to disentangle, deconstruct, and tease out how taken-for-granted moral concepts, social categories, and intellectual discourses are formulated in the first place (DeVries & Subedi, 1998).

Discussions and research studies by individuals such as Hoffmaster (1992), Anspach (1987, 1993), Chambliss (1996), Zussman (1992), and Ceci (2004) all pose relevant lessons for nursing ethics from a sociological perspective. Chambliss, for example, sees ethical problems as a function of the organization, and believes that traditional medical ethics does not pay adequate attention to the role of nurses or that of patients and families. He sees bioethics as not necessarily describing the dilemmas that nurses face, since the profession does not reflect the powerful, atomized, individualistic group. In Anspach's work, she sees nurses and physicians as having different views of reality, resulting from their position within the culture and structure of a medical setting like the technologically driven neonatal intensive care unit

(NICU). She provides examples of how the social context and institutional social positions influence the definition and framing of informed consent.

The production and legitimization of knowledge is a political act influenced by one's social position in an institution (Gustafson, 2005, 2007). This sociopolitical process of knowledge and the legitimation of knowledge are clearly articulated in Joan Liaschenko's essay. She raises critical questions pertaining to the process by which nurses are discredited and dismissed as not credible knowers. Ceci (2004) notes that nurses were consistently concerned about the competence of the surgeon and made complaints to this effect. However, their concerns were ignored and not taken seriously. She argues that it is important to understand how knowledge is created, legitimized, and negotiated within social context of the health care system. Nursing, being a predominately female profession, and one that occupies a lower status than physicians, has a challenging task in attaining professional credibility for itself within the social context of the organization (Ceci; Davies, 1995).

Changes within the nursing profession are bound to exacerbate problems within nursing ethics. Nurses are faced with increasing corporatization, managed care, deskilling and bureaucratization of their work, and organizational downsizing. Will these affect nursing ethics (Chambliss, 1996; Zussman, 1992)? Carol Taylor and other seminar participants point to the many changes, including the commodification of health care, technological advances, and the deprofessionalization of nursing and other health care professions as important factors that will influence the future of nursing and nurse ethics.

Multiple Axes of Subordination within the Nursing Profession

Nurse ethicists would do well to turn the ethical lens inward on nursing itself to understand the class, and race/ethnic biases (in addition to issues of gender subordination), that exist within the profession, and critically examine the historical and current systems of prejudice and institutional discrimination that continue to support, inform, and reproduce current nursing practice and research (Barbee, 1993; Duffy, 2007; Gustafson, 2007; Hine, 1989). Are such issues of subordination and discrimination necessarily conceptualized as "ethical" issues? Whose voices are seen as being legitimate within nursing? Is the nursing and nursing ethics discourse a reflection of the "hegemonic but unmarked white discourse that informs the research knowledge and institutional structures that guide nursing practice" (Gustafson, 2007, p. 154)?

Legacy Seminar participants represented a reflection of the profession of nursing and nursing ethics as a whole, and, interestingly, involved all but one nurse of color. This begs a broader question: Are there no nurses of color interested in nursing ethics, or perhaps, who define themselves as "nurse ethicists," and are different social classes of nurses represented in nursing ethics? Using an ethical lens, perhaps, nursing can examine factors within the profession that may have caused the "chilling out" of nurses of color from ethical discourses and debates. Also, has the framing of ethical issues within nursing, by predominately white, well-educated, middle-class nurses, either consciously or unconsciously steered away from defining difficult, yet necessary issues of institutional discrimination as ethical issues? In her essay, Joan Liaschenko states that denying feminist theory might serve to protect nurses from confronting the damage done by gendered, classed, and raced divisions of labor. An open and critical examination of the concept and politics of "unearned white privilege" (Rothenberg, 2005), and how it plays out at multiple levels in nursing and nursing ethics, is the first step toward reducing the institutional process of marginalization that exists within the profession. (See Gustafson, 2005, 2007.)

An intersectional analysis focuses on how the different dimensions of inequality (social class, gender, race/ethnicity, sexual orientation, etc.) influence structural arrangements and distribution of rewards and sanctions in society (Collins, 2004; Dillaway & Clifford, 2001; Duffy, 2007; hooks, 1989; Sokoloff & Dupont, 2005). Within the context of nursing and nursing ethics, how do these multiple dimensions of subordination and oppression influence nursing ethics? While Legacy Seminar participants rightly pointed out that caring is at the core of nursing, Glenn (1992, 2002) and Roberts (1997) have suggested that white women tend to be the "public face" or the "spiritual" face of nurturant care, and are overrepresented in those jobs that require nurturance, emotional skill, and social interaction, while women of color are relegated to the more menial and backroom tasks with lower pay. If this is the case in nursing, then does this constitute an "ethical" problem worthy of further exploration by nurse ethicists?

Duffy (2005) points out that the conceptualization of care as nurturant care serves to "racialize" the discourse, and excludes the experience of women of color and poor women. She states, "A theoretical focus on nurturance certainly appears to privilege the experiences of white women over the more varied care work experiences of women of color" (p. 78). Besides, with caring and care-related activities being devalued in society, as underscored by seminar participants, how does the "care deficit" as described by Hochschild (1989) contribute to the social status of nurses and the different levels of nurses in the health care labor market (Duffy, 2005)? On the other hand, will the care movement (England, 1992; England, Budig, & Folbre, 2002) reassert and revalue nurturance and the importance and value of care, and thus serve to further render these backroom jobs as invisible and marginalized? While the subordination of women within the nursing profession is not the only problem, the issues of race/ethnicity, social class, age, and sexual orientation are important factors that might require further analysis by nurse ethicists.

Conclusion

Nursing ethics is at an important crossroads, and has the unique opportunity to lead the way in clarifying the field and making a case for why nursing ethics is tremendously important for the dignity, health, and well-being of people. Nursing ethics can "seize the moment" and provide leadership for the nursing profession in redefining the importance of caring work within a medical care framework, for social justice within the profession itself, and a broader societal and global framework. Legacy Seminar participants appeared to be doing a stellar job in trying to articulate the uniqueness of nursing and nursing ethics. A critical examination of the profession is essential to uncover biases, and institutional processes of oppression and domination—both conscious and unconscious—that exist within the hierarchy of nursing. Before attempting to gain credibility through applying moral theories, principles, and frameworks to determine the appropriate course of action, the nurse will do well to take the lead in deconstructing the underlying sociological and political processes that result in framing and naming of ethical problems within the health care context. This knowledge and skill will serve nurses and nurse ethicists well in trying to further refine the need for and the uniqueness of nursing ethics. It is only through a critical stance that nurses can continue to serve as patient advocates and carry out the job of caring, and be true to their profession.

References

Anspach, R. (1987). Prognostic conflict in life and death decisions: The organization as ecology of knowledge. *Journal of Health and Social Behavior, 28*(3), 215–231.

Anspach, R. (1993). *Deciding who lives: Fateful choices in the intensive care nursery.* Berkley: University of California Press.

Atkinson, P., Delamont, S., Coffey, A., Lofland, J., & Lofland, L. (2007). *Handbook of ethnography.* Thousand Oaks, CA: Sage Publications.

Barbee, E. L. (1993). Racism in U.S. nursing. *Medical Anthropology Quarterly, 7*(4), 346–362.

Berger, P. (1963). *Invitation to sociology: A humanistic perspective.* Garden City, NY: Doubleday.

Ceci, C. (2004). Nursing knowledge and power: A case analysis. *Social Science and Medicine, 59*(9), 1879–1889.

Chambliss, D. F. (1996). *Beyond caring: Hospitals, nurses, and the social organization of ethics.* Chicago: University of Chicago Press.

Collins, P. H. (2004). *Black sexual politics. African-Americans, gender and the new racism.* New York: Routledge.

Cooley, C. H. (1962). *Social organization: A study of the larger mind.* New York: Schocken Books.

Davies, C. (1995). *Gender and the professional predicament in nursing.* Philadelphia: Open University Press.

Denzin, N., & Lincoln, Y. (2005). *The Sage handbook of qualitative research* (3rd ed.). Thousand Oaks, CA: Sage Publications.

DeVries, R., & Subedi, J. (1998). Why bioethics needs sociology. In R. DeVries & J. Subedi (Eds.), *Bioethics and society: Constructing the ethical enterprise* (pp. 233–257). Upper Saddle River, NJ: Prentice Hall.

Dillaway, H., & Clifford, B. (2001). Race, class, and gender difference in marital satisfaction and divisions of household labor among dual earner couples: A case for intersectional analysis. *Journal of Family Issues, 22*(3), 309–327.

Duffy, M. (2005). Reproducing labor inequalities: Challenges for feminists conceptualizing care at the intersections of gender, race, and class. *Gender and Society, 19*(1), 66–82.

Duffy, M. (2007). Doing the dirty work: Gender, race and the reproductive labor in historical perspective. *Gender and Society, 21*(3), 313–336.

England, P. (1992). *Comparable worth: Theories and evidence.* New York: Aldine De Gruyter.

England, P., Budig, M., & Folbre, N. (2002). Wages of virtue: The relative pay of care work. *Social Problems, 49,* 455–473.

Glenn, E. N. (1992). From servitude to service work: Historical continuities in the racial division of paid reproductive labor. *Signs: Journal of Women in Culture and Society, 18*(1), 1–43.

Glenn, E. N. (2002). *Unequal freedom: How race and gender shaped American citizenship and labor.* Cambridge, MA: Harvard University Press.

Gustafson, D. L. (2005). Transcultural nursing theory from a critical cultural perspective. *Advances in Nursing Science, 28*(1), 2–16.

Gustafson, D. L. (2007). White on whiteness: Becoming radicalized about race. *Nursing Inquiry, 14*(2), 153–161.

Hine, D. C. (1989). *Black women in white: Racial conflict and cooperation in the nursing profession, 1890–1950.* Bloomington, IN: Indiana University Press.

Hochschild, A. R. (1989). *The second shift*. New York: Avon Books.

Hoffmaster, B. (1992). Can ethnography save the life of medical ethics? *Social Science and Medicine, 35*(12), 1421–1431.

hooks, b. (1989). *Talking back: Thinking feminist, thinking black*. Toronto, ON: Between the Lines.

Mead, G. H. (1959). *Mind, self and society from the standpoint of a social behaviorist*. Chicago: Chicago University Press.

Mills, C. W. (1959). *The sociological imagination*. New York: Oxford University Press.

Roberts, D. (1997). Spiritual and menial household. *Yale Journal of Law and Feminism, 9*(1), 51–80.

Rothenberg, P. S. (2005). *White privilege: Essential readings on the other side of racism* (2nd ed.). New York: Worth Publishers.

Smith, D. (1990). *Texts, facts and femininity. Exploring the relations of ruling*. New York: Routledge.

Sokoloff, N., & Dupont, I. (2005). Domestic violence at the intersections of race, class, and gender. *Violence Against Women, 11*(1), 38–64.

Thomas, W. I. (1966). The relation of research to the social process. In M. Janowitz (Ed.), *W. I. Thomas on social organization and social personality*. Chicago: University of Chicago Press.

Zussman, R. (1992). *Intensive care: Medical ethics and the medical profession*. Chicago: University of Chicago Press.

Zussman, R. (1997). Sociological perspectives on medical ethics and decision-making. *Annual Review of Sociology, 23*(1), 171–89.

Shireen S. Rajaram is a Professor of Sociology at the University of Nebraska at Omaha (UNO). She is the chair of the Department of Sociology and Anthropology at UNO. She has a courtesy joint-appointment with the College of Public Health at the University of Nebraska Medical Center. She is a member of the Women's Studies, Latino and Latin American Studies, and Environmental Studies programs at UNO. She received her PhD in Medical Sociology from the University of Kentucky and has a Certificate in Medical Behavioral Science from the Department of Behavioral Sciences at the University of Kentucky. Her main areas of interest are women's health, minority health, and environmental health.

She has done research in breast and cervical cancer, diabetes, and childhood lead poisoning. She has published extensively in journals such as *Women and Health, Health Care for Women International, Preventive Medicine,* and *Sociology of Health and Illness.* She teaches graduate and undergraduate classes on Women's Health, Ethnicity and Health, and Society and Health.

CRITICAL THINKING ACTIVITIES

Nursing Ethics and Sociology

+ Retrieve a study from the nursing literature in which the investigators used an ethnographic design. What sorts of ethics research questions could be answered using an ethnographic design?

+ Rajaram states, "The sociologist's approach to nursing ethics is grounded in a social context perspective which acknowledges a hierarchal organizational structure of health care. Understanding this lack of power, perhaps, adopting a broader sociological perspective related to power might help." How do you think this sociological perspective might help?

SECTION II

Philosophical and Theoretical Issues

Theories, principles, and propositions and concepts which comprise the epistemology of nursing ethics and the possible paradigm shift in nursing ethics from those postulated in medical ethics.

The Body Flute

Cortney Davis

O my body! I dare not desert the likes of you in other men
and women, nor the likes of the parts of you.
Walt Whitman

I go on loving the flesh
after you die.
I close your eyes
bathe your bruised limbs
press down the edges of tape
sealing your dry wounds.

I walk with you to the morgue
and pillow your head
against the metal drawer. To me
this is your final resting place.
Your time with me
is the sum of your life.

I have met your husbands and wives
but I know who loved you most,
who owned the sum
of your visible parts.
The doctor and his theory
never owned you.

Nor did "medicine" or "hospital"
ever own you.
Couldn't you, didn't you
refuse tests, refuse to take your medicine?

But I am the nurse
of childhood's sounds in the night,
nurse of the washrag's sting
nurse of needle and sleep
nurse of lotion and hands on skin
nurse of sheets and nightmares
nurse of the flashlight beam at 3 a.m.

I know the privacy of vagina and rectum
I slip catheters into openings
I clean you like a mother does.
That which you allow no one,
you allow me.

Who sat with you that night?
Your doctor was asleep,

your husband was driving in.
Your wife took a few things

home to wash, poor timing,
but she had been by your side for days.

Your kids? They could be anywhere
even out with the vending machines

working out just how much
you did or didn't do for them.

You waited
until you were alone
with me. You trusted
that I could wait and not be
frightened away.
That I would not expect

anything of you—
not bravery or anger, not even
a good fight.

At death
you become wholly mine.

∽   ∽   ∽

Your last glance, your last
sensation of touch,
your breath

I inhale, incorporating you
into memory.
Your body

silvery and still on the bed,
your lips fluttering into blue.
I pull your hand away from mine.

My other hand lingers, traces
your finger from the knucklebone
to the sheets

into which your body sinks,
my lips over yours,
my cheek near the blue

absence of your breath,
my hands closing
the silver stops of your eyelid.

Sara T. Fry

CHAPTER 5

Philosophical and Theoretical Issues in Nursing Ethics

Framing the Issues/Themes

There are a number of philosophical and theoretical issues in nursing ethics. Some issues concern the "moral phenomena of nursing practice." For example, we might ask: What are the moral phenomena that nurses encounter in the practice of nursing? How are they recognized, and how do nurses name and address them? How should these phenomena be understood? A second group of issues concerns "patients' rights and nurses' moral duties and responsibilities." For example, we might ask: How are patients' basic rights recognized and respected by the nurse? How do we understand nurses' moral duties in response to patients' rights? Which moral goods and values ought to guide the nurse-patient relationship?

A third group of issues concerns the "moral language of nursing." For example: What do we mean by terms such as "moral concepts," "rights," "duties," "goods," and "values" in relation to nursing practice? What are the moral concepts that guide nursing practice and what are their origins? What do we mean by "patient good," and how do nurses contribute to this "good"? Which moral values guide the nurse-patient relationship?

A last set of questions involves the "nature and type of theory needed for ethical nursing practice." For example: What role should a theory of care play in nurses' ethical judgments, and is care a necessary and/or sufficient condition for any theory of nursing ethics? To what extent should theories of bioethics or theories of medical ethics influence theories of nursing ethics? What type of theory is needed for nurses' ethical practices for the 21st century?

Where ethical judgments of the nurse are concerned, there is a diverse body of literature addressing the usefulness of rational systems of thought and the application of ethical principles, justice-oriented and care-oriented patterns of reasoning, and the care perspective in nursing practice. All of these approaches are laden with different theoretical presuppositions, and may potentially influence the way that the nurse recognizes ethical conflict, names and addresses it, as part of the clinical judgment process.

Raising questions about these presuppositions and articulating the role of ethical reasoning in nurses' clinical judgments are essential aspects of doing the philosophy of nursing. For example, some philosophical discussions about nurses' ethical judgments have explored the relationships among experience, expertise, context, and nurses' "skilled ethical comportment" (Benner, 1991), and promoted caring as a way of knowing and not knowing (Benner, 1994). Other scholars are exploring questions about the meaning of moral concepts and principles in terms of culture as a necessary step to the development of nursing ethics theory (Lutzen, 1997; Lutzen & Nordin, 1993). As I have argued elsewhere (Fry, 2004a), the care perspective means different things to different people. For example, some assert that the care perspective is a necessary basis for nurses' ethical judgments (Nortvedt, 1996). Some claim that it promises a theoretical foundation for a nursing ethic (Fry, 1989) and can be formally classified for its use in clinical judgment (Ray, 1984). Others, however, criticize the care perspective as a basis for nurses' ethical judgments, because (a) the current focus on care attempts to explain a complex process with conceptual similarities to teaching, in terms of behavioral categories and structures (Phillips, 1993); (b) it emphasizes the caring relationship between nursing and patient, rather than the individuals in that relationship (Omery, 1995; Warelow, 1996); and (c) the caring ideal is a vice rather than a virtue in that it promotes dependency, sexism, unfairness, emotional attachment, and burnout (Curzer, 1993).

The philosophy of nursing is an emerging type of inquiry and not a new field—indeed, it has developed alongside the development of nursing science over the past 150 years. Only recently, however, has there been evidence of increased productivity and interest in the field. It is now possible to (a) identify the ontological, epistemological, and ethical issues that comprise the field of inquiry, (b) provide an overview of current work in the philosophy of nursing, and (c) anticipate the areas of discourse that will require further development in the 21st century.

Background and Influences

My background and influences have prepared me to make contributions to the philosophy of nursing and to address some of the particular issues identified above. I was in clinical nursing practice for about 15 years, I pursued higher education in philosophy both at the undergraduate and graduate levels, and focused my professional work specifically on the philosophy of nursing and nursing ethics.

My professional work is based on several basic presuppositions and understandings. For example, I understand that the philosophy of nursing is not a well-defined field of inquiry with a coherent structure. Philosophy, itself, is a type of inquiry that uses critical analysis to describe, evaluate, and understand various phenomena in the universe or the world of human affairs. The forms of the inquiry can be speculative, normative, or logical. Nursing, on the other hand, can be defined differently, depending on whether one focuses on its social construction, purpose, activities, or outcomes. Regardless of how nursing is defined, most people understand that nursing includes activities that are supported by the sciences and the humanities, and is oriented "to the provision of care that promotes well-being in the people served" (American Nurses Association [ANA], 1995, p. 6). Unlike medicine, which is concerned with diagnosing, treating, and preventing disease, nursing is concerned with promoting health, preventing illness, restoring health, and alleviating suffering (International Council of Nurses [ICN], 2006). In addressing these concerns, nursing focuses on "human experiences and responses to birth, health, illness, and death" (ANA, 1995, p. 8).

With these definitions of "philosophy" and "nursing" in mind, the philosophy of nursing can be understood as philosophical inquiry about nursing's social and humanitarian role, its forms of thought, nature, scope, purpose, methods, language, moral presuppositions, and knowledge claims. The philosophy of nursing is an activity that one does. It is not an entity that is created by one type of investigation or another. It is a type of inquiry that uses philosophical methods and raises questions about the aspects of nursing listed above. This is a broad view of the field of inquiry and is influenced by my own study of the philosophy of medicine as well as discussions with colleagues over the years. Other views of the philosophy of nursing probably exist and may or may not be in agreement with this view.

Impact of My Work on Health Care Ethics

Most of my professional work has been concerned with identifying and analyzing (a) the beginning discussions of philosophy of nursing in the scholarship of nurse leaders, in general, and (b) the development of nursing ethics throughout nursing's short history, in particular. I have also contributed to discussions about the moral concepts and language of nursing and conducted research about ethical issues experienced by practicing nurses. An overview of some of this work is described below.

Philosophical Questions Addressed by Others

As I have discussed elsewhere (Fry, 1999), a number of nurse leaders and scholars have, over the years raised philosophical questions about nursing. Some of the ontological questions they have posed are: What is the nature of nursing practice? Is it an art, a science, or a type of presence? Asking these types of questions is important because it helps us to identify the objects of nursing knowledge and, as Kikuchi points out, "without the direction provided by nursing knowledge, the end result of our efforts at inquiry would be chaos" (1992, p. 35). Metaphysical or ontological questions about the nature of nursing are not new. Nightingale (1860/1969) asked such questions, and concluded that the nature of nursing was assisting reparative processes brought about by disease by putting the patient in the best condition for nature to act upon him.

Some 90 years later, Peplau (1952) asked similar questions and offered the view that the nature of nursing is to "function in cooperation with internal and external human processes" (p. 13). More recently, the nature of nursing has been described as (a) "existential advocacy," where the nurse participates with the patient in determining the unique meaning that the experience of health, illness, suffering, or dying has for that individual (Gadow, 1980); (b) an art that is associated with expressive, creative, and intuitive activities (Johnson, 1994, 1996; Katims, 1993); (c) a moral practice that is characterized by "good nursing" and caring relationships between nurse and patient (Gastmans, Dierckx de Casterle, & Schotsmans, 1998); and (d) a professional practice with affective, cognitive, volitional, imaginative, motivational, and action-expressive conditions that are both necessary and sufficient (Taylor, 1997, 1998).

Epistemological issues in the philosophy of nursing have received a lot of attention from nurse scholars. One reason for this may be related to the functions of philosophy, especially its function as an analytical tool that can display the structures of reasoning in clinical judgment. Epistemological issues include the nature, scope, and objects of nursing knowledge (Kikuchi, 1992). Some of the questions asked are the following: Is there knowledge used by nurses that is unique to nursing? If so, what is its nature and structure, and how is its truth evaluated? If the knowledge that nurses use is shared with other disciplines, what does it consist of and how is the truth of that knowledge evaluated?

Philosophical Questions that Need to be Addressed

One of the issues that ought to be addressed about the nature of nursing knowledge is whether a conceptualist-realist or an ontological view of human responses is more appropriate to the practice of nursing. Are human responses merely the ways in which actual or potential health problems manifest themselves in people and that can be ameliorated by nursing interventions (realist view)? Or do human responses have etiological and pathophysiological causes that are amenable to nursing interventions (ontological view)? This issue has been extensively discussed in the philosophy of medicine literature (Englehardt & Erde, 1980). It is missing, however, in the discussion of nursing diagnosis and its taxonomy (nosology) that blends both perspectives together, and that may make it harder to design, test, and evaluate the effectiveness of nursing interventions in terms of measurable outcomes. The blending phenomenon also tends to blur the boundaries of the nurse's focus in making nursing diagnoses.

A similar question concerns whether the human responses that nurses diagnose are grounded in underlying pathological, physiological, and psychological processes or are socially determined and therefore part of a social construct (Foucault, 1973). The present forms of nursing diagnoses do not consider the social construction of the human responses that nurses address and therefore miss environmental and intervening variables that may be involved in their manifestation and the reason for their recognition. Discussion of these last two issues might shed new light on how nurses "know" and recognize patterns of human responses. The world of human responses might even appear quite different to nurses if their theoretical assumptions or concepts change.

The role of theory in what is known about the patient is a metatheoretical issue that should be philosophically addressed. We might, for example, question whether the "thought style" of the nursing research community influences the character of the human responses that are recognized by nurses. The interrelatedness of theory and fact has been demonstrated in other sciences (Fleck, 1979) but has not been adequately addressed in nursing. The recent trend in the use of more formalized systems of clinical judgment, including the usefulness of probability reasoning to rationally construct the process of clinical judgment, might also be questioned for its influence on what is known about the patient.

The Development of Nursing Ethics

Most of my early work concerned the ethic of nursing and the moral concepts and values of nursing. Where the ethic of nursing was concerned, I was aware that there are many views about the nursing ethic, and that some have argued that the nursing ethic is a role-specific and "derived" ethic, based on an ethic of medicine and its tradition of paternalism (Veatch, 1981). In my opinion, the nursing ethic is still evolving; therefore, we should let the ethic speak for itself and not try to cast it into one form or another at the present time. I am still letting it speak to me, so I do not claim to have the final word on the topic. But I do have a few thoughts on how it has been formed and the central values of this ethic.

Early interpretations of the nursing ethic tend to be associated with the image of the nurse as a chaste, good woman in Christian service to others; also, as an obedient, dutiful servant (Fry, 2004b). The nursing ethic was practicing forms of etiquette and keeping one's duty. The nurse demonstrated her acceptance of the moral duties of nursing by following the rules of etiquette and by being loyal and obedient to the physician (Robb, 1921). Textbooks in nursing described nursing ethics as the ideals, customs, and habits associated with the general characteristics of a nurse (Aikens, 1916), and as doing one's duty with skill and moral perfection (Gladwin, 1930). The rules of etiquette were followed in order to promote professional harmony in patient care.

Following World War II, however, the nurse's role in patient care changed. Keeping the rules of etiquette became less important than meeting standards for nurses' moral behavior and following the science of ethics. The nurse was expected to do good for the patient and was beginning to define "doing good." Being competent, having compassion, protecting the patient's dignity, and doing for others were the central elements of what was beginning to be understood as the nursing ethic. This was an obligation model of the nursing ethic and was based on duties of the nurse as expressed in the nursing code of ethics.

It was not until the patients' rights movement during the 1950s that the nursing ethic evolved to an ethic based on the service nature of the nurse-patient relationship. The image of the nurse as the physician's obedient helper carrying out her duties was replaced by an image of the nurse as an independent practitioner who could be held accountable for what had been done, or not done, in providing nursing care. Rather than someone who carried out the decisions made by others, the nurse now claimed authority and moral responsibility for specific clinical judgments in patient care.

As the ethic of nursing developed, discussion about the moral concepts and values of nursing likewise developed. They support a moral foundation for nursing practice and have important implications for understanding what characterizes nurses' ethical practices. The concept of cooperation stems from early conceptions of the relationship of the nurse to the physician and other health care workers. The concept of accountability developed out of the moral responsibility of the nurse as an independent nurse practitioner after World War II.

The concept of caring developed from the perceived need for the nurse to perform caring behaviors as health care delivery became a highly impersonalized and complex system of multiple health care workers. The nurse is the one health care worker who still maintains a close relationship with the patient despite these changes. Thus, caring behaviors, while always expected of the nurse, have a new importance and meaning in modern health care delivery. One new concept, advocacy, has emerged in recent years in response to trends in the protections of patients' rights in health care and the roles that nurses have in helping patients to exercise these rights. Together, these four moral concepts provide a starting point for nursing ethics inquiry in the 21st century and help us understand the "good" nurse and the nature of nurses' ethical practices. Because there is consensus among nurses throughout the world that these four concepts provide a moral foundation for the work of nursing and shape the nursing ethic, there is remarkable agreement, as well, on the moral values of nursing. These values are honesty (or truthfulness), compassion, respect for others, doing good for others, competence, and keeping commitments.

These values indicate that the nursing care relationship is truly a covenantal one and not just a relationship of obligations or duty (Raines, 1997). I use the term "covenant" to mean that the nursing care relationship has certain elements that make it more than a contracted relationship within which code behaviors or certain services are obliged to take place (May, 1975; Stenberg, 1979). This is what nurses offer to patients and to the public—a covenantal relationship responsive to patients' needs. As I have written elsewhere (Fry, 2000), it includes a promise to be faithful in providing nursing services to those who need them. Essentially, this is the nursing ethic—a promise to serve or provide nursing care, and fidelity to the promise (May).

Broader Significance beyond the Discipline of Nursing

Unfortunately, the nursing ethic is an endangered ethic for several reasons. First, nurses are currently doing more good with fewer resources than ever before. As a 1996 study (Shindul-Rothschild, Berry, & Long-Middleton, 1996) of over 7,000 nurses found, part-time or temporary Registered Nurses (RNs) and unlicensed personnel are being substituted for full-time RNs throughout the United States. They are taking care of more patients, are being cross-trained to take on more nursing responsibilities, and have substantially less time to provide all aspects of nursing care. A major reason for these changes is cutbacks and alterations in how health care is delivered. What does this say about the service of nursing care and how nurses understand their commitment to doing good?

A second reason that the nursing ethic is endangered is that nurses are now expected to do limited good, or do good within prescribed limits. Many nurses leave patient interactions feeling that they did not "do good," where good is interpreted as quality care or what the patient actually needs in order to remain healthy and not be at risk for more health care problems. As Mohr and Mahon (1996) point out, these types of problems are "dirty hands" situations in that the nurse has been required to take part in or implement an immoral project. A third reason for an endangered ethic is profit-driven incentives that can compromise clinical judgments about patient care needs. Such incentives make it difficult for nurses to exercise their judgments about patients' nursing care needs. A fourth reason is that nurses are taking on more responsibilities in the health care environment than direct patient care. They may be supervising a variety of health care workers, doing budgets, arranging in-service education for these workers, and so forth. Finally, many nurses report that they need other skills in order to be an ethical nurse. Knowing the professional code of ethics, using good clinical judgment, and understanding how to apply ethical principles to patient care situations are no longer sufficient skills for one to be an ethical nurse. Nurses need to have superior communication skills in order to raise ethical questions about a patient's care with physicians and other staff who often do not value the nurse's information about the patient. They need assertiveness training in order to defend patients' rights within a health care system that is increasingly unresponsive to patients' rights. They need to have good negotiation skills in order to work with for-profit, managed-care case managers. They need skills of persuasion in order to bring different members of the health care team to consensus about what to do for the patient. They need to know how to use the techniques of ethical compromise so that members of the health care team can agree on a plan of care for the patient, and not feel that they have lost their integrity in doing so (Fry, 1989).

These are all reasons why the nursing ethic is presently endangered. The climate for the delivery of health care in the past 15 years has changed in much the same way that the climate changed in the 1950s—the cost of health care has dramatically increased while the pattern of health care delivery has changed. These changes have the potential to change the future of nursing care and how it is provided.

References

Aikens, C. S. (1916). *Studies in ethics for nurses.* Philadelphia: W. B. Saunders.

American Nurses Association. (1995). *Nursing's social policy statement.* Washington, DC: Author.

Benner, P. (1991). The role of experience, narrative, and community in skilled ethical comportment. *Advances in Nursing Science, 14*(2), 1–21.

Benner, P. (1994). Caring as a way of knowing and not knowing. In S. S. Phillips & P. Benner (Eds.), *The crisis of care: Affirming and restoring caring practices in the helping professions* (pp. 42–62). Washington, DC: Georgetown University.

Curzer, H. J. (1993). Is care a virtue for health care professionals? *Journal of Medicine and Philosophy, 18*(1), 51–69.

Englehardt, H. T., & Erde, E. L. (1980). Philosophy of medicine. In P. T. Durbin (Ed.), *A guide to the culture of science, technology, and medicine* (pp. 364–461). New York: Free Press.

Fleck, L. (1979). *Genesis and development of a scientific fact.* (T.J. Trenn & R. K. Merton, Eds.; F. Bradley, Trans.). Chicago: University of Chicago Press. (Originally published as Entstehung und entwicklung: Einer wissenschaften tatsache. Basel, Switzerland: Benno Schwabe, 1935).

Foucault, M. (1973). *The birth of the clinic: An archaeology of medical perception.* (A. M. Sheridan Smith, Trans.). New York: Pantheon Books.

Fry, S. T. (1989). Toward a theory of nursing ethics. *Advances in Nursing Science, 11*(4), 9–22.

Fry, S. T. (1999). The philosophy of nursing. *Scholarly Inquiry for Nursing Practice, 13*(1), 5–15.

Fry, S. T. (2000). Doing good: From paternalism to a nursing ethic. In A.B. McBride (Ed.), *Nursing & philanthropy: An energizing metaphor for the 21st century* (pp. 17–30). Indianapolis, IN: Center Nursing Press, Sigma Theta Tau International.

Fry, S. T. (2004a). Nursing ethics. In G. Khushf (Ed.), *Handbook of bioethics: Taking stock of the field from a philosophical perspective* (pp. 489–505). Dordrecht, Netherlands: Kluwer Academic.

Fry, S. T. (2004b). Nursing ethics. In S. G. Post (Ed.), *Encyclopedia of bioethics* (3rd Ed.). New York: Macmillan Reference, USA.

Gadow, S. (1980). Existential advocacy: Philosophical foundation of nursing. In S. F. Spicker & S. Gadow (Eds.), *Nursing, images and ideals: Opening dialogue with the humanities* (pp. 79–101). New York: Springer.

Gastmans, C., Dierckx de Casterle, B., and Schotsmans, P. (1998). Nursing considered as moral practice: A philosophical-ethical interpretation of nursing. *Kennedy Institute of Ethics Journal, 8*(1), 43–69.

Gladwin, M. E. (1930). *Ethics: Talks to nurses.* Philadelphia: W. B. Saunders.

International Council of Nurses [ICN]. (2006). *The ICN Code of Ethics for nurses.* Retrieved November 13, 2007, from http://www.icn.ch/icncode.pdf.

Johnson, J. (1994). Toward a clearer understanding of the art of nursing. *AARN Newsletter, 50*(1), 18.

Johnson, J. (1996). Dialectical analysis concerning the rational aspect of the art of nursing. *Image: Journal of Nursing Scholarship, 28*(2), 169–175.

Katims, I. (1993). Nursing as aesthetic experience and the notion of practice. *Scholarly Inquiry for Nursing Practice, 7*(4), 269–282.

Kikuchi, J. F. (1992). Nursing questions that science cannot answer. In J. F. Kikuchi & H. Simmons (Eds.), *Philosophic inquiry in nursing* (pp. 26–37). Newbury Park, CA: Sage Publications.

Lutzen, K. (1997). Nursing ethics into the next millennium: A context-sensitive approach for nursing ethics. *Nursing Ethics, 4*(3), 218–226.

Lutzen, K., & Nordin, C. (1993). Structuring moral meaning in psychiatric nursing practice. *Scandinavian Journal of Caring Sciences, 7*(3), 175–180.

May, W. (1975). Code, covenant, contract or philanthropy. *Hastings Center Report, 5*(6), 29–38.

Mohr, W. K., & Mahon, M. M. (1996). Dirty hands: The underside of marketplace health care. *Advances in Nursing Science, 19*(1), 28–37.

Nightingale, F. (1969). *Notes on nursing: What it is, and what it is not.* New York: Dover. (Original work published in 1860).

Nortvedt, P. (1996). *Sensitive judgment: Nursing, moral philosophy, and an ethics of care.* Oslo, Norway: Tano Achehoug.

Omery, A. (1995). Care: The basis for a nursing ethic? *Journal of Cardiovascular Nursing, 9*(3), 1–10.

Peplau, H. E. (1952). *Interpersonal relations in nursing.* New York: G. P. Putnam.

Phillips, P. (1993). A deconstruction of caring. *Journal of Advanced Nursing, 18*(10), 1554–1558.

Raines, D. A. (1997). From covenant to contract: How managed care is changing provider/patient relationships. *AWHONN Lifelines, 1*(4), 41–45.

Ray, M. A. (1984). The development of a classification system of caring. In M. M. Leininger (Ed.), *Care: The essence of nursing* (pp. 95–112). Thorofare, NJ: Slack.

Robb, I. H. (1921). *Nursing ethics: For hospital and private use.* Cleveland, OH: E. C. Koeckert.

Shindul-Rothschild, J., Berry, D., and Long-Middleton, E. (1996). Where have all the nurses gone? Final results of our patient care survey. *American Journal of Nursing, 96*(11), 24–39.

Stenberg, M. J. (1979). The search for a conceptual framework as a philosophical basis for nursing ethics: An examination of code, contract, context, and covenant. *Military Medicine, 144*(1), 9–22.

Taylor, C. R. (1997). *The morality internal to the practice of nursing.* Unpublished doctoral dissertation. Georgetown University, Washington, DC.

Taylor, C. R. (1998). Reflections on "nursing considered as moral practice." *Kennedy Institute of Ethics Journal, 8*(1), 71–82.

Veatch, R. M. (1981). Nursing ethics, physician ethics, and medical ethics. *Law, Medicine, and Health Care, 9*(5), 17–19.

Warelow, P. J. (1996). Is caring the ethical ideal? *Journal of Advanced Nursing, 24*(4), 655–661.

Sara T. Fry, BS, MS, MA, PhD, RN, is former Henry R. Luce Professor of Nursing Ethics at the Boston College School of Nursing, Chestnut Hill, MA. Her education includes degrees at Georgetown University (MA and PhD in philosophy), University of North Carolina, Chapel Hill (MS), University of South Carolina, Columbia (BS) and The Johns Hopkins Hospital School of Nursing. She is co-author with Dr. Robert Veatch of *Case Studies in Nursing Ethics.* Dr. Fry's role in nursing ethics covers a broad spectrum of experiences and contributions to the field including but not limited to funded and unfunded research projects, consultations and other professional services, editorial and scholarly review functions, positions in various professional organizations and committees, presentations and publications (books, book chapters, journal articles, reviews, and letters).

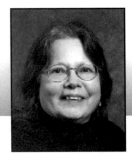

Mary Ellen Wurzbach

CHAPTER 6

Moral Conviction, Moral Regret, and Moral Comfort— Theoretical Perspectives

Moral knowledge is seen, by some, as the epitome of rational thought about ethical issues, whereas the same philosophical theorists see emotion as the greatest impediment to the thoughtful resolution of ethical dilemmas. This debate about the role of reason and emotion in ethics goes back to the time of Plato (trans. 2007), who created and argued for the three concepts he considered essential to the soul—cognition, emotion, and conation (motivation). The disagreement continues today. My work is grounded in this debate, emphasizing the role of moral conviction (moral certainty and uncertainty), moral comfort, and moral regret in ethical decision-making.

Until recently, the role of emotion in and the psychological aspects of ethical decision-making were infrequently studied. Ethical decision-making was seen as a rational, evaluative, cognitive process of choosing options or alternatives from a variety of possibilities. Choices were presumed to be based on the consequences of the action, or on a standard or principle. Despite this belief that ethical decision-making was more like scientific thought and was thus more palatable to the philosopher/scientist, emotion could not be ignored.

I have followed many paths in nursing ethics. Most of my work examines the interface between rational, ethical decision-making and moral emotions based on the qualitative study of nurses' thoughts, beliefs, and experiences. My research involved the exploration of moral certainty/uncertainty (moral conviction), moral regret in ethical decision-making, and comfort as a moral principle in nursing ethics, but I have also written about other ethical issues which affect Advanced Practice Nurses (nurse practitioners), such as ethical conflict in managed care (Wurzbach, 1998), practitioner-assisted suicide (Wurzbach, 2000), and risk and trust as they impact patients in our health care system. My most frequently cited work describes the "moral metaphors of nursing" (Wurzbach, 1999b). In all cases I have tried to write from a nursing perspective, rather than simply following principlism as a medical model of bioethics. In my experience nurses have a unique experiential position in the health care system and in many cases a unique vision of ethical issues. My research is most strongly related to the issues of withholding or withdrawing artificial nutrition and hydration. Through the years I have also personally experienced the ethical dilemmas that many ethicists discuss but never live through, thereby grounding my personal perspective in nursing theory and philosophy.

My Context

Over the years I have held a Durable Power of Attorney for Health Care (DPOA-HC) or served as guardian for six family members and had the opportunity to not only study moral certainty, moral uncertainty, moral regret in ethical decision-making, and comfort as an ethical principle in nursing ethics, but have also lived these many nursing ethical concepts. When I began as my uncle's guardian, I held the moral conviction that withholding the feeding tube was the "right" thing to do. Withholding would keep him from dying slowly over many years without being able to recognize members of his family, unable to communicate or eat or retain any other characteristics of a quality of life. As the situation went on, I became more uncertain about whether I was doing the "right" thing or whether I was making a decision that I ought not to be making. The decision was taken out of my hands within a week when he died.

During this episode I learned several things that I think require research. In almost all cases the doctors and nurses refused to give me any advice; they indicated to me that they were just there to support my decisions. This is what I called the "influence taboo" in my own research (Wurzbach, 1996b). The second aspect of the situation that struck me was that there seemed to be as much uncertainty about withholding a gastrostomy tube now as there was about refusing a nasogastric tube 17 years ago. The staff (both at the nursing home and in the hospital) was more amenable to the idea today than years ago, but still told me that if a gastrostomy tube were put in it would not be removed until my uncle's death. Many years ago the Hastings Center working group (1987) came to the conclusion that there was no moral difference between withholding or withdrawing a feeding tube, and that "trials" of a tube were morally permissible, yet here, probably 20 years later, there was still the belief that if a feeding tube was put in, it could not come out until death. This led me to the conclusion that although there is no moral difference between withholding or withdrawing, the psychological aspects of withholding and withdrawing are as different from the moral aspects today as they were so many years ago. There was no belief that a trial of the tube was permissible, leaving me in the situation of having to make an all-or-nothing decision (Wurzbach, 1990, 1991, 1992, 2002).

My Work in Health Care Ethics

According to Quinn and Smith (1987), a lack of ethical knowledge, situational uniqueness, insufficient precedents, questions about the applications of principles, and a difference in basic values or principles, lead to moral conflict. Moral conflict is comprised of conflict between principles, conflict between two moral actions, conflict between the demand for action and the need for reflection, conflict of equally unsatisfactory alternatives, conflicts of value, and conflicts of principles and role obligations (Davis & Smith, 1980).

My work fits into the area of personality and social psychological theory of bioethics and is based on the qualitative study of nurses' thoughts, beliefs, and experiences. I concentrate on nurses' experiences of moral certainty, moral uncertainty with moral regret, and comfort as an ethical principle for nurses. Because I "grew up" in nursing at a time when the study of the conceptual basis of nursing was taught and studied, I have continued to pursue this aspect of nursing—the concepts of ethical theory.

Moral Uncertainty

Moral uncertainty and moral certainty, if discussed at all in the nursing ethics or research literature, are in reference to an ethical dilemma. Moral uncertainty results in indecision and feelings of loss of control (Crisham, 1981; Quinn & Smith, 1987). Moral certainty can come from moral knowledge, principles, virtue or character, contextual variables, or one's own experience. In my own research, the nurse's experience with an issue and the situation surrounding the decision were the primary sources of moral certainty. Consensus arose from moral uncertainty with its questioning, investigating, and delving deeply into a moral dilemma—all essential aspects of moral behavior.

Moral uncertainty as defined in my studies is an inability to determine the "right" course of action to pursue. Possible responses to uncertainty include acknowledging this condition and dialoguing about possible options to make moral uncertainty a moral opportunity. Acceptance or tolerance of uncertainty might lead to indifference (Quinn & Smith, 1987). Another option is choosing the status quo, which involves less responsibility. Delay can make it possible to inspect further alternatives but can also result in a failure to perceive an occasion for choice (Corbin, 1980). Some argue that making "no" choice is a viable choice (Quinn & Smith).

For centuries the theoretical model for dealing with uncertainty was the expected utility model (EU) first suggested by John Stuart Mill (1859/2007). Persons were assumed to weigh the utility or desirability of each option available to them, the possible outcomes, and their probability of occurring. This was the consequentialist approach to ethics. In my research, nurses' moral uncertainty prompted them to seek information, look for consensus, and required structured preplanning (advance directives) and documentation of the resident's choice. I believe they could not gauge the probabilities, so they sought more information and in almost all cases either abdicated decision-making in favor of the "influence taboo" or contributed to a consensus among the decision-makers. In either event, there was no individual choice for the nurse to make (Wurzbach, 1995).

One of the consequences of moral uncertainty found in my research is moral regret (looking back). This consequence, discussed later, was the most frequent and long-lasting experienced by nurse caregivers. Despite this negative consequence of moral uncertainty, I found that it may also provide the opportunity to search for new information, consult others, and provide time for a thoughtful response (Wurzbach, 1995).

Moral Certainty

In contrast to moral uncertainty, moral certainty is based upon absolute conviction, psychological commitment, and the absence of doubt (Klein, 1981; Miller, 1978). This conviction is based upon indubitable evidence that the belief is "right" and no strong counterevidence is perceived (Odegard, 1982). I concurred with this definition (Wurzbach, 1995). Moral certainty or clarity can be positive and admirable. How does one differentiate between justifiable action (reflective moral conviction) and unjustifiable action (unfounded zeal or self-deception), however?

Moral certainty may have different results, depending upon the nurse's potential to act upon the belief. If there are no institutional constraints, the nurse may experience a feeling of security. In addition, nurses may be able to direct their course of action, thus translating intention into action (Wurzbach, 1995). Conversely, if there are institutional constraints which make action impossible, moral distress may result (Jameton, 1984).

My research on moral conviction demonstrated that moral conviction supported by strong emotion may be positive, in that nurses who are morally convinced speak up, stand up, and/or refuse to participate, but may also be compelled to act and seek very little or no advice from others before acting (Wurzbach, 1996b). Based on their results, researchers suggest that some emotions, such as those of loss or injustice, contain "action tendencies" which prompt action. Intense emotions carry with them these tendencies (moral certainty) (Frijda, 1986; Frijda & Mesquita, 1994). Some scientists believe adding affect to decision-making models greatly improves their explanatory potential (Clore, 1992; Forgas, 1995; Isen, 1993; Lerner & Keltner, 2000; Lowenstein & Lerner, 2003). Emotions thus simplify cognitive processing, because people respond in predetermined ways to loss, injustice, and threat but emotions can also be a possible source of "biased judgment" and "reckless action" (Loewenstein & Lerner).

On the other hand, moderate conviction with the ability to make ethical decisions allows persons to respond with courage to dilemmas and issues which require a decision. Advocacy is possible. A converse argument can be provided in situations where possibly only one viewpoint is heard and the person, agency, and society are benefited. Yet, absolute conviction also has a negative aspect, which is the inability to question oneself.

Since experience seems to make moral certainty more likely, bioethicists convey to decision-makers that sometimes reserving judgment is more prudent, allowing for the possibility of revising recommendations. One aspect of moral certainty is insensitivity to new information, or a failure to hear alternative solutions. One of my research participants observed that "continuous dialogue leads to less moral certainty and also less moral uncertainty" (Wurzbach, 2005b).

Moral Comfort

Comfort as an aspect of nursing care has been cited as a desired goal or outcome for over a century. References to comfort may be found in historical nursing texts, in nursing diagnoses, and measures of quality care. One nursing theorist has made comfort an integral concept (Kolcaba, 1992, 2003). However, little has been written about comfort as an ethical principle and little research has been conducted. In my studies of long-term care nurses' convictions, comfort for all individuals was a prominent theme in end-of-life care of the elderly (Wurzbach, 1996b). In fact, comfort rose to the level of an ethical principle more commonly in the nurses' stories than the most often-cited bioethical principles of autonomy, beneficence, nonmaleficence, and justice. Comfort for the dying person, the family, and nursing caregivers was the ultimate test (both ethically and clinically) of the efficacy of final interventions.

Comfort as an ethical principle in the care of the dying entails both "doing" and "feeling" (Wurzbach, 1996a). "Doing" means meeting the needs of both the dying and their families and promoting their comfort. "Feeling" means experiencing comfort as a sense of peace. Long-term care nurses provided comfort by looking at everyone's wishes in order to come to the best decision about an issue. They shared "common ground" with their residents, tried to be nonjudgmental, gave residents options, and provided comfort for residents and families by being ready to listen. Promoting the resident's and family's comfort was one of the primary moral choices these nurses made. Comfort led to the belief that a right decision had been made and formed the basis for their subsequent sense of serenity and peace (Wurzbach 2004, 2005a).

Conversely, moral discomfort arose when these nurses believed they had not done what the "good" nurse would have done—their mental ideal. I also found an "influence taboo" which was almost universal and resulted in great moral discomfort for nurses (Wurzbach, 1995). Sharing personal beliefs with the family, which might influence the family or resident's end-of-life decisions, violated this influence taboo.

Moral discomfort was also caused by perceived ethical infractions by peers, treatments done but not ordered, staff disagreements with a decision, reversal of a decision by a superior, and futile treatments. This resulted in difficulty sleeping, feeling badly, anger, and feelings of not being at peace (Wurzbach, 1996a). Many long-term care nurses "looked back" (moral regret) at decisions they had made years earlier with regret (Wurzbach, 1995).

Moral Regret (Looking Back)

Nurses who were the most uncertain or who had the least time to plan a response to an ethical event experienced a long-term response—moral regret (Wurzbach, 2007). One of the primary psychological purposes of looking back is psychological undoing. Individuals in their search for the causes of events tend to use counterfactual thinking, that is, they reflect on how past events might have been different if some aspect of the situation or their own behavior had been different (Niedenthal, Tangney, & Gavanski, 1994). Counterfactual thinking helps to shape the emotions an individual experiences in reaction to a situation. Two emotions associated with attempted mental undoing were shame and guilt. Persons who look back and consider alternatives may actually amplify feelings of guilt or shame (Niedenthal, et al.). In shame the failure is failure of the self and in guilt the failure is failure of a particular behavior (Tangney, 1991). Shame was much more devastating to the person because it involved undoing something about the self, whereas guilt involved changing previous behavior (Niedenthal, et al.).

Moral regret is usually found in choices that have deep salience for the decision-maker (Zeelenberg & Beattie, 1997; Zeelenberg, Beattie, van der Plight, & de Vries, 1996). There seems to be agreement that it may be intensified after the consequence of one's decision is experienced. Some scientists believe in order to influence the decision, the regret must be anticipated prior to making the decision. The most damaging outcome is recrimination, which is regret accompanied by a feeling that one should have known better (Sugden, 1986).

Several studies considered moral regret as the result of the decision-maker's self-evaluation of competence and intelligence (Josephs, Larrick, Steele, & Nisbett, 1992; Larrick, 1993). Moral uncertainty accompanied by moral regret and/or moral recriminations may contribute to nurses' moral distress because their perceived moral or professional competence is being questioned, which has profound implications for nursing practice.

Meaning of My Work for the Future

My work will invite debate about the aspects of nursing ethics and bioethics that address "how" ethical decisions are made, the difference between medical and nursing concepts or principles (promoting comfort is a primary value, concept, or principle of nurses), and the aftermath of ethical decision-making. My studies indicate that moral certainty, moral uncertainty, and a somewhere-in-between moral conviction are very common psychological reactions to ethical dilemmas. Those who are morally certain take action without consultation, questioning, or in some cases thought. Those who are uncertain seek consensus and many times feel moral regret, often for many years after the decision. Many nurses do not want to influence the decisions of others ("influence taboo"). In addition, one of the principles of ethical decision-making that nurses follow is that of promoting the comfort of every party to the ethical decision. The belief is that the choice made by the nurse, doctor, patient, or family "ought" to make them comfortable. Many authors in nursing and bioethics have called the difference between this moral comfort and moral discomfort "moral distress."

The nurses I have studied can be either morally certain or uncertain (Wurzbach, 1999a). Their experience with the dilemma (the more experience, the more likely that the nurse will be morally certain) determines whether they will be certain or uncertain. In my writing I have tried to walk a path between totally discouraging moral convictions (moderate conviction), which some would say prompts courageous action, and cautioning ethical decision-makers to avoid absolute certainty without doubt, because this absolute conviction can lead to precipitous, dangerous, and regretted decisions.

References

Clore, G. L. (1992). Cognitive phenomenology: Feelings and the construction of judgment. In L. L. Martin & A. Tesser (Eds.), *The construction of social judgments* (pp. 133–163). Hillsdale, NJ: Erlbaum.

Corbin, R. M. (1980). Decisions that might not get made. In T. Wallsten (Ed.), *Cognitive processes in choice and decision behavior.* Hillsdale, NJ: Lawrence Erlbaum Associates.

Crisham, P. (1981). Measuring moral judgment in nursing dilemmas. *Nursing Research, 30*(2), 104–110.

Davis, A., & Smith, M. (1980). Ethical dilemmas: Conflicts among rights, duties, and obligations. *American Journal of Nursing, 80*(8), 1463–1466.

Forgas, J. P. (1995). Mood and judgment: The affect infusion model (AIM). *Psychological Bulletin, 117,* 39–66.

Frijda, N. H. (1986). *The emotions.* Cambridge, U.K.: Cambridge University Press.

Frijda, N. H., & Mesquita, B. (1994). The social roles and functions of emotions. In S. Kitayama & H. R. Markus (Eds.), *Emotion and culture: Empirical studies of mutual influence* (pp. 51–87). Washington, DC: American Psychological Association.

Hastings Center. (1987). *Guidelines on the termination of life-sustaining treatment and the care of the dying.* Briarcliff, NY: The Hastings Center.

Isen, A. M. (1993). Positive affect and decision making. In M. Lewis & J. M. Haviland (Eds.), *Handbook of emotions* (pp. 261–277). New York: Guilford Press.

Jameton, A. (1984). *Nursing practice: The ethical issues.* Englewood Cliffs, NJ: Prentice-Hall.

Josephs, R. A., Larrick, R. P., Steele, C. M., & Nisbett, R. E. (1992). Protecting the self from the negative consequences of risky decisions. *Journal of Personality and Social Psychology, 62*(1), 26–37.

Klein, P. D. (1981). *Certainty: A refutation of scepticism.* Minneapolis: University of Minnesota Press.

Kolcaba, K. Y. (1992). Holistic comfort: Operationalizing the construct as a nurse-sensitive outcome. *Advances in Nursing Science, 15*(1), 1–10.

Kolcaba, K. Y. (2003). *Comfort theory and practice: A vision for holistic health care and research.* New York: Springer.

Larrick, R. P. (1993). Motivational factors in decision theories: The role of self-protection. *Psychological Bulletin, 113*(3), 440–450.

Lerner, J. S., & Keltner, D. (2000). Beyond valence: Toward a model of emotion-specific influences on judgment and choice. *Cognition and Emotion, 14*(4), 473–493.

Loewenstein, G., & Lerner, J. S. (2003). The role of affect in decision-making. In R. J. Davidson, K. R. Scherer, & H. H. Goldsmith (Eds.), *Handbook of affective sciences* (pp. 619–642). Oxford, U.K.: Oxford University Press.

Mill, J. S. (2007). *On liberty.* Vancouver, BC: Emerald Knight Publishers. (Originally published in 1859).

Miller, R.W. (1978). Absolute certainty. *Mind, 87*(1), 46–65.

Niedenthal, P. M., Tangney, J. P., & Gavanski, I. (1994). "If only I weren't" versus "if only I hadn't:" Distinguishing shame and guilt in counterfactual thinking. *Journal of Personality and Social Psychology, 67*(4), 585–595.

Odegaard, D. (1982). *Knowledge and scepticism.* Totowa, NJ: Rowman and Littlefield.

Plato. (2007). *The dialogues of Plato.* (R. E. Allen, Trans.). New Haven, CT: Yale University Press. (Originally written approximately 360 BC.)

Quinn, C. A., & Smith, M. D. (1987). *The professional commitment: Issues and ethics in nursing.* Philadelphia: W. B. Saunders Company.

Sugden, R. (1986). Regret, recrimination and rationality. In L. E. Daboni, A. E. Montesano & M. Lines (Eds.), *Recent developments in the foundations of utility and risk theory* (Vol. 47, pp. 67–80). Dordrecht, Netherlands: Reidel.

Tangney, J. P. (1991). Moral affect: The good, the bad and the ugly. *Journal of Personality and Social Psychology, 61*(4), 598–607.

Wurzbach, M. E. (1990). The dilemma of withholding or withdrawing nutrition. *Image: Journal of Nursing Scholarship, 22*(4), 226–230.

Wurzbach, M. E. (1991). Judgment under conditions of uncertainty. *Nursing Forum, 26*(3), 27–34.

Wurzbach, M. E. (1992). An assessment and intervention for certainty and uncertainty. *Nursing Forum, 27*(2), 29–35.

Wurzbach, M. E. (1995). Long-term care nurses' moral convictions. *Journal of Advanced Nursing, 21*(6), 1059–1064.

Wurzbach, M. E. (1996a). Comfort and nurses' moral choices. *Journal of Advanced Nursing, 24*(2), 260–264.

Wurzbach, M. E. (1996b). Long-term care nurses' ethical convictions about tube-feeding. *Western Journal of Nursing Research, 18*(1), 63–76.

Wurzbach, M. E. (1998). Managed care: Moral conflicts for primary health care nurses. *Nursing Outlook, 46*(2), 62–66.

Wurzbach, M. E. (1999a). Acute care nurses' experiences of moral certainty. *Journal of Advanced Nursing, 30*(2), 287–293.

Wurzbach, M. E. (1999b). The moral metaphors of nursing. *Journal of Advanced Nursing, 30*(1), 94–99.

Wurzbach, M. E. (2000). Nursing perspectives on practitioner-assisted suicide. *Nursing Outlook, 48*(3), 116–119.

Wurzbach, M. E. (2002). End-of-Life treatment decisions in long-term care. *The Journal of Gerontological Nursing, 28*(6), 14–21.

Wurzbach, M. E. (2004). Comfort and RNs moral choices. *Delaware State Nurses Association Newsletter, 30*(2), 14.

Wurzbach, M. E. (2005a). Comfort: An essential ethical principle for palliative nursing care. *ASBH Exchange, 8*(3), 9.

Wurzbach, M. E. (2005b). Spring 2003 Commencement Speech at University of Wisconsin-Oshkosh. Nursing ethics and Hagar the Horrible. *Reflections on Nursing Leadership 3rd Quarter, 31*(3), 18–19, 28.

Wurzbach, M. E. (2007). Acute care nurses' experiences of moral uncertainty: Unpublished manuscript.

Zeelenberg, M., & Beattie, J. (1997). Consequences of regret aversion: Additional evidence for effects of feedback on decision-making. *Organizational Behavior and Human Decision Processes, 72*(1), 64–78.

Zeelenberg, M., Beattie, J., van der Plight, J., & de Vries, N. K. (1996). Consequences of regret aversion: Effects of expected feedback on risky decision-making. *Organizational Behavior and Human Decision Processes, 65*(2), 148–158.

~ SECTION II ~
CRITICAL THINKING ACTIVITIES

Philosophical and Theoretical Issues

✦ Each theme begins with a poem written by poet Cortney Davis, who is also a nurse. The following general questions can be applied to each poem:

  • What did you like about the poem? What didn't you like and why?

  • How does the poem relate to the theme?

  • What does the poem allow you to see about the theme that the essays do not? How is this helpful in understanding ethics, if at all?

✦ Fry argues that endangerment of a nursing ethic comes (partly) from the health care system and its problems. Do you agree or disagree? Explain why.

✦ Fry cites Patricia Benner's research (see Benner, P. [1983] Uncovering the knowledge embedded in clinical practice. *Image: The Journal of Nursing Scholarship, 15*(2), 36-41, for example). Generally speaking, Benner's work frames nursing practice from the perspective of what nursing is and does in the context of clinical practice. How does this differ from the philosophical questions that Fry raises about nursing such as "What is the nature of nursing practice?"

✦ Choose one of Wurzbach's research publications. Read the study. Then go to a library resource that will assist you in obtaining citations for a selected author, in this case Wurzbach, such as Web of Science or Science Direct to find at least two other research publications in which the investigator(s) has/have referenced Wurzbach's work. How do the studies build on Wurzbach's work? How do they utilize or criticize Wurzbach's conceptual models?

✦ Think about the concept "influence taboo" that Wurzbach describes. Are nurses unwilling to share information and opinions with patients and families because they don't want to overly influence decisions or do they lack the skills to do so? Prescribe a strategy to remedy lack of will or skill.

Mary Ellen Wurzbach is a Professor of Nursing at the University of Wisconsin-Oshkosh, where she was recently named a Triss Endowed Professor. She is a graduate of the University of Wisconsin-Oshkosh (BSN), University of Wisconsin-Oshkosh (MSN), and the University of Minnesota (PhD). Bioethics has been the focus of her teaching and research since 1980, beginning with her graduation from the Primary Health Care Nursing Masters Program at UW-Oshkosh. Special interests include the role moral conviction plays in nurses' ethical decision-making, comfort as an ethical principle utilized by nurses to make ethical decisions, and moral theory and philosophy.

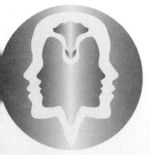

SECTION III

Political, Administrative, and Systems Aspects

Regulation and governing as affected by and affecting the profession of nursing and its ethical implications. Moral freedom and privacy are two relevant considerations.

continued

There Are No Poems at Hospital Management Meetings

Cortney Davis

The CEO has a wary gaze; the executive women
wear pearls. We nurses
settle in the audience like small change.

Poems hide on other floors—
rooms where we measure cost
in milligrams of morphine, liters of blood;

where *how many more treatments* or *how many more days*
are the only questions on the agenda.
What does this say about management meetings, or poems?

That there are different ways of thinking
about the same thing? Black and white *vs.* metaphor—
or sometimes you save, and sometimes you spend?

Like today, management talks about fiscal responsibility,
how to cut costs to yield better growth. I
mishear, think they say *bitter* but hold my tongue.

The poems recoil, a slithering sound.
All day, patients polish their diamonds of pain.
Soon, we will pry the dimes from their eyes.

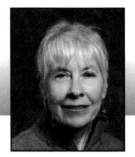

Mila Ann Aroskar

CHAPTER 7

Three Decades at the Interface of Nursing Ethics and Policy in Health Care Settings

...try to love the *questions themselves*
...*Live* the questions now.

Rainer Maria Rilke

Living in the worlds of nursing and health care ethics is to dwell on a daily basis with profound questions of birth and death, sickness and health, pain and suffering, joy and sorrow. Often these questions yield no ready-made answers and involve moral struggles. We are required to create individual, organizational, and public policy responses to these moral struggles through a process of ethical reflection and discernment.

Perplexing questions and decision-making at the interface of nursing ethics and health care policy from patient care settings to organizational and public policy arenas were a major focus of my writing and teaching over the past three decades. My practice areas of professional nursing and public health represent these areas of human concern and action in critical and consequential ways for individuals, families, organizations, and society. The ethical questions inherent in the domains of clinical practice, research, education, and administration in nursing and health care are difficult to view without taking this interface into account.

The American Nurses Association (ANA) Codes (1976, 1985, 2001) of the past three decades include ethical obligations to work collaboratively with others to meet health needs of the public, an obvious connection of ethics and policy in nursing. A duty to shape social policy is made even more explicit in the 2001 Code. Reflection and action on these ethical obligations involve moral questions about the right decisions in or responses to complex situations often involving conflicting interests and groups, a domain of politics. Even difficult ethical choices and policy development involved in the care of an individual patient may, and often do, involve conflicting interests and parties. The Terri Schiavo case is but one example—from the bedside to the highest levels of government.

My writing about the interface of ethics and policy in nursing and health care systems was inspired by Florence Nightingale, Annie Goodrich, Virginia Henderson, and other leading thinkers of modern nursing who identified both the social and ethical obligations of the nursing profession and its practitioners to protect individual patients, to create healthy environments, and to change what needs to be changed. Hence, nurses are obligated not only to address ethical questions at the hospital bedside but also in community health settings and beyond, whether their domain of practice and decision-making is at the level of the individual nurse-patient-family system, organizational systems, or government systems.

The 1970s—Beginnings

How did I, as a Community/Public Health Nursing faculty member, become immersed in the study and teaching of the ethical questions in nursing and health care to the extent that this challenging area became the focus of my professional life? I first discovered health care ethics in the early 1970s while reading an article about the work of the Hastings Center, then known as the Institute of Society, Ethics and the Life Sciences. It was such a source of interest and fascination for me that I immediately signed up for a Hastings Center workshop on ethical theories and was excited to hear some of the preeminent thinkers in medical ethics and ethical theory such as Paul Ramsey, Sissela Bok, Ruth Macklin, Daniel Callahan, Willard Gaylin, Robert Veatch, and others. Upon returning to my faculty position in the School of Nursing, State University of New York (SUNY)/Buffalo, I obtained support for a multidisciplinary Conversation in the Disciplines Program from the SUNY, entitled, "Ethical Dilemmas and Health Care Delivery." This multidisciplinary conference held in 1975 was the first health care ethics conference in the Buffalo area, to my knowledge. Presentations and discussion covered challenging topics such as competing priorities in health care; patient rights and responsibilities; genetics, politics, and medicine; the right to die; consent to research; accountability of the health team; and issues of distributive justice in health care. Several of these topics provided questions and content for my teaching and writing over the past three decades. This conference led to coteaching a multidisciplinary course in ethics and health care with philosopher Richard Hull, a colleague at SUNY/Buffalo.

In the 1970s, the Joseph P. Kennedy, Jr., Foundation opened its postdoctoral fellowships in medical ethics to nurse educators for the first time. Three different faculty colleagues urged me to apply for the fellowship. Much to the delight of myself and my dean, Jeanne Spero, I received one of the fellowships and was privileged to attend the interdisciplinary program at Harvard University, where I met Anne Davis, who was to become a treasured colleague and friend sharing my journey in nursing ethics and bioethics. A project of national import was a requirement of the fellowship in addition to taking relevant courses at Harvard, so Anne and I decided to write a book using our courses such as ethical theory, medical ethics, human rights, and a theory of justice taught by John Rawls as resources. The manuscript for the first edition of *Ethical Dilemmas and Nursing Practice* was completed in 1977, just before the end of our fellowship year and the return to our faculty positions in Schools of Nursing.

One of my challenges in the first edition was writing the chapter on public policy and health care delivery (Davis & Aroskar, 1978). Public policy was viewed in the chapter as those principles guiding actions of society as a whole and determined by federal, state, and local governmental bodies. I saw the chapter as a call to nurses and the profession to participate more actively in policy arenas and to raise awareness that health policy development and resource allocation decisions involved ethical dimensions that are often not discussed in focusing on economic factors, political factors, and competing societal priorities such as education and social welfare. Economist E. F. Schumacher (1973) warned his readers even then that judgments based solely on economics are fragmentary, and that other values need to be considered in policy decisions and implementation.

Political and power dimensions of policy development were briefly discussed in questions about who actually makes allocation of economic and social resource decisions as evidenced by consumer unrest, the patients' rights movement, and the development of the National Commission for the Protection of Human Subjects of Biomedical and Behavioral Research in the 1970s. Jonsen and Butler wrote in the 1970s that ethical and value considerations as part of public policy debate raise problems that make such discussion difficult (1975). Two examples of such obstacles to public dialogue include the special language of ethics and the common idea that ethics has to do primarily with individual values and behavior, even though policy-makers are accustomed to using the technical expertise of others in policy development.

Ethical and political dimensions of policy development and implementation such as issues of distributive justice in the allocation of finite societal resources were discussed, with specific examples of Medicare legislation for care and treatment of the elderly and patients with end-stage renal disease, as opposed to legislation and funding for other catastrophic diseases. Ethical questions to be addressed included: What criteria should be used to set priorities in delivering the benefits of health care? and How can our society meet a goal of fairness for all when not all can get care? Examples of criteria of distributive justice to be considered in responding to such questions included ability to pay, need, and John Rawls' idea that inequalities may be allowed only to improve the condition of the least advantaged (or most vulnerable), e.g., the elderly and the incapacitated. Medical need has often been used in managed care organizations to develop and implement policy, but not without significant challenges. Issues remain to this day of who determines the criteria and priorities for medical need after general agreement on provision of emergency life-saving care as the top priority. Eventually the state of Oregon held open public forums to debate and develop priorities for use of public monies in delivery of health care services.

In searching for resources to write the ethics and policy chapter, I discovered what I consider to be a "classic" article written by social scientists, Warwick and Kelman (1973), on the ethics of social intervention. They viewed social intervention as any planned or unplanned action(s) that changes characteristics in the pattern of relationships between individuals on a continuum from national policy to policy-making in neighborhood programs and use of human subjects in research. This perspective fit with development and implementation of any organizational or public policy related to health care and provided a way to consider ethical and value questions and nurses' obligations in policy work.

Four major aspects or questions to be addressed in any social intervention were identified in the Warwick and Kelman (1973) article that became a touchstone for later writing about ethics and politics in policy development beyond "the book" (Aroskar, 1987, 1995). The four questions to be addressed by policy-makers in the development of organizational and governmental health policies are:

1. What values are maximized or minimized by the choice of policy goals?

2. Who or what is the target of change in policy proposals?

3. What are the means or methods that will be used to develop and implement a proposed policy?

4. What are the direct and indirect consequences of a proposed policy, including all types of costs?

Again, this assessment should be done to the extent possible before policies are developed and implemented (Warwick & Kelman).

Addressing the Warwick and Kelman (1973) questions in health policy development leads to what might be called an ethical impact statement that also incorporates political considerations as doing public ethics. The practice of public ethics incorporates acting on obligations to meet the common and often conflicting needs of the public. Such a document has some of the features of environmental impact statements required prior to development of industrial complexes, housing developments, placement of landfills, nuclear waste, and so on. Given the obstacles discussed by Jonsen and Butler (1975), this is a difficult, but not impossible, task. These questions address ethical concerns without explicitly using the language of ethics. Responding to these questions has the potential to move public dialogue beyond the notion that ethics is strictly a personal matter, to a way of viewing policy work as doing public ethics in the spirit of prevention. Public ethics is concerned primarily with ethical relations and duties of governments and other social organizations focused on the conflicting interests of groups rather than individuals and their families, a more traditional focus of professional ethics in nursing and health care.

In the 1978 edition of the public policy chapter, reflective practices related to nurses' ethical obligations were compared to the nursing assessment process in an attempt to incorporate nursing's ethical values and obligations in a familiar process. The use of "needs" by nurses was discussed briefly as a basis for considering justice as fairness in the distribution of the benefits of nursing and health care. Needs were considered on a continuum that ranged from the individual with a serious illness through consideration of needs that arise in the social and physical environments as they are related to physical and mental health. While consideration of nursing and health care needs is not a panacea in the competition for finite societal resources, it is one way to make ethics and values more explicit. Nurses and nursing organizations were urged to participate in and provide leadership in the articulation of health needs on a broad basis in influencing the development and implementation of health policy (Davis & Aroskar, 1978).

At the time, it was also recognized that many nurses were ill-prepared to participate in development of public policy. Hence, the need to look at educational preparation of nurses was recognized as key to their effective participation in public policy arenas. Other influences on nurses' participation in policy work include the position of nurses in health care hierarchies and nurses' views of the goals and values of health care. The following views have consequences for practice and policy development: health care as medical cases or scientific projects with cure of disease as the most important goal and nursing practice as following physician orders; health care as a commodity to be sold for profit in the health care marketplace; health care as a patient's right to relief from pain and suffering and a nursing focus on patient advocacy; or health care as the promotion, maintenance, and restoration of health within a moral community with respect for all participants' values in decision-making (Aroskar, 1982).

The Kennedy Fellowship and "the book," as Anne and I fondly called it, were the entrée to many experiences that expanded my own thinking and professional experiences in untold ways locally, nationally, and internationally—teaching professional ethics courses to health professionals, writing, speaking, and research. Shortly after the Kennedy Fellowship year, I left SUNY/Buffalo and joined the Public Health Nursing faculty in the School of Public Health at the University of Minnesota, where I began teaching a course on Ethical Issues in Public Health Nursing, based on publications about issues in ethics and community health nursing (Aroskar, 1977, 1979).

The 1980s and 1990s—Attention to the Interface in Writing and Teaching

Supported by the ethical codes of the nursing profession and leaders of the profession, beginning with Nightingale, I wrote about nurses' ethical obligations to act as advocates in the development of organizational and public health policy that incorporates ethical considerations, and to participate in the world of politics as doing public ethics, that is, acting on the obligation to meet the common and often conflicting needs of the public. This focus of obligation and action expands the Code's foundational emphasis on respect for meeting the health needs of individuals and the importance of individual autonomy and personal rights in our society, to include the wider interests of public health concerns and issues of justice (Davis & Aroskar, 1983).

In the last two editions of *Ethical Dilemmas and Nursing Practice,* nurses and professional nursing organizations are viewed as both actual and potential players in health policy arenas as nurses are better prepared in educational curricula for participation in policy development (Davis, Aroskar, Fowler, & Fry 1991; Davis, Aroskar, Liaschenko, & Drought, 1997; also see Mason, Talbott, & Leavitt, 1993). Nurses and nursing organizations are viewed as having an important role in the practice of what may be called "preventive ethics" in development of policy. The practice of preventive ethics focuses on use of processes to mitigate or even prevent the occurrence of ethical crises and can be carried out at various levels of decision-making. It occurs when there is proactive discussion prior to decision-making that involves all individuals, parties, and groups affected by the consequences of policies. An important resource for the health policy chapter in the 1991 and 1997 editions of *Ethical Dilemmas and Nursing Practice* was the work of the President's Commission for the Study of Ethical Problems in Medicine and Biomedical and Behavioral Research, specifically the report on access to health care (1983).

During the 1990s, I organized and taught a course in ethics in health care administration and a multidisciplinary course entitled, "Public Ethics/Politics and Public Health." My writing and research ranged across various areas of nursing and health care. Some examples included nurses' ethical dilemmas in intensive care and community health settings, managed care and ethical decision-making, role of nursing administration on ethics committees, a survey of ethics teaching in health care administration, and nursing ethics and policy. From my perspective in 2007, these varied activities were reflective of my location in two different divisions in the School of Public Health (Healthcare Administration and Health Services Research & Policy), and my grounding in the nursing profession. These activities also reflect my own professional stance as a generalist rather than a specialist and my interest in multidisciplinary education and practice in health care—this in a world of increasing specialization, and at the same time, a growing recognition that the challenges such as safe water and food supplies, AIDS, and bioterrorism in health care and society require conversation, cooperation, and even collaboration among disciplines that have their own specialized languages.

As I contemplated a concluding chapter to my formal professional life in nursing and health care ethics at the University of Minnesota, I decided to conduct a small project on Minnesota nurses' voices in policy, practice, and ethics (Aroskar, Moldow, & Good, 2004) funded by the University of Minnesota Center for Bioethics. When I think about this endeavor, it was definitely a project of the heart that reflected my professional interests and activities of 30 years at the interface of nursing ethics and policy. Major themes in the findings encompassed primarily negative effects of policy, focused on cost containment, effects on quality of care, effects on patient education and access to needed services, and effects on nurses and nursing.

The major ethical concerns identified were the inability to provide needed care and to meet their ethical obligations and values as professional nurses. The nurses in this project were prepared and ready to participate in policy development and implementation, an exciting reality quite different from the impressions of the 1970s.

Impact of My Work in Nursing and Health Care Ethics

Reflecting on the impact of my professional activities has two aspects. One is the more tangible aspect reflected in the numbers of publications, citations of one's work in the publications of others, courses taught to nursing students and others, presentations given to a variety of audiences, including retired members of a steelworkers' union and participation, on ethics committees in hospitals and other health care organizations. The second is more intangible: that is, the hope that one's work has not been in vain and has some meaning in the lives that one has touched in nursing and other disciplines over three decades through teaching, writing, and even possibly in chance remarks.

A most exciting and humbling reality for me is the fact that the Davis/Aroskar book is going into its 5th edition this year, with Anne Davis and Marsha Fowler as coauthors and this author again updating the health policy chapter. Various editions of "the book" have been published in more than 10 countries. I hope that this book as a representation of thinking in nursing ethics from the Western world may serve as encouragement and as a point of departure for our nursing colleagues in other countries to explore their cultural and ethical values and perspectives on patient care and health care policy.

Another great challenge for the future is to gain, or at least maintain, explicit attention to the ethics and values of nursing and health care, whether it is in direct patient care, in research, administrative, or policy circles. Economic and political values are important realities, but not adequate by themselves to guide the work of nursing and delivery of health care services in any society that considers itself to be civilized and humane. Whether we learn to love the perplexing questions of nursing and health care ethics as Rilke (1934) suggests to the young poet is a point to ponder as nurses, health care organizations, and our society live the questions and respond to them.

References

American Nurses Association. (1976). *Code for nurses with interpretive statements.* Kansas City, MO: American Nurses Publishing.

American Nurses Association. (1985). *Code for nurses with interpretive statements.* Kansas City, MO: American Nurses Publishing.

American Nurses Association. (2001). *Code of ethics for nurses with interpretive statements.* Nursebooks.org.

Aroskar, M. A. (1977). Ethical dilemmas in community health nursing. *Linacre Quarterly, 44*(4), 340–346.

Aroskar, M. A. (1979). Ethical issues in community health nursing. *Nursing Clinics of North America, 14*(1), 35–44.

Aroskar, M. A. (1982). Are nurses' mind sets compatible with ethical practice? *Topics in Clinical Nursing, 4,* 22–32.

Aroskar, M. A. (1987). The interface of ethics and politics in nursing. *Nursing Outlook, 35*(6), 268–272.

Aroskar, M. A. (1995). Exploring ethical terrain in public health. *Journal of Public Health Management and Practice, 1*(3), 16–22.

Aroskar, M. A., Moldow, D. G., & Good, C. M. (2004). Nurses' voices: Policy, practice and ethics. *Nursing Ethics, 11*(3), 266–276.

Davis, A. J., & Aroskar, M. A. (1978). *Ethical dilemmas and nursing practice.* New York: Appleton-Century-Crofts.

Davis, A. J., & Aroskar, M. A. (1983). *Ethical dilemmas and nursing practice* (2nd ed.). Norwalk, CT: Appleton-Century-Crofts.

Davis, A. J., Aroskar, M. A., Fowler, M., & Fry, S. (1991). *Ethical dilemmas and nursing practice* (3rd ed.). Norwalk, CT: Appleton & Lange.

Davis, A. J., Aroskar, M. A., Liaschenko, J., & Drought, T. S. (1997). *Ethical dilemmas and nursing practice* (4th ed.). Stamford, CT: Appleton & Lange.

Jonsen, A. R., & Butler, L. H. (1975). Public ethics and policy making. *Hastings Center Report, 5*(4), 19–31.

Mason, D. J., Talbott, S. W., & Leavitt, J. K. (Eds.). (1993). *Policy and politics for nurses: Action and change in the workplace, government, organizations and community* (2nd ed.). Philadelphia: W. B. Saunders.

President's Commission for the Study of Ethical Problems in Medicine and Biomedical and Behavioral Research. (1983). *Securing access to health care,* Report (Vol. 1). Washington, DC: Author.

Rilke, R. M. (1934). *Letters to a young poet* (M. D. Herter Norton, Trans.). New York: W. W. Norton & Company.

Schumacher, E. F. (1973). *Small is beautiful.* New York: Harper & Row.

Warwick, D. P., & Kelman, H. C. (1973). Ethical issues in social intervention. In G. Zaltman, (Ed.), *Processes and phenomena of social change* (p. 377–449). New York: J. Wiley.

Mila Ann Aroskar, retired Associate Professor, School of Public Health Adjunct Associate Professor, School of Nursing, is an emeritus Faculty Associate, Center for Bioethics, University of Minnesota, Minneapolis, MN. She is a graduate of the College of Wooster (BA); Columbia University School of Nursing (BS); Teachers College, Columbia University (MEd); State University of New York at Buffalo (EdD), and has an honorary DSc from Creighton University. Her career in bioethics and professional ethics spanned three decades in nursing, patient care, health care administration, public health, and health policy.

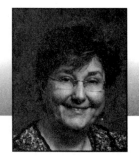

Leah L. Curtin

CHAPTER 8

Ethics in Everyday Language for Nurses in Everyday Practice

My work in "nursing ethics" began, as so many things do, with a struggle to understand my own experiences. For example, as a new graduate, I was asked to pass medications on a 50-bed ward. One of the resident physicians ordered many unusual drugs—and extraordinarily high doses of the drugs. None of the other nurses questioned them. I did—continually. Late one afternoon, this physician demanded that I give him two vials of an experimental drug rather than the usual one vial. When I questioned him, he assured me that he needed to test one for its stability and the other he would give to the patient. I gave him both vials about 3:00 p.m. The patient was dead by the time I returned to work at 10:30 p.m. for the night shift. In a discussion with numerous officials, I voiced my concerns. After that discussion, my work hours became very erratic. I worked all three shifts—sometimes on the same day. I worked weeks without a day off. I was routinely doubled back, and I had to check my schedule daily because it changed daily. As a new graduate, I did not know that staff nurses usually were not treated this badly. Several years passed before I understood what went on, and then I knew that nurses in leadership had helped force me to resign.

When I left this position, I accepted employment as a visiting nurse, working for the Visiting Nurses Association of Cincinnati. I had many adventures and learned just how unfair society was to those who had little or no money. My district included tens of thousands of people, and I "saw it all," from inner city fights to racial riots to children dying in the hills of Kentucky because they could not get antibiotics. And then there were the babies, so many of them, so poor, so undernourished. And the abused children; one I found hanging from the back of a door with a wire around his penis because he had wet the bed; another who was burned with cigarettes and irons and beaten with electric cords; still another who was stomped by his mother's boyfriend (the child died later in the hospital). How could one live through these days and *not* become interested in ethics?

By the mid-1970s, I went back to school to study philosophy, majoring in medical ethics. As part of this experience, I became a clinical intern at the Cincinnati Center for Developmental Disabilities (CCDD). The Center's Founder and Medical Director, Dr. Karl Rubenstein, arranged for me to sit in on all committees—including an ethics committee and a sterilization committee—to help me learn why and how decisions were made. I was not permitted to participate in the decisions—only to observe, and then to discuss my perceptions with Dr. Rubenstein and with the Center's Director of Nursing, Barbara Engstrom. While still an intern, Dr. Rubenstein asked me to teach what may have been the first, certainly one of the first, interdisciplinary courses in ethics actually conducted in a clinical facility. For many participants, this was the first time they had heard ethics discussed at all—no less in an interdisciplinary setting. Getting them to speak up was a challenge.

In 1975, at the National Spina Bifida Association meeting in Cincinnati, Barbara Engstrom introduced me to the audience as the "Director of the National Center for Nursing Ethics." I was stunned, primarily because I was not—and it was not either. That is, I had talked about the need for such a center with nurses who attended many of the workshops offered by the Hastings Center, and at the College of Mount St. Joseph's yearly, weeklong "International Institute of Bioethics and Human Values." But that was all it was, an idea! Nonetheless, following this talk, I was inundated with requests for information about the "Center," and people seemed unwilling to accept, "there is no such 'Center'." So I called some of the nurses I had met at ethics institutes and seminars—Mila Aroskar, Anne Davis, Josephine Flaherty, Sr. Eileen Kantz, Helen Creighton, Luther Christman, Barbara Engstrom, and Gina Giavinco—and the "Center" was born. Its goals were ambitious: to raise awareness of ethical issues in nursing and health care; to encourage the American Nurses Association (ANA) to ratify a genuine Code for Nurses (not a code of etiquette!); to encourage the National League for Nursing (NLN) to mandate ethics in the nursing curriculum; to encourage the Joint Commission on Accreditation of Healthcare Organizations (JCAHO) to mandate ethics committees for hospitals; and to assure that nurses' ethical concerns could be voiced.

The "Center's" resources were pathetic; we had no money, no office, no secretary, and no standing. Much of the time, our activities were funded with money I scrounged from my food budget. Yet we "met" by phone, published a newsletter called *Update on Ethics* (which we later discontinued in favor of publishing in mainstream nursing journals so that we could influence a wider audience), and sponsored booths at conventions of the ANA and the NLN. We even sponsored a daylong institute for high school teachers on "Ethics at the End of Life." As the Hastings Center (Facing death, 1974) had just published an entire issue devoted to this topic, I contacted the Hastings Center and ordered several hundred back issues.

Running the "Center" was fun and very challenging, but by 1988 most of our goals were achieved. This is not to say that the goals were achieved solely or even primarily because of "The Center," for this is simply not true...but nonetheless, the goals were achieved, and because they were achieved, the "Center" had fulfilled its purposes and died a good and timely death.

Framing the Issues

During the mid- to late 1970s, I became embroiled in the abortion controversy for a variety of reasons, perhaps most importantly because of my concern for the place of conscience in professional decision-making. From the late 1950s onward, nurses were taught that they must always consider two patients when caring for the pregnant woman: mother and fetus. Thus, when the Supreme Court legalized abortion and state laws were changed literally overnight, many nurses were caught unaware— as were many hospitals and clinics. The surge in demand for abortions was overwhelming and immediate. Many nurses felt conflicted, but by virtue of their status as employees, they were forced to assist in abortions or to lose their jobs for insubordination. Even though the Supreme Court included a conscience provision in Roe v. Wade (1973), many institutions interpreted this provision to apply "only" to physicians; nurses were simply the instruments of their decisions.

These matters came to a head in a case that originated in Kentucky. Despite the fact that the Kentucky abortion statute included a severability clause, a federal district court "went further than it had to," and invalidated Kentucky's "individual conscience" clause in Wolfe v. Schroering (1976). This was particularly remarkable because the individual conscience clause had not even been challenged. In the appeal from that decision, I recruited, organized, and funded a brief "amicus curiae" on behalf of Kentucky Registered Nurses, in which we claimed that nurses were not simply the instruments of the orders of others—physicians, employers, or patients— but rather moral persons who were responsible for their own decisions. In part we based the claim on the legally recognized status of conscientious objectors to war, in part on freedom of religion, and in part on the education and preparation of nurses.

This brief had nothing to do with the legalization of abortion "per se," but rather it addressed the right of the nurses to freedom of conscience in regard to their participation in the abortion procedure. It is notable that the American Civil Liberties Union and several state nurses associations joined us in this effort. In 1976, the U.S. Court of Appeals for the Sixth Circuit reversed the district court's decision in regard to both private institutions and private individuals—but upheld the district court in regard to public institutions (Wolfe v. Schroering).

What this meant was that nurses (and other health care personnel as well) now had a "clearly defined right to freedom of conscience"—a right that soon was supported by conscience clause legislation in almost all states. For the first time, nurses were recognized in law as persons who exercised judgments "independent" from those of a physician or an employer. No longer were nurses merely instruments of the order of others. Freedom of conscience is the "sine qua non" of any profession "and it extends well beyond any one issue." Publishing a Code of Ethics, licensing the practitioner, defining practice, setting standards, and so forth does not make a group a profession "unless" its practitioners can make decisions about "their" practice within "their" role and within "their" workplace.

I fully believed then, and still believe, that the most pervasive ethical problem for nurses is that they are not able to practice nursing the way they were taught to practice it and in the way they believe it should be practiced. It is, in fact, the most pervasive ethical problem for nurses. Ethics in the professional context truly is the practical application of a philosophy that permeates practice and structures relationships. Nursing practice, its ethos and ethical problems, was also the focus of the text that M. Josephine Flaherty, Principal Nursing Officer of Canada, and I published in 1982 (Curtin & Flaherty). Fully half of the book was devoted to analysis of the ethical problems "nurses encountered" in practice—not as adjuncts to physicians and their problems, or even as adjuncts to patients and their problems, but as professionals faced with problems "unique to their own practice."

Ethics, Nursing Leadership, and the Work Environment

To address the problems of practicing nurses through a professional association is critically important. To address them philosophically gives direction and focus to nursing practice. To assure some legal basis for autonomous decision-making also is essential. However, while all of these are necessary, they "are not enough." The work environment dramatically affects nurses' professional autonomy and also the consequences they face for making ethical and moral decisions that are distinctly different. Ethics as a discipline involves the identification, clarification, and analysis of a problem by applying certain principles to determine what is the right thing to do in a given situation, while morality, on the other hand, deals with what you choose to do about what you think is right. The insight related to the effect of work environment on practice led me to an enduring interest in nursing leadership: how leaders make ethical decisions and the impact their decisions have on staff nurses, their work environment, and nurses' ability to exercise moral judgment. For this reason, I was delighted when publisher John Harling invited me to be editor-in-chief of *Supervisor Nurse* in 1978. Harling was concerned that I might try to turn *Supervisor Nurse* into an ethics journal. I did not. Instead, after extensive consultation with him, I turned it into the journal of *Nursing Management*—and addressed many of the ethical and moral aspects of nursing leadership, as well as professional, social, and political issues in my editorials.

In April of 1979, I wrote an editorial entitled "The Prostitution of CPR," in which I cited the policies at Massachusetts General Hospital (MGH) as being particularly humane. As a result, the MGH was so inundated with requests for copies of its cardiopulmonary resuscitation (CPR) policy that they complained about the time it was taking and asked that the journal take over the job of responding to inquiries and sending out copies of MGH's policy. So, we did. The editorial addressed the nurse's need for a clear, rational, and humane CPR policy (Curtin, 1979).

Eventually (it took 14 years!), Harling himself asked me to design and write an ethics column—which, as you may imagine, I happily agreed to do. I explored the impact of the workplace on moral decision-making in some detail in the ethics columns that appeared in *Nursing Management* from 1993 through 1998, including one editorial exploring the concept of intention and the various factors which influence the context of decision-making and the consequences of that process (Curtin, 1996).

Several years later, Barbara Brown, the editor-in-chief of *Nursing Administration Quarterly (NAQ),* invited me to write two articles on ethics. In these articles I specifically addressed the role-related responsibilities of the chief nurse on a variety of levels. The first targeted a need for discretionary professional judgment and independence in practice (Curtin, 1993). The second, for *NAQ's* 25th Anniversary Edition, published my thinking as it evolved in this area. I proposed a set of ethical principles for nurse administrators and suggested that "... ethical behavior—walking your talk—establishes long-term relations of trust and cooperation, which in turn promote consistency and stability in an unstable world. Predictability in this realm is essential: it provides security where certainty is not possible..." (Curtin, 2000).

Understanding the Interplay between Leadership and Politics

A natural extension of my interest in nursing leadership and nurses' work environments is the impact of politics and law on both. This led me to explore the parallels between ethics in nursing and ethics in politics, as the two often intersect—particularly since the advent of Medicare and Medicaid (and cost overruns!). Thus, I wrote "Ethics and Politics are Not Oxymorons!" (Curtin, 2001). In 2003, the American Academy of Nursing asked me to address some of the social, economic, and ethical issues of aging in America, issues of grave concern to all people but particularly to health care leaders as they grapple with greater demand and lower reimbursements (Curtin, 2004).

I have a number of concerns as the pendulum swings away from the absolutes of the past that placed power solely in the hands of physicians toward a future that places that power solely in the hands of payers—or even of patients. While I believe in diversity and in patients' rights, I also believe that nurses and other health professionals are human beings too—and they have values and rights also.

What nurses choose to do every day in everyday practice, for better or for worse, "is" the profession. Thus, the most important ethical decisions—the ones that create the profession—are made every day, by nurses in everyday practice…which is precisely why I have devoted most of my career to discussing ethics in everyday language for nurses in everyday practice!

References

Curtin, L. (1979). The prostitution of CPR. *Supervisor Nurse, 10*(4), 7.

Curtin, L. (1993). Keepers of the keys: Economics, ethics and nursing administrators. *Nursing Administration Quarterly, 17*(4), 1–10.

Curtin, L. (1996). Why good people do bad things. *Nursing Management, 27*(7), 63–65.

Curtin, L. (2000). The first ten principles for the ethical administration of nursing services. *Nursing Administration Quarterly, 25*(1), 7–13.

Curtin, L. (2001). Ethics and politics are not oxymorons! *Policy, Politics and Nursing Practice, 2*(1), 6–8.

Curtin, L. (2004). The coming gerontocracy: Social and ethical ramifications. *Policy, Politics and Nursing Practice, 5*(3), 196–204.

Curtin, L., & Flaherty, M. J. (1982). *Nursing ethics: Theories and pragmatics.* Bowie, MD: Brady Communications.

Facing death. (1974). *Hastings Center Studies, 2*(2), 3–80.

Roe v. Wade, 410 U.S. 113 (1973).

Wolfe v. Schroering, 541 F.2d 523 (6th Cir. 1976).

Leah L. Curtin, Clinical Professor of Nursing at the University of Cincinnati College of Nursing and Health, is a managing partner in Metier Consultants. A graduate of the University of Cincinnati (BS and MS), and the Athenaeum of Ohio (MA), she was awarded two honorary doctorates: one from the State University of New York at Utica for her work in ethics and one from the Medical College of Ohio for humanitarian services following the publication of her work on the impact of war on children. A Fellow of the American Academy of Nursing since 1982, Curtin's interest in ethics arose out of her experiences in clinical practice and its intersections with social justice, workplace environment—particularly autonomous decision-making for nurses—and the impact of laws and social and/or institutional policies on patients and nursing practice.

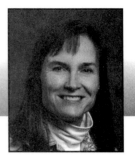

Sarah E. Shannon

CHAPTER 9
Ethics for Neighbors

Everything I know about confidentiality, I learned in the grocery store in Juneau, Alaska. My first nursing position was as a staff nurse in the 65-bed general hospital for this town of approximately 19,000. Juneau is bound on one side by Gastineau Straits and on the other by glaciers. The hospital served Juneau, the capital of Alaska, and a much larger geographical area. When hospice patients could no longer be cared for in their small bush communities accessible only by boat or float plane, they arrived with their families in tow to spend their final weeks of life. The hospital had the only lock-up room for mentally ill patients in many miles. We utilized a walking blood bank: local donors were phoned whenever blood was needed. A local prison and the town's jail admitted inmates to the hospital, sending a guard to sit by patients secured to their beds. Pediatric admissions were frequent to all areas of the hospital. When parents were unable to room in, we found a "grandmother," admitted for deep vein thrombosis treatment or the like, to be the child's roommate and assist us with monitoring.

In the urban world, clinicians work under an illusion of anonymity. Signs in hospital elevators remind professionals not to discuss patients in public places, to prevent what is perceived as the rare event when the person overhearing the conversation would know the patient being discussed. I learned about confidentiality while grocery shopping as I ran a gauntlet of questions from other shoppers about patients, roommates of patients, or the person they saw admitted as they left the hospital. Privacy was a concept that we considered every day in making room and staffing assignments.

Fidelity also was a principle we lived by as a small community. If the nurse who was scheduled to relieve you could not get to work due to weather, illness, or because he or she had boat trouble returning from fishing, there was no float or agency nurse to call. If you left, you would literally abandon your patients. One evening I was asked to work a double shift because we had had multiple emergency room (ER) admissions, a nurse had been unable to get into work, and the entire hospital was busy. Just as I was nearing the end of that 16-hour shift, the supervisor came by and asked, "What's your blood type?" I am O-negative—the universal donor. A woman in the maternity ward with placenta abruptio had ruptured, was hemorrhaging, and we had run out of blood. Could I donate a unit of blood on my way home? This was a patient I had cared for, laughed about the food with, hoped with for a better outcome. In a rural community, duty to your colleague who will work 16 hours, to your patient who is bleeding, is personal. It requires that you ask not, "What should someone else do?" but rather, "What should I do?" and "What can I do?" I donated the unit and went home with a new definition for exhausted.

The cases that captivated me, and eventually directed my career path, were those of dying patients. Later, as a critical care nurse in Seattle, end-of-life (EOL) cases were often characterized by conflict among the health care team over the aggressiveness of treatment, whether the patient's wishes were being honored, or whether the patient's family should be allowed more decision-making authority. But in Juneau, the cases were qualitatively different. I was the learner. The patients and their family members, and sometimes my physician and nurse colleagues, were my teachers. Conflict was the exception rather than the rule. Not all cases were good stories, happy endings. But we, as clinicians, did not sit in a position of judgment in the same way as I later experienced in an urban setting. Or if we did, we were wise enough to be embarrassed by our biases.

One patient was a little boy. He was born "perfect," but contracted a streptococcus infection during the birth process. A nursing colleague had assisted with the lumbar puncture when he was only a few days old—she recalled that his cerebrospinal fluid had been "like butter." Sammy was profoundly neurologically devastated by the infection. He had cerebral palsy, a shunt, and feeding tube. The first time I cared for Sammy, he was admitted for a blocked shunt secondary to an infection that started with a simple cold. He was having seizures, vomiting, and would need to be airlifted to Seattle for his third shunt revision. I went in to talk with his mother about EOL decision-making. She listened to my opening salvo and then sighed deeply. She patiently explained to me how she and her husband had needed to make a decision early in Sammy's life to either let him go, or to treat him as they would have treated any other child. They had chosen the latter and they could not revisit that decision every time Sammy got a cold. She talked about how when she visited Sammy after work when he was hospitalized, nurses were never with him as they were with the other children. Her gentle criticism changed my practice. I quit thinking about what she needed to do differently, and focused on what I needed to do so that Sammy's parents could feel confident that he was cared for and cared about. A year later, Sammy asphyxiated from a mucus plug one night at home, and died. His parents invited me to his wake and introduced me to their friends as "Sammy's favorite nurse." I learned from Sammy's family that by supporting the tough choices that families have needed to make, we provide them with the space to grieve. There were many other lessons like this, in which I learned that death could be welcomed, but that families may need help to uphold promises and need to be forgiven when they were not able to do so. I learned how to nurture young colleagues in their continued learning and moral growth as professionals. First experiences with ethics cases are opportunities to develop clear thinking based on clinical facts, rather than emotional reactions to human tragedies.

I left Alaska and moved to Seattle with the dual goals of getting critical care experience and going to graduate school. The cases I had found compelling were those like Sammy and others. I wanted to go into ethics and this required a terminal degree. After exploring several options, including law, philosophy, anthropology, or sociology, I opted to apply to the doctoral program at the University of Washington School of Nursing. Two factors drove this decision. First, for practical reasons I wanted my doctoral education to include data-generating research methods that would allow funding through grants. Second, I wanted to maintain my clinical identity and roots by obtaining my doctoral degree within nursing. I had the good fortune of quickly identifying a champion for my interest in ethics, Dr. Rheba deTornyay, who had just stepped down as the dean of the School of Nursing and taught the required undergraduate ethics course. Her agreement to serve as my dissertation chair was instrumental to my focus on ethics. The next stroke of luck was that Dr. Albert Jonsen accepted the chairmanship of the Department of Medical History and Ethics in the School of Medicine at UW the year I began doctoral study. He agreed to be a member of my dissertation committee and became my mentor and guide to the larger bioethics community.

My scholarship and teaching in ethics reflect my rural roots. The "other" in the health care interaction—whether the patient, the family of a dying patient, or a colleague—is also a neighbor. Ethics for neighbors are different than ethics for strangers—one's relationship to one's neighbor is personal and immediate, while that to a stranger may be hypothetical, distant, or arbitrary.

Communication: Linking Nursing and Ethics, Neighbors and Strangers

My scholarship developed around several themes: supporting families of critically ill patients, communication around EOL care, interprofessional communication, negotiations between nurses and patients around provision of nursing care, and professionals' claims of futility in response to patient requests for aggressive care at the EOL. The overarching theme is communication under challenging situations.

Communication around difficult topics challenges health care professionals on a regular basis. Challenging communication situations include supporting families of dying patients, discussing EOL care options, disclosing errors to patients, team analysis of ethics cases, handling interprofessional conflict, and responding to families' requests for treatments with which we disagree. How nurses and physicians approach these situations may differ, but I have chosen to illuminate interprofessional commonalities. This has been an intentional and nuanced position rather than a naïve wish for interprofessional collaboration. Health care professionals yield enormous power in their relationship to patients and their families. They can stand apart from patients—as strangers—or beside them—as neighbors. In choosing to highlight our similarities as health care professionals, my goal has been to focus attention on the shared power we hold as professionals in comparison to our patients or their families, and to help health care teams function more effectively around ethics.

Supporting Families of Critically Ill Patients

My dissertation was a qualitative study examining the nurse's role in EOL decision-making for critically ill patients (Shannon, 1992). The experience of critical illness was often like a roller coaster, and nurses reported that they rode the roller coaster with the family. In order for decisions to be made, hopes needed to match realities and perceptions needed to match physiological situations. Nurses reported that the process of making connections was essentially a communication process comprised of three components: knowing, facilitating, and guiding. The nurses in this study provided the foundation for how I began to see the relationship between health care professionals and patients and their families. These nurses spoke to the importance of their communication and their compassion and respect for families' perspectives of their loved ones' condition, prognosis, and treatment plan.

Helping families of critically ill patients prepare for and cope with the death of a loved one is a critical skill for all intensive care unit (ICU) practitioners. Families need to be supported as context for the dying patient, as surrogate decision-makers for the patient, and as recipients of our care for their own needs (Shannon, 2001). Strategies for supporting families can be divided into four categories: general support strategies, support for surrogate decision-making, support during the dying process, and support following the patient's death. Specific strategies for each category have been identified through prior research and through identification of best practices (Shannon, 2001).

End-of-life Communication

In collaboration with several research teams, my colleagues and I have conducted studies with the goal of understanding EOL communication between health care teams and patients and families of critically ill patients. One study involved patients with chronic conditions; family members of patients who had recently died of a chronic disease; nurses and social workers from hospice or acute care settings; or physicians with expertise in EOL care (Curtis et al., 2001). We identified 12 domains of skills for physicians caring for patients at the EOL, which we mapped into five conceptual categories: (a) patient-centered care systems, (b) communication skills, (c) cognitive skills, (d) affective skills, and (e) patient-centered values.

Perhaps not surprising, in this study, patients and family members most frequently identified the domains of emotional support and communication with the patient as important. Specifically, patients and families valued health care teams talking with patients in an honest and straightforward way, being willing to talk about dying, giving bad news in a sensitive way, listening to patients, encouraging questions from patients, and being sensitive to when patients are ready to talk about death (Wenrich et al., 2001). Providing emotional support and personalization of care was qualitatively and quantitatively more important to patients and family members than other domains (Wenrich et al., 2003). We also examined differences in the occurrence of themes among the three disease groups (chronic obstructive pulmonary disease [COPD], AIDS, and cancer) (Curtis, Wenrich et al., 2002). Patients were similar in what they valued; however for each disease group, a unique theme emerged. For example, COPD patients focused on education, including wanting to know what dying might be like.

Overall, the analyses of these data yielded several important contributions for health care ethics. First, these data represented the perspectives of patients, family members, nurses, social workers, and physicians, lending an important empirical perspective. Second, while this research was conceptualized as an exploration of physicians' skills for EOL care, I believe it has—and we continue to explore—applicability to nurses' practice. Third, the importance of communication and emotional support were paramount to patients and families in these focus groups.

In collaboration with a related team, we explored the communication that occurs between the health care team and families of critically ill patients by audiotaping conferences about withholding or withdrawing life-sustaining treatments or breaking bad news (Curtis, Engelberg et al., 2002). We found that in nearly a third of the conferences, clinicians missed opportunities to listen and respond to families; to acknowledge and address family members' emotions; and to pursue key principles in medical ethics and palliative care, including exploration of patient values or explanation of surrogate decision-making, or affirm that patients would not be abandoned (Curtis et al., 2005). Several publications resulted from these data, including a quantitative analysis of these data comparing the length of time the family spoke during the conferences to the length of time clinicians spoke with families, and survey ratings of clinician communication skills; for example (McDonagh et al., 2004). The take-home message was that the more we listen to families, the higher they rate our communication skills. A qualitative analysis of the same data set *de novo* (Hsieh & Shannon, 2005) found that we may avoid discussing a key issue for some families of whether withdrawal of life support constitutes active killing.

Interprofessional Communication

Differences in perceptions among patients, nurses, and physicians, such as on quality of ICU care, have been documented (Shannon, Mitchell, & Cain, 2002). Ethics cases often seem to exaggerate these differences in perceptions and bring to the surface or exacerbate interprofessional conflicts. Drawing on 10 years of experiences on interprofessional ethics committees, I reflected on the roots of interprofessional conflict around ethics in an article whose greatest impact may be in teaching interprofessionalism (Shannon, 1997). By recognizing the roots of interprofessional differences, professionals can avoid having ethics cases exacerbate conflict and instead capitalize on their different perspectives. With a colleague, I commented in an invited editorial on the importance of interprofessional communication and care in the critical care environment, particularly around EOL (Curtis & Shannon, 2006). The positive impact of increased interprofessional collaboration on patient, family, and professional outcomes makes the case for focusing research and professional efforts on this worthwhile goal.

My work in the area of interprofessional communication has been critiqued heavily. Some nurse colleagues have felt that I did not champion nurses and their unique contributions enough. Some have felt that I ignored issues of gender too much in my work. Others have simply accused me of being a hopeless optimist. I prefer to be labeled a pragmatist. Health care will continue to be delivered by multiple professional groups, each with its own gendered history, to patients and families who are forced because of the nature of illness to believe in our fidelity to them. Yet, because of our power (whether we are physicians or nurses), we are challenged daily in whether we honor that fiduciary relationship—or abuse it.

Marginalized Cases, Marginalized Groups: Justice and Ethics

Published ethics cases have tended to ignore those that concern refusals of nursing care. Some would claim that patients have no right to refuse "just" nursing care, though they can refuse life support. A case occurred that an ethics colleague and I felt was important to publish to help develop a taxonomy of cases involving refusals of nursing care similar to the taxonomies that exist for refusal of tube feeding, blood products, or mechanical ventilation, so that ethics committees and consultants would begin to build expertise in this area (Dudzinski & Shannon, 2006; Dudzinski, Shannon, & Tong, 2006).

A similar type of case is that of a patient who is viewed as "bad" for social reasons, such as a patient who is a convicted sex offender (Schonfeld, Romberger, Hester, & Shannon, 2007). When patients such as these want aggressive care at the EOL, it is easier for care providers, including nurses, to judge treatment as futile. Yet I question whether it is patients' physiologic conditions, or social situations, that are being judged futile. This type of case illustrates how the new language of "futility" can reinforce the unequal power relationship between care providers and patients.

I have become increasingly concerned about the growth of medical futility as a professional response to patients' and families' requests for aggressive EOL care (Shannon, 2006a; Shannon, 2006b). While the cases of the 60s, 70s, and 80s primarily concerned patients' rights to refuse beneficial but unwanted therapies, more recently clinicians have been challenged by patients and families who want more aggressive treatment at the EOL than many clinicians believe to be effective, cost-efficient, or humane.

I am opposed to a due process approach to requests for what is viewed as futile therapy, such as the 1999 Texas Advance Directives Act. While not a perfect solution, I believe that we should focus on communication solutions to right-to-live cases that treat patients and families as our neighbors rather than as strangers. My reasons are threefold. First, right-to-live cases are not randomly distributed across Americans, but rather occur in two groups in particular: African-Americans and those with greater religiosity (Shannon, 2006a; 2006b). Early data from Texas confirmed that African-Americans were being disproportionately affected by futility policies, potentially exacerbating long-standing trust issues among this community. Similarly, a due process solution is likely to disproportionately affect those with greater religiosity, exacerbating the cultural divide around religion already occurring within United States (Teno et al., 1994). Simple communication interventions around EOL decision-making have been found to have remarkably powerful effects on both economic factors such as length of stay (Lilly et al., 2000; Schneiderman, Gilmer, & Teetzel, 2000) and family outcomes (Lautrette et al., 2007).

Beyond Communication, Beyond Nursing: A View to the Future

Communication around difficult situations is the overarching theme of my collaborative research. Nursing has focused on teaching broad, generalizable communication skills. In contrast, medicine has focused on teaching communication techniques for particular situations, such as obtaining informed consent. Our research helps to illuminate the black box of communication in more detail. Three outcomes studies have shown communication interventions to be successful—usually with an interprofessional component (Lautrette et al., 2007; Lilly et al., 2000; Schneiderman et al., 2000). Yet, the specifics of how the communication is improved, or how interprofessional interactions are strengthened, remain relatively opaque.

A potential benefit for nursing and medicine would be to create a common platform for teaching and evaluating communication skills for all health care clinicians. By doing research that looks at nurses' and physicians' communication skills concurrently, patterns and similarities emerge in addition to unique qualities and differences. These commonalities create the opportunities for interprofessional teaching, practice, collaboration, and evaluation.

Communication, Health Care Professionals, Justice, Nursing, and Ethics: How Does It All Fit Together?

I have taught bioethics for 10 years, primarily for nursing students. My research on communication is visible in my teaching. In addition to teaching ethics content, I focus on the historical and legal context and the social topography of key topics in bioethics. Content and context alone are inadequate to engage and prepare future clinicians; it is crucial to teach skills. I teach how to analyze ethics cases that involve treatment decisions (e.g., refusal of nursing care) versus cases that involve professional values (e.g., what to do if you witness a colleague lie to a patient).

My work on futility, due process solutions, and the impact on disparities in health care is important to bioethics. The dominant voices in ethics are in support of futility policies, due process solutions, and legal safe harbors for clinicians and health care organizations. Yet the social determinants of health make these seemingly fair options suspect. There are relatively few people in bioethics speaking out against due process solutions to futility. I believe right-to-live cases will dominate the legal landscape during the next decade or more. Nurses and nursing, bioethicists and bioethics, will benefit from continuing to hear divergent views on these cases because these issues are far from settled.

Finally, my recent collaborations around cases of refusal of nursing care represent a needed contribution. These cases are missing from the mainstream bioethics literature. My collaborator and I hope that nurses will receive more targeted and helpful guidance from ethics committees around cases of refusal of nursing care, and that ethics committees will recognize these cases as valid and refer to a growing literature base when providing guidance.

Growing up in a rural community in a rural state, later practicing as a new nurse in a small Alaskan town, I first experienced ethics from a position of personal duty and nearness, rather than from a position of privilege and distance. Ethics for neighbors requires us to talk to the "other" in the health care relationship, to negotiate and to compromise. The lessons I learned from Sammy's mother and others have been enduring in my career. Everything I truly know about ethics, I learned from these neighbors.

References

Curtis, J. R., Engelberg, R. A., Wenrich, M. D., Nielsen, E. L., Shannon, S. E., Treece, P. D., et al. (2002). Studying communication about end-of-life care during the ICU family conference: Development of a framework. *Journal of Critical Care, 17*(3), 147–160.

Curtis, J. R., Engelberg, R. A., Wenrich, M. D., Shannon, S. E., Treece, P. D., & Rubenfeld, G. D. (2005). Missed opportunities during family conferences about end-of-life care in the intensive care unit. *American Journal of Respiratory & Critical Care Medicine, 171*(8), 844–849.

Curtis, J. R., & Shannon, S. E. (2006). Transcending the silos: Toward an interdisciplinary approach to end-of-life care in the ICU. *Intensive Care Medicine, 32*(1), 15–17.

Curtis, J. R., Wenrich, M. D., Carline, J. D., Shannon, S. E, Ambrozy, D. M., & Ramsey, P. G. (2001). Understanding physicians' skills at providing end-of-life care: Perspectives of patients, families, and health care workers. *Journal of General Internal Medicine, 16*, 41–49.

Curtis, J. R., Wenrich, M. D., Carline, J. D., Shannon, S. E., Ambrozy, D. M., & Ramsey, P. G. (2002). Patients' perspectives on physicians' skill at end-of-life care: Differences between patients with COPD, cancer, and AIDS. *Chest, 122*(1), 356–362.

Dudzinski, D. M., & Shannon, S. E. (2006). Competent patients' refusal of nursing care: What is the best ethical response? *Nursing Ethics, 13*(6), 608–621.

Dudzinski, D. M., Shannon, S. E., & Tong, R. (2006). Case commentary: Competent refusal of nursing care. *Hastings Center Report, 36*(2), 14–15.

Hsieh, H. F., & Shannon, S. E. (2005). Three approaches to qualitative content analysis. *Qualitative Health Research, 15*(19), 1277–1288.

Lautrette, A., Darmon, M., Megarbane, B., Joly, L. M., Chevret, S., Adrie, C., et al. (2007). A communication strategy and brochure for relatives of patients dying in the ICU. *New England Journal of Medicine, 356*(5), 469–478.

Lilly, C. M., De Meo, D. L., Sonna, L. A., Haley, K. J., Massaro, A. F., Wallace, R. F., & Cody, S. (2000). An intensive communication intervention for the critically ill. *American Journal of Medicine, 109*(6), 469–475.

McDonagh, J. R., Elliott, T. B., Engelberg, R. A., Treece, P. D., Shannon, S. E., Rubenfeld, G. D., et al. (2004). Family satisfaction with family conferences about end-of-life care in the ICU: Increased proportion of family speech is associated with increased satisfaction. *Critical Care Medicine, 32*(7), 1484–1488.

Schneiderman, L. J., Gilmer, T., & Teetzel, H. D. (2000). Impact of ethics consultations in the intensive care setting: A randomized, controlled trial. *Critical Care Medicine, 28*(12), 3920–3924.

Schonfeld, T. L., Romberger, D. J., Hester, D. M., & Shannon, S. E. (2007). Resuscitating a bad patient. *Hastings Center Report, 37*(1), 14–16.

Shannon, S. E. (1992). Caring for the critically ill patient receiving life-sustaining therapy: combining descriptive and normative research in ethics. *Dissertations Abstracts International,* 53.09B:4594.

Shannon, S. E. (1997). The roots of interdisciplinary conflict around ethical issues. *Critical Care Nursing Clinics of North America, 9,* 13–28.

Shannon, S. E. (2001). Helping families prepare for and cope with a death in the ICU. In J. R. Curtis & G. D. Rubenfeld (Eds.), *The transition from cure to comfort: Managing death in the intensive care unit* (pp. 165–182). Oxford, U.K.: Oxford University Press.

Shannon, S. E. (2006a). Damage compounded or damage lessened? Disparate impact or the compromises of multiculturalism? *American Journal of Bioethics, 6*(5), 27–28.

Shannon, S. E. (2006b, Spring). Medical futility and professional integrity, religious tolerance and social justice. *ASBH Exchange, 9,* pp. 5, 10.

Shannon, S. E., Mitchell, P. K., & Cain, K. (2002). Patients, nurses, and physicians have differing views of quality in critical care. *Journal of Nursing Scholarship, 34*(2), 173–179.

Teno, J. M., Murphy, D., Lynn, J., Tosteson, A., Desbiens, N., Connors, A. F., Jr., Hamel, M. B., Wu, A., Phillips, R., Wenger, N., et al. (1994). Prognosis-based futility guidelines: Does anyone win? SUPPORT Investigators. Study to Understand Prognoses and Preferences for Outcomes and Risks of Treatment. *Journal of the American Geriatrics Society, 42*(11), 1202–1207.

Texas Advance Directives Act. (1999). Retrieved November 10, 2006, from http://www.tapm. Org/vault/Texas%20Advance%20Directives%20Act.pdf

Wenrich, M. D., Curtis, J. R., Ambrozy, D. A., Carline, J., Shannon, S. E., & Ramsey, P. G. (2003). Dying patients' need for emotional support and personalized care from physicians: Perspectives of patients with terminal illness, families, and health care providers. *Journal of Pain and Symptom Management, 25*(3), 236–246.

Wenrich, M. D., Curtis, J. R., Shannon, S. E., Carline, J. D., Ambrozy, D. M., & Ramsey, P. G. (2001). Communicating with dying patients within the spectrum of medical care from terminal diagnosis to death. *Archives of Internal Medicine, 161*, 868–874.

Sarah E. Shannon is an Associate Professor in the Department of Biobehavioral Nursing and Health Systems, School of Nursing, and Adjunct in Department of Medical History and Ethics, School of Medicine, at the University of Washington in Seattle. She is a graduate of the University of Arizona (BSN) and University of Washington (PhD and MS). Her research focus has been primarily in improving the care of dying ICU patients through improving team communication around end-of-life decision-making with patients and their families. More recently she has collaborated on looking at team disclosure of medical errors to patients. Dr. Shannon's teaching and service has also been focused in bioethics.

✑ SECTION III ✑
CRITICAL THINKING ACTIVITIES

Political, Administrative, and Systems Aspects

✦ Cortney Davis writes in the poem "There Are No Poems at Hospital Management Meetings," "Poems hide on the floors." Take a moment and write about an image that won't go away from any of the chapters in this book or your own practice. Don't worry about structure or trying to write a poem. Just write down words that convey the look and feel of the image. Now look at your words. What appears that was hidden before?

✦ Apply the steps of the ethical impact statement that Aroskar proposes to a proposed health policy on a federal, state, or county level.

✦ Nurse managers are often caught between several conflicting obligations such as loyalty to the institution, nursing, and other staff members and patients. Additionally, Curtin raises external factors that impact nurse managers' ethical conduct. Name these factors, add others, and describe methods to balance these competing demands.

✦ Shannon embeds her research in ethics into the contexts in which she has worked as a nurse. Choose one of Shannon's publications. Read it, then describe how the context in which Shannon practiced at the time it was written had an impact on the development of the research question.

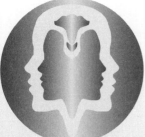

SECTION IV

Perspectives on Advocacy

Active support, recommendation, or defense of persons or policies is included. Persons particularly include patients, but professional members of nursing themselves are also considered. Relevant policies include those affecting the ethical practice of nurses, health, and health care.

Every Day, the Pregnant Teenagers

Cortney Davis

assemble at my desk, backpacks
jingling, beepers on their belts like hand grenades,
and inside, their babies
swirl like multicolored pinwheels in a hurricane.

The girls raise too-big smocks, show me
the stretched-tight skin
from under which a foot or hand thumps,
knocks, makes the belly wobble.

A girl strokes her invisible child,
recites all possible names, as if a name
might carry laundry down the street or fix
a Chevrolet. I measure months

with a paper tape, maneuver the cold stethoscope
that lifts a fetal heart (swoosh) into air.
Then, shirts billowing like parachutes,
the girls fly to Filene's where infant shoes,

on sale, have neon strobes and satin bows—*oh,*
Renee, Shalika, Blanca, Marie,
the places you'll go, the places you'll go!

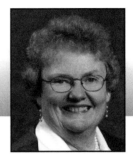

Joyce E. Beebe Thompson

CHAPTER 10

Advocacy for the Voices of Women, Nurses, and Midwives

Ihave been driven by a compelling vision that views girls and women everywhere as persons worthy of respect by all, as fully human. Women deserve better health and health services than they are receiving, and I can do something about this! I am challenged by innumerable factors and tremendous barriers that keep women, including many nurses and midwives, without either choices or voices in their lives. My life is dedicated to advocating that all persons listen "to" and "hear" the voices of women; and once heard, to empower women to speak up and contribute to the development of themselves and their societies.

Framing the Issue

My primary issue is advocacy for and by nurses and midwives as they take their rightful place at decision tables in health and illness care, with a special emphasis on working with vulnerable populations of women, nationally and internationally. My concept of advocacy includes active support, defense of persons, risk-taking, changing behaviors, and consideration of the context within which advocacy occurs—primarily the daily challenges for nurses and midwives in caring for others. Advocacy also focuses on giving voices to those who can knowledgeably speak for themselves, demand their human rights, and contribute to their communities and their world through teaching, supporting, modeling, and promoting ethical understanding and reasoning. Knowing how to make ethical decisions in life and one's professional practice is as important as knowing what constitutes ethics, and why health professionals need to be ethical persons.

The Journey

Three questions framed my journey into values, ethics, moral reasoning, and ethical decision-making. They were: (a) How can I best use my talents in service to others throughout the world? (b) What does it mean to be born female in various societies? and (c) How can I help nurses and midwives make good, that is, ethical decisions, in their daily practice, especially for themselves and when working with girls and women?

My introduction to nursing came during childhood when my mother went to work in a family doctor's office every day, resulting in my decision to become a nurse in the 7th grade. My introduction to the importance of healthy and strong women came from my maternal grandmother and my parents, who instilled in me the confidence to be and do whatever I chose in my life, with instructions to always do my best. My core values of faith, family, love, and service to others culminated in my response to an altar call in the 11th grade, where I dedicated my entire life to the service of God and others. When I applied for mission service at the end of my baccalaureate nursing program, the mission board suggested that I seek midwifery education before going overseas, which I did. I thought my life complete when as a nurse and a midwife I was sent to southern Chile for 3 years of mission work. This was just the beginning of my life's work, and I had much to learn about what it means to be a human being, to be respected as a person, and to make good decisions in both my personal and professional lives.

My introduction to questions about ethics, especially the meaning and value of life and what it meant to be a woman in a Latin society, began in earnest during my missionary days in southern Chile in the latter half of the 1960s. I was privileged to work with Arucanian (Mapuche) Indian women and families on remote hillsides, river islands, and in rural villages. I cared for women having their 15th pregnancy, with only three or four living children—this I questioned. I experienced my first maternal death in a rural hospital in Nueva Imperial, and I questioned this. Little did I know that advocating for women would become my destiny.

I continued to question what it meant to be a woman in society—questions that intensified when I began working in sub-Saharan Africa in the 1970s—and realized that many of my nursing and midwifery colleagues were "voiceless" in their societies.

Women were treated as objects, not persons. Though nurses and midwives were the essence of professional staff throughout Africa, they were mistreated, paid little, and expected to give of their services freely and not complain. They were dedicated to caring for everyone, even under the most difficult of circumstances. I experienced affective dissonance related to my core religious teachings of honesty, loving one's neighbor, and respect for others—values that appeared not often shared by those in power. My values were tested, held fast, and were strengthened—a fact that led to my interest in and writing about how we gain our core values and how values influence what we do and say. I began to understand how culture and cultural norms can be harmful to members of that same cultural group. This understanding formed part of my work in developing codes of ethics for midwives.

My continuing development as a person and as a student of human nature took a huge leap forward in the fall of 1972 when I met an amazing man, the Rev. Dr. Henry O. Thompson, my future husband. Hank was an ordained clergyman, an Old Testament scholar, Biblical archaeologist, school psychologist, and pastoral counselor. In the early years of our courtship, Hank suggested we take advantage of our different disciplines to do something scholarly together. That "something" became our ethics thinking, teaching, writing, and consultations, both nationally and internationally, until his death in 1997.

My particular interest in working within the field of bioethics was in helping nursing students (later medicine and other health disciplines) understand "how" to make ethical decisions in practice. Hank's particular interest was in helping health professionals understand the ethical "why" of making good decisions in health and illness care. As a team, we combined a strong theoretical foundation for understanding health care ethics (nursing in particular), based on moral philosophy, moral theology, human psychology (behavior), values, moral development, and decision theory, with a practical approach to making decisions in daily nursing practice. We focused primarily on the day-to-day and minute-to-minute decisions that nurses were called upon to make, recognizing that each had an ethical component based on the interaction with other human beings, which was captured in our first book (Thompson, J. B., & Thompson, 1981). Our value perspectives were highlighted so that those with different values, cultural traditions, or thought patterns could understand where we were coming from and decide if our thinking was congruent with theirs, and if not, why not. The translation of this ethics text into Spanish (1984) and its continued use throughout Latin America suggest that our approach was helpful in other cultures.

Hank and I held a strong position that if nurses understood both the why and how of moral reasoning and ethical decision-making, they would be empowered to contribute their unique nursing expertise and improve decision-making processes and outcomes. We advocated for, encouraged, and supported nurses as they began to understand their valuable role in ethical decision-making and became more willing to participate in such efforts in spite of bureaucratic constraints (Thompson, 1982). When nurses contributed to shared decision-making with the care team, along with the patient and family, the patient received care that more closely met the patient's needs/values. We jointly explored ethical theory and nursing practice, and wrote about ways to expand one's knowledge of personal and professional values, levels of moral development à la Kohlberg and Gilligan, and how this understanding influenced one's ability to make ethical decisions in practice (Thompson, J. E., & Thompson, 1985).

Hank brought the thinking of moral philosophy, moral theology, and moral development to my scientific preparation in nursing and midwifery and my interest in values and decision-making. I used my personal experiences in learning about morals, moral development, and ethics as positive encouragement and reinforcement for nurses and midwives as they learned about these topics. In addition, I took on the investigation of personal and professional values and how they become a part of an individual's development and life choices, which led to our important contributions to codes of professional behavior.

The definition of values that I developed over the years and use in my teaching and writing about ethics is based on the works of Raths, Simon, Uustal, Steele, and Harmon, among others. Values are attitudes and beliefs we put into practice in our daily lives. We have far more attitudes and beliefs, but fewer values that direct our choices and actions. Psychologist Morris Massey greatly influenced my thinking about personal values in the early 1980s with his discussion of "gut-level" values that are 90% programmed into us by the age of 10. I am a strong advocate for nursing and midwifery students understanding the core values of the professions and the standards of behavior they are expected to uphold. I was part of the American Nurses Association (ANA) ethics committee during the 1980s, reviewing the code and revising its interpretive statements. Hank and I also contributed to two additional codes (International Confederation of Midwives [ICM], 1993; Thompson, H. O., & Thompson, 1987; Thompson, J. E., & Thompson, 1986).

We started teaching ethics to graduate students in nurse-midwifery at Columbia University in the late 1970s, where I was director of the graduate nurse-midwifery program. This was a time when nursing ethics was rarely a discrete course in nursing curricula. In fact, it was a time when nurses and midwives were not viewed as participants in ethical decision-making by many bioethicists and physicians. We focused our teaching on such questions as why nurses and midwives should bother with the study of ethics (Beebe & Thompson, 1976, 1978; Thompson, H. O., & Thompson, 1981; Thompson, J. E., & Thompson, 1984), and whether this study would make a difference in the way they practiced their profession.

Over the years, Hank and I taught many courses in health care ethics, primarily at the University of Pennsylvania. Those courses included our separate definitions of "morals" and "ethics" (Beebe & Thompson, 1976; Thompson, J. B., & Thompson, 1981). We found it helpful to define "morals" as the shoulds and oughts of life—what one should do or ought to do. We then defined "ethics" as the reasons why one should or ought to do something.

Hank and I developed an approach to our ethics teaching that was grounded in Western philosophical ethical theories, moral theology, moral development, human values, and critical thinking (Thompson, J. E., & Thompson, 1983; 1985). We used this knowledge to understand the variety of human behavior faced on a daily basis. We then urged the students to apply this knowledge in making ethical decisions in nursing and midwifery practice. I learned that one cannot understand the ethical "why" unless one understands ethics. I valued self-determination, I liked to think for myself, and I modeled those aspects of personhood to my fellow nurses and midwives as they struggled with the language, content, and application of ethics.

Our initial articles were based on our early teaching efforts and grounded in our understanding that the great majority of ethical concerns raised in health and illness care can arise when working with women and families of childbearing age experiencing amniocentesis, electronic fetal monitoring, abortion, and contraception (Beebe & Thompson, 1976, 1978; Thompson, J. E., & Thompson, 1989). Likewise, using a principle-centered approach (autonomy) to sharing knowledge or information so that women/partners could make informed decisions about their childbearing care was grounded in the ethical concept of informed consent (Thompson, H. O., & Thompson, 1980).

Impact of Ethics Work

The biggest impact Hank and I have had on nursing ethics is centered on our decision model and my ongoing work on advocacy for social justice that focuses on improving health outcomes for the most vulnerable of any society—especially women, nurses, and midwives.

Early in our ethics teaching and consultations in hospital and academic nursing settings, we received increasing requests for help in knowing how to make good decisions in practice. These requests led to our exploration of decision models from mathematics to engineering, comparing them to the scientific method and the nursing process. The results of our exploration and thinking culminated in the development of the TnT decision model (Thompson, H. O., & Thompson, 1981, Thompson, J. B., & Thompson, 1981). Though the 10 steps of the model have not changed, some of the items under each step have been refined over the past 30 years of use with a variety of groups—both lay and professional (see Figure 10.1). We continued to explore why humans act as they do and what criteria or factors influence and contribute to making "good" or "correct" decisions, whether for the self or for others. Understanding values as distinct from morals and ethics, moral reasoning, and moral development added to our teaching effectiveness and ethical reasoning.

Step 1 of the model helps to focus the ethical analysis by clearly identifying key individuals in the situation and defining the health or illness condition under discussion. The emphasis in Step 2 is understanding not only what information is available to consider in decision-making, but what information is not available and what potential influence that lack of information (e.g., prognosis) might have on the decision process and outcome. The influence of historical roots of ethical issue(s) and societal views (culture, norms) on each is evident in Step 3.

Steps 4, 5, and 6, with the focus on values and levels of moral development (descriptive ethics), most distinguish this decision model from others in the nursing ethics literature. The importance of the consideration of values and value conflicts when faced with ethical decisions in our lives is based on the fact that values give direction to our daily living. We need to know ourselves well before we participate in decisions about others. Our own values lens often clouds what we see and hear others say, especially if that information is dissonant with our own experiences or values. Sometimes our personal values must give way to what is ethical action, especially when the decision needed affects another person, as most health care decisions do.

We understood that in nursing practice there is an ethical dimension to any decision involving other human beings, and we offered a guideline for making ethical decisions in one's professional work. We empowered nurses to take an active role in the ethical decisions with and for their patients—to be educated in ethics and to use their "voices" responsibly. Nurses know more than other health professionals about patients and their responses to health, illness, and hospitalizations. And it is that very information about the patient that is needed in order to make the best decisions about care, especially when the patient cannot speak for himself/herself.

Aroskar's sentinel article (1982) helped us understand the perceived apathy we found in many nurses who seemed unwilling to take an active role in decisions that

Figure 10.1

Thompson & Thompson Bioethical Decision-Making Model

Adapted from Thompson & Thompson, 1985.
Updated January 2005

Step 1: Review the situation to determine:
- Health problems—physical, spiritual, mental, psychosocial.
- Decision/actions needed immediately & in near future.
- Ethical components of situation and decision/action.
- Key individuals potentially affected by the decision/action & outcomes.
- Any potential human rights violations in situation.

Step 2: Gather additional information to clarify and understand:
- Legal constraints, if any.
- Limited time to thoroughly explore.
- Decision capacity of individual(s).
- Institutional policies that affect choices in situation.
- Values inherent in choice of information.

Step 3: Identify the ethical issues or concerns in the situation:
- Name the ethical concern.
- Explore historical roots of each.
- Identify current philosophical/religious positions on each issue.
- Discuss societal/cultural views on each issue.

Step 4: Define personal and professional moral positions on ethical concerns:
- Review personal biases/constraints on issues raised.
- Understand personal values affected by situation/ethical issues raised.
- Review professional codes of ethics (moral behavior) for guidance.
- Identify any conflicting loyalties and/or obligations of professionals and family in the situation.
- Think about your level of moral development operant in this situation.
- Identify the virtues needed for professional action.

Step 5: Identify moral positions of key individuals in the situation:
- Think about levels of moral development operant in each participant.
- Identify any communication gaps or misunderstandings.
- Provide guidance in clarifying varying levels of moral development.

(continued)

Figure 10.1 (Continued)

Step 6: Identify value conflicts, if any:
- Provide guidance in identifying potential conflicts, interests, competing values.
- Work toward possible resolution of conflict based on respect for differences.
- Seek consultation if needed to resolve key conflicts.

Step 7: Determine who should make needed decision:
- Clarify your role in the situation.
- Who "owns" the problem/decision?
- Who stands to lose or gain the most from the decision/action?
- Is the decision to be made by single individual or group?

Step 8: Identify the range of actions with anticipated outcomes of each:
- Determine the moral justification for each potential action.
- Identify the ethical theory that supports each action.
- Apply concepts of beneficence and fairness to each potential action.
- Attach outcomes to each potential action and determine best outcome.
- Are additional actions/decisions required as a result of each action?

Step 9: Decide on a course of action and carry it out:
- Understand why a given action was chosen.
- Help all involved understand these reasons.
- Establish a time frame for review of the decision/action and expected outcomes.
- Determine who can best carry out the chosen action/decision.

Step 10: Evaluate/review outcomes of decisions/actions:
- Determine whether expected outcomes occurred.
- Is a new decision or action needed?
- Was the decision process fair and complete?
- What was the response to the action by each key individual?
- What did you learn from this situation?

affected their patients, not wanting to "rock the boat" of the system or risk losing their jobs. In addition, we were heavily influenced by writings that exposed physicians and other health workers who used clinical "judgment" as an excuse to cover their own value biases when selecting the option that they would have made for themselves in a similar situation.

Hank and I were strong advocates of responsible decision-making that included not only making good decisions, but also taking responsibility for the outcomes of those decisions. We recognized that following a particular framework for making decisions was "not" synonymous with making an ethical decision. We reinforced that critical thinking was required, along with time, respect for differing points of views, mutual trust, and involvement of key individuals.

Another aspect of empowering nurses to use their knowledge and voices for ethical care relates to our leadership in developing an ethics consultation committee in a large academic health center in the earlier 1980s. We convinced this medical center to accept the proposal that the committee would consist of equal numbers of physicians and nurses, with representatives from social work, pastoral care, and the public. The cochairs of the committee would be a nurse and a physician. As nurses gained understanding of ethics and moral reasoning, they were better able to care for individuals, even when the plan of care was not one thought best by the nurse (Thompson, J. E., & Thompson, 1988).

Broader Significance of Ethics Work

A new area of ethics expertise has evolved from my international work focusing on advocacy for the ethical concepts of social justice, personhood, and human rights for women. Helping women find their "voices" to speak out against oppression, harmful cultural traditions, systems, and structures that render them "voiceless" begins the process, while also clearly identifying the personal and professional risks they may have to take to make needed changes in their family, their community, or their nation. The essence of practicing ethically in whatever situation nurses or midwives find themselves is based on understanding the interrelationships of culture, values, moral development, and ethics. Using that understanding to advocate for ethical care and treatment of the most vulnerable groups in any society supports full human rights for all.

The expansion of my ethics expertise into human rights has had a definite impact globally. I still struggle with the occurrence of gender-based violence and discrimination evident in many resource-poor nations. I have channeled my anger into a stronger voice advocating for change, for social justice, for the ethical treatment of all individuals (Thompson, J. E., & Thompson, 1997). This has resulted in several international presentations and publications (Thompson, 2002, 2004, 2007).

The influence of my expertise and publications on ethics and human rights carried over to my leadership role with the ICM as Director of the Board of Management (1999–2005), where I continued to assist with its Code revision. In my role (2005–2007) as a member of the interim Steering Committee of the global Partnership for Maternal, Newborn, and Child Health, I contributed to the development of the conceptual framework that recognizes the value of women and their right to fair treatment, wherever they live and work.

My Legacy

Hank and I were a successful ethics team. The primary focus of our ethics efforts was on promoting understanding of what it means to be a professional (Thompson, J. B., & Thompson, 1981; Thompson, J. E., & Thompson, 1984). Hank's significant contribution was the inclusion of the concept of covenant fidelity as an integral part of the relationship between self and others, especially the professional self of the nurse. This covenantal relationship goes well beyond being paid to nurse others—it goes to the very core of how human beings should relate to one another. My significant contribution was/is a focus on values and decision-making within the context of human rights and social justice. Together we promoted an ethic of "care" based on competence, compassion, and covenant fidelity.

Through our teaching and consultations, we advocated that nurses accept and be accepted as valued participants in moral reasoning and ethical decision-making. And through our sharing of ethics thought and examples, we empowered nurses and midwives to take an active role in ethics education themselves. Together we published numerous articles, ethics columns, books, and several book chapters and monographs. With this grounding in sharing our ethics thinking with others for over two decades, I continued to present, teach, and write about health care ethics after Hank's death in 1997.

I will close as I began. I, for one, can do something about the health of women, primarily by giving voices and choices to women, to nurses and midwives, and continuing to speak out for the ethical treatment of all people. That is my contribution to nursing ethics. That is my legacy for future nurses and midwives. That is my contribution to women and families of the world.

References

Aroskar, M. (1982). Are nurses' mind sets compatible with ethical nursing practice? *Topics in Clinical Nursing, 4,* 22–32.

Beebe, J. E., & Thompson, H. O. (1976). Nurse midwifery and ethics—A beginning. *Journal of Nurse Midwifery, 21*(4), 7–11.

Beebe, J. E., & Thompson, H. O. (1978). Teaching ethics to nurse midwives. *Journal of Nurse Midwifery, 23,* 31–35.

International Confederation of Midwives (ICM). (1993). *International code of ethics for midwives.* London: Author.

Thompson, H. O., & Thompson, J. E. (1980). The ethics of being a female patient and a female care provider in a male dominated health-illness system. *Issues in Health Care of Women, 2*(3–4), 25–54.

Thompson, H. O., & Thompson, J. E. (1981). Ethical decision making in nursing. *MCN: The American Journal of Maternal Child Nursing, 6*(1), 21–23; 60.

Thompson, H. O., & Thompson, J. E. (1987). Toward a professional ethic. *Journal of Nurse Midwifery, 32*(2), 105–110.

Thompson, J. B., & Thompson, H. O. (1981). *Ethics in nursing.* New York: Macmillan. Spanish language edition, Spring, 1983. Reprinted by University Press of America, Lanham, MD, 1992. Translated into Japanese, 2005.

Thompson, J. E. (1982). Conflicting loyalties of nurses working in bureaucratic settings. In *Professionalism and the empowerment of nursing* (pp. 27–37). Kansas City, MO: ANA Publication G 157, 2M.

Thompson, J. E. (2002). Midwives and human rights: Dream or reality? *Midwifery, 18*(3), 188–192.

Thompson, J. E. (2004). A human rights framework for midwifery care. *Journal of Midwifery & Women's Health, 49*(3), 175–181.

Thompson, J. E. (2007). Professional ethics. In L. A. Ament, *Professional issues in midwifery* (Chapter 14, pp. 277–300). Sudbury, MA: Jones & Bartlett.

Thompson, J. E., & Thompson, H. O. (1983). Nursing, ethics, and moral development. *International Social Science Review, 58*(3), 155–158.

Thompson, J. E., & Thompson, H. O. (1984). Ethical decision making is an integral part of nursing. *AORN Journal, 39*(2), 157–159.

Thompson, J. E., & Thompson, H. O. (1985). *Bioethical decision making for nurses.* Norwalk, CT: Appleton Century Crofts. Reprinted by University Press of America, Lanham, MD, 1992. Translated into Japanese, Spring 2003.

Thompson, J. E., & Thompson, H. O. (1986). Code of ethics for nurse-midwives. *Journal of Nurse-Midwifery, 31*(2), 99–102.

Thompson, J. E., & Thompson, H. (1988). Living with ethical decisions with which you disagree. *MCN: The American Journal of Maternal Child Nursing, 13,* 245–250.

Thompson, J. E., & Thompson, H. (1989). Teaching ethics to nursing students. *Nursing Outlook, 37*(2), 84–88.

Thompson, J. E., & Thompson, H. O. (1997). Ethics and midwifery. *World Health, 2*(2), 14–15.

Joyce E. Beebe Thompson, RN, CNM, DrPH, FAAN, FACNM is currently the Lacey Professor of Community Health Nursing at the Bronson School of Nursing, Western Michigan University, and Professor Emerita of Nursing at the University of Pennsylvania. She is a graduate of the University of Michigan (BSN, MPH), Maternity Center Association (CNM) and Columbia University (DrPH). In 1983 she completed the Intensive Bioethics Course at the Kennedy Institute of Ethics, Georgetown University. She has taught health care ethics since 1975 at Columbia, Penn, and in Japan, sub-Saharan Africa, and Latin America. Most of her ethics teaching and writing was with Rev. Dr. Henry O. Thompson until his death in 1997. She continues to write and teach ethics in the relatively new PhD program in Interdisciplinary Health Studies at WMU and within the community-based BSN and MSN programs. Her particular interest in health care ethics is helping professionals make ethical decisions in practice, informed by understanding the importance of values and moral development on decision-making. She has also contributed to the revision of the ANA code and development of the first codes of ethics for the American College of Nurse-Midwives and the International Confederation of Midwives. Her life passion is helping girls and women of the world be viewed as fully human, as persons, with full human rights.

Beverly J. McElmurry

CHAPTER 11

Transitions to Global Health Perspectives through an Advocacy Lens

One of my favorite sayings is "seize the opportunity of a lifetime in the lifetime of the opportunity." Thus, I have endeavored to use this paper as an opportunity to integrate the lived and living experience of enacting advocacy to achieve global primary health care goals over multiple transitions in a professional career. How do we identify characteristics of just or fair health systems? The answer usually relies on the components of advocacy—"trying to figure out the right thing to do within the constraints of a particular situation."

Context

At some point after high school, I began to notice that not all things were treated or created equal. I now attribute this to growing up in a small town—a protected environment where the larger world did not intrude on children and youth. However, going off to Chicago to study nursing introduced me to a new world. Although I was doing everything wrong (according to current educational standards) by attending a diploma program, my course of study had most of the basic and behavioral sciences offered by professors from the University of Chicago and the Illinois Institute of Technology. The teaching staff at the time included Ingeborg and Hans Mauksch, who were both sociologists, and Ingeborg was also a nurse. Hans loaded us on a bus and gave a tour of Chicago that was exquisite. Migration, neighborhoods, poverty, and wealth were vividly imprinted. There were several times as a beginning student when I went home for the weekend determined not to return to school. My father always responded that these times were a "challenge." He would drive me back into the city rather than have me return by train, stopping along the way for a corned beef sandwich and a pep talk.

Over time, I began to ponder physiological expressions of emotion. There were a few times as a student when I could not absorb what I was seeing or asked to do, and had to excuse myself, as I knew that I was about to faint or otherwise embarrass myself. Survival in basic training was based on bonding with classmates and mutual support. In my final year of the nursing diploma program, a former high school administrator/counselor contacted me and offered me a scholarship to pursue baccalaureate education. This was a "no strings attached" offer, based on the assumption that I would in turn find a means to help someone else go to school. The offers of scholarships and encouragement were enough for me to decide to go to the University of Minnesota, as it had a special program for registered nurses, and this award—supplemented by a nursing traineeship and part-time work—would make it possible for me to study. The opportunity for baccalaureate study was freeing. Over time, I have seen the ideas I was exposed to incorporated into a personal perspective on being. Ideas like advocacy start with small things near at hand and evolve (or spiral) as the complexity and richness of experiences develop into a frame of reference.

The Minnesota program had many giants over the years and produced numerous leaders in nursing education and administration, as well as international health care. Carol Lindeman became a mentor for my student teaching experience. Carol made many contributions to nursing and her sense of humor was also instructive—I quote her often when it is time to change my ideas about a topic—"If the horse is dead, I suggest that you dismount."

A Transition

After completing my bachelor's degree, I was offered a teaching position at St. Mary's Hospital Diploma program by Sister Anne Joachim Moore, a dynamite nun with a law degree and aspirations to develop an innovative associate degree program (LaBelle, 1974; LaBelle & Egan, 1975). I became chair of the faculty group that was to devise the experimental curriculum and I completed a master's degree.

After several years at St. Mary's, I moved from Minneapolis to the University of Wisconsin-Madison. After 2 years I came to the conclusion that if I wanted to continue to work in university settings, I would have to go back to school. I had also had an epiphany of sorts one day when I looked around and asked why I was caring for so many sick people. I wondered what had happened to health and why there was so little literature on the subject. So, as students protested activities in Cambodia and Vietnam, the National Guard patrolled campus, pepper spray filled the air, and the math building blew up, I left Madison for Northern Illinois University (NIU) to obtain a doctoral degree in education.

More Education

As I approached the end of my doctoral study, the NIU administration indicated an interest in hiring me as faculty in the community health nursing area. Working in community health was totally new, and it was great fun to take on the challenge of providing community health experiences in an area that I considered more rural than any place I had ever worked (Ashley & LaBelle, 1976). With a car as a mobile office, I met students in jails, schools, clinics, migrant centers, and public aid offices, for example, and toured the countryside (Dewar, Helgeson, & McElmurry, 1977; McElmurry, 1979). I also served on the board of a local hospital as it converted to a long-term care facility, chaired the county Tuberculosis Association, helped establish a local chapter of Sigma Theta Tau International (the nursing honor society), and was active in state nursing research and ethics activities (McElmurry, 1978).

By the late 1970s I was working half time at the University of Illinois at Chicago (UIC), and half time at Northern (Egan, McElmurry, & Jameson, 1981; LaBelle, Pender, & Goodman, 1976; McElmurry, Krueger, & Parsons, 1982; McElmurry, & Newcomb, 1980). Eventually, the NIU nursing administrators refused to release me for further participation as the Illinois representative in the six state regional studies of school, occupational, and public health nursing, led by Beverly Flynn at Indiana University. I resigned from NIU and moved to UIC. The transition was a logistical challenge for a while, given that I was expecting a baby and had to adjust to a new job, physical relocation, and find child care in a new setting.

At this time I met a young philosopher from the University of Chicago, Rod Yarling, with whom I eventually collaborated on several nursing ethics activities. Rod and I (and others) tried to obtain funding for a state-of-the-art conference on nursing ethics, and a training program built on the development of nursing ethics teaching models. We developed a concept paper describing the desired "Institute for the Study of Social Issues in Nursing," and circulated a prospectus to establish a nursing ethics journal. We did not succeed. From our perspective, nurses had to be recognized as having a moral, legal, and institutional base to advocate for patients. As primarily hospital employees, nurses often found themselves in conflict if they advocated for the patient against hospital or physician directives. Liberation from professional and institutional pressures is a necessity if nurses are to be free to be moral. A community of moral discourse is only possible where all participants are free to be moral agents. Our position was that nurses were not free to be moral, and were instead defined by the situations of employment and practice (Yarling & McElmurry, 1986).

This position was confirmed by research Sue Swider led, in which we surveyed students, practicing nurses, and administrators (Swider, McElmurry, & Yarling, 1985). Students were oriented to patient and family advocacy, but by the time they became full-fledged nurses, the practice bureaucracy trumped what they had learned in education. Although we published this study, it was never cited to any extent as far as I know. Likewise, we were appalled that most hospitals did not recognize patients' Do Not Resuscitate wishes when they had been related to nurses and duly recorded (Yarling & McElmurry, 1983). Risk management strategies required a physician's order to be taken seriously, but not nurses' notes detailing patients' wishes. Such practices dehumanize health care. Interestingly, there has been little change in my perspective that nursing ethics could be the ethics of health care reform. To paraphrase Carol Lindeman, this horse is not dead. The practice of nursing ethics is dependent upon the reflective and critical thinking of the person who "is" the nurse. Revolution or reform starts in the head.

One of the immediate areas of interest for me when I moved to UIC was women's health, as I had started research at NIU on tool development for assessing the health of older women (McElmurry, 1986; McElmurry & LiBrizzi, 1986) that later incorporated evaluation of the research base for health care of older women (McElmurry & Zabrocki, 1989; Zabrocki & McElmurry, 1989, 1990), and research related to midlife women's self-care response to menopause (Huddleston & McElmurry, 1990; McElmurry & Huddleston, 1991a, 1991b). By 1984, my colleagues (Denny Benton, Diane Boyer, Diana Biordi, Alice Dan) and I were joined by others in an effort to obtain a special projects grant from the Division of Nursing to develop a graduate concentration in women's health—a 5-year endeavor (McElmurry & Newcomb, 1995). We developed a position on women's health that was operationalized as the Women's Health Exchange (Webster, et al., 1986a; 1986b). It struck us that if women helped us advance our practice, teaching, and research, in exchange we owed them information about what was learned. The women's health training grant helped us launch a graduate concentration in women's health that cut across all departments of the UIC College of Nursing, and incorporated colleagues from the community and other campus departments. It was also a time when we questioned whether the voices of women's health scholars were muffled by existing manuscript review processes (Blank & McElmurry, 1988; McElmurry, Newcomb, Barnfather, & Lynch, 1981), classification systems for women's health knowledge, and retrieval index systems (McElmurry & Parker, 1993, 1995, 1996). In 2006, a campus-wide multidisciplinary graduate concentration in women's health was formally approved. Again, this sort of activity—"advocacy" if you will—is not an individual accomplishment, but one that requires a community of participants. The list of students who participated in the doctoral program in women's health is extensive, and their current contribution to nursing science is not only a terrific gift for faculty, but a real legacy to the profession.

I began community projects with urban women in 1982 via a project funded by the Chicago Mayor's Office titled, "Urban Women's Health Advocacy." This was followed by a period of funding that launched the nurse-health advocate demonstration projects in the Chicago communities of West Town (Latino) and Grand Boulevard (African-American). The transition from the women's health grant to these demonstration projects was a natural evolution for me (McElmurry, Swider, Bless, et al., 1990; McElmurry, Swider, & Norr, 1991; McElmurry, Swider, & Watanakij, 1992; Swider & McElmurry, 1990; Watanakij & McElmurry, 1995). Because of a million-dollar grant received from The Chicago Community Trust to undertake advocacy for a revitalization of health services in Chicago, we soon moved into spheres of activity at the city and national health levels. For us, health advocacy was a means of giving voice to women's participation in the health of their community, wherever they defined their community. Thus, the later 1980s and early 1990s was an immersion in community-based initiatives within a primary health care (PHC) framework, with special emphasis on community participation in health care that is affordable, acceptable, culturally sensitive, and concerned about essential health care for all (McElmurry & Keeney, 1999, 2006). Basically, we wanted to change the health care delivery system and recognize the work in health care that was community based and more than disease focused. The women we recruited as health advocates needed to learn to process their understanding and approach to work and problem resolution. Likewise, the nurses needed to understand how to work with community people.

In one of our projects for leadership training, we pooled a mix of health professionals and low-income advocates to learn about primary health care and health systems delivery, for example, and then to use what they had learned in developing a program for the community (McElmurry, Tyska, Gugenheim, Misner, & Poslusny, 1995). A vivid memory is of the first attempts of a male physician who served a

Latino clientele and an African-American woman with General Educational Development (GED) learning to communicate with each other. So much of it was reflective of the fact they had not walked or talked in the other's world. They made progress through food. When they had to develop a community project, he expressed amazement at what she could do at little cost to serve a good meal to a large group and she found herself praised by him. A good deal of what we learned in bringing diverse people together had to do with helping them learn to negotiate communication and role clarification.

There were books, videos, articles, and presentations that came from all of this activity, and today the use of health advocates in various settings is not at all unusual. We contributed to the sustainability of this idea. Some of the original funders wanted to know how our projects would achieve sustainability of the health advocacy model. While they have long ago retired, I can now look back and see that it was a very long process (McElmurry, Tyska, & Parker, 1999). There is now a technical college in Chicago that offers a training program for health advocates, provides credit that can be applied toward an associate degree, and has built-in support for low-income women to have their tuition costs covered.

About the time that we recognized we could not continue to produce health advocates for community-based health education without a steady source of income from foundations or the university, we turned to programs developed by the Corporation for National Service. In 1994 we began an AmeriCorps program, using many of the training strategies that we had developed to prepare health advocates (McElmurry, Buseh, & Dublin, 1999; McElmurry, Park, & Buseh, 2003; McElmurry, Wansley, Gugenheim, Gombe, & Dublin, 1997). This initiative allowed the recruitment of participants for 1 or 2 years of community service at a minimal stipend with an educational benefit. Mixed funding from the government, foundations, and community agencies, as well as the support of the university, have kept this program alive. Participants recruited from local communities were provided sufficient time to develop some skills for the workforce as well as confidence in what they had to offer their community agencies, and they contributed to the health of their communities.

Primary Health Care (PHC) is the theme of the World Health Organization (WHO) Collaborating Center that I direct, and the premise (especially as it has been applied to nursing) incorporates a systems perspective, participation of community members, engagement of nurses and other health professionals in health promotion and maintenance, as well as sick care (McElmurry & Keeney, 1998, 1999, 2006). For PHC to ever really be adopted in the United States, a conversion to minimal or basic health care for the entire population will be required.

Transition to Senior Faculty Role

I acquired an international perspective by virtue of being director of the UIC WHO Collaborating Center. The HIV/AIDS crisis in Africa became a major focus. When Sheila Tlou (one of my advisees) returned to Botswana following the completion of her doctorate, she enjoined several of us from Illinois to examine how our PHC model with lay community health workers combined with health professionals could be used to mobilize local women in HIV/AIDS prevention (Norr, McElmurry, Moeti & Tlou, 1992, 1994; Norr, Norr, Tlou, McElmurry, & Moeti, 2004; Norr, Tlou, & McElmurry, 1996). That request resulted in the introduction of a PHC Community Health Worker intervention in Botswana. This disease prevention, health promotion model (introduced before Botswana HIV figures exploded) demonstrated success via changes in peoples' attitudes, knowledge, and behavior. The same type of intervention was later tried with similar success via a low-budget model in Lithuania, where staff nurses were taught outreach health education for HIV/AIDS prevention (Norr, McElmurry, et al., 2001). Over the years, there have been many HIV/AIDS-related activities with the support of multiple public and private funding. The combined PHC, women's health, and HIV programs have included work with collaborators in nine other countries (Keeney, Cassata, & McElmurry, 2004; Lin, McElmurry, & Christiansen, 2007; McElmurry, Marks, & Cianelli, 2002; Thongpriwan & McElmurry, 2006; Yang, McElmurry, & Park, 2006).

Many have discussed changes in women's health scholarship and activity over the years, but the appalling conditions for low-income, underserved people have not gone away (McElmurry, McCreary et al., 2008 in press). To advocate for better health care for women, there have been many opportunities to advance awareness of their health situations via publications on current research-based knowledge and country assessments to highlight gender inequalities that limit the economic development of countries (Lin, et al., 2007; McElmurry, Norr, & Parker, 1993). Ethics has been a part of the course requirements for our PHC trainees, as well as many others outside the PHC concentration. The course continues to be fun and has stimulated many publications by students as well as staff (Dresden, McElmurry, & McCreary, 2003; McElmurry, Solheim, et al., 2006). PHC requires development of a community ethics focus.

The Minority International Research Trainee (MIRT) program was a 10-year endeavor that provided an enormous payoff for the participants (Buseh, Glass, & McElmurry, 2002; McElmurry, Kim, & Al Gasseer, 2000; McElmurry & Misner, 1996; McElmurry, Misner, & Buseh, 2003; McElmurry, Misner, Dresden, et al., 2003). The intent was to provide nursing science undergraduates from underrepresented ethnic/racial groups with an opportunity to go abroad for 8–10 weeks (all expenses paid), and participate in ongoing international nursing research. The process of matching students with foreign nurse investigators and projects provided another learning opportunity for the staff. There were many ways in which we brought ethics to the attention of the MIRT trainees. Once accepted, the MIRT scholars were required to complete the federal training certificate ("IRB 101") and a four-module instructional program on professional, research, community, and cultural ethics. In addition, they learned about dual IRB reviews (United States and host country site), and the history of the country they would visit. Upon completion of the 8–10 weeks abroad, they presented their research to a host site audience. Many MIRT scholars also participated in a publication with their host researcher. Overall, it was a life-altering experience for participants.

The last 15 years have continued to amaze and discourage me. There are many times when I tend to go back to early problem-solving strategies with the basic questions—what is the real problem here, and what will work in this situation to realize some improvements. Poverty and gender inequalities seem as intractable as corruption. While there is some dialogue about globalization, there remains little clarity and inadequate development of what can be accomplished in health globalization. In particular, how do we blend traditional approaches to nursing ethics with community and cultural components that are so much a part of international health practice?

Perhaps one of the most vexing issues to be faced at this point is the management of manipulated nurse migration (McElmurry, Solheim, et al., 2006). This type of migration is distinguished from the normal movement of people. While we tried to raise ethical concerns and issues in our migration article, it is not an issue that is receiving sufficient attention. Manipulated economic markets, such as those occurring in the "forced" migration of nurses, are nothing short of human trafficking. The enormous sums that are paid to nurse finders and brokers are a financial burden to the migrating nurses. The decimation of the nurse workforce in the home countries of the migrating nurses harms the global health infrastructure. Resistance to participating with those who want to buy a curriculum for their profitable export nursing schools is sometimes viewed as quaint. After all, do not the financial contributions the foreign nurses remit to their home countries make the practice mutually beneficial? I find this manipulation of the global professional market wrong. Perhaps I will eventually "see the light." Right now, I see red lights and danger signs for global nursing.

What Does It All Mean?

The struggle to examine advocacy as a personal experience or way of being has been an interesting challenge. Interpretation of the lived experience as a way of being and enacting advocacy becomes easier as one gains more distance from the experience. Being embedded in the work, it is sometimes a struggle to clearly grasp the big picture. Global health advocacy is complex, chaotic, and fascinating. There are many ways for nursing to enact global health advocacy. There is some truth in the view that one needs to think globally and act locally to make sense of it.

References

Ashley, J., & LaBelle, B. M. (1976). Breakthrough to ideas: Education for freeing minds. In J. Williamson (Ed.), *Current perspectives in nursing: The changing scene* (pp. 50–65). St. Louis, MO: Mosby.

Blank, J. J., & McElmurry, B. J. (1988). Editors of nursing journals. *Nursing Outlook, 36*(4), 179–181.

Buseh, A. G., Glass, L. K., & McElmurry, B. M. (2002). Cultural and gender issues related to HIV/AIDS prevention in Swaziland: A focus group analysis. *Health Care for Women International, 23*(2), 173–184.

Dewar, M., Helgeson, R., & McElmurry, B. J. (1977). Many scars and me: One victim's story of growth with multiple sclerosis. *Health Values: Achieving High Level Wellness, 1*(6) 274–282.

Dresden, E., McElmurry, B. J., & McCreary, L. M. (2003). Approaching ethical reasoning in nursing research through a communitarian perspective. *Journal of Professional Nursing, 19*(5), 295–304.

Egan, E. C., McElmurry, B. J., & Jameson, H. (1981). Practice-based research: Assessing your department's readiness. *Journal of Nursing Administration, 11*(10), 26–32.

Huddleston, D., & McElmurry, B. J. (1990). A women's health perspective of the natural menopause. In C. Leppa (Ed.), *Women's health perspectives: An annual review* (Vol. 3, pp. 210–228), Phoenix, AZ: Oryx Press.

Keeney, G. B., Cassata, L., & McElmurry, B. J. (2004). *Adolescent health and development in nursing and midwifery education.* Geneva: World Health Organization.

LaBelle, B. M. (1974). Creative problem-solving techniques in nursing. *Journal of Creative Behavior, 8*(1), 55–66.

LaBelle, B. M., & Egan, E. C. (1975). Follow-up studies in nursing: A case for determining whether program objectives are met. *Journal of Nursing Education, 14*(3), 7–13.

LaBelle, B. M., Pender, N. J., & Goodman, E. S. (1976). *Midwest directory of resources for graduate education in nursing.* Evanston, IL: Committee on Institutional Cooperation.

Lin, K., McElmurry, B. J., & Christiansen, C. (2007). Women and HIV/AIDS in China: Gender and vulnerability. *Health Care for Women International, 28*(8), 680–699.

McElmurry, B. J. (1978). Illinois: State-wide council for nursing research. *International Journal of Nursing Studies, 15*(1), 17–22.

McElmurry, B. J. (1979). Health appraisal of low-income women. In D. Kjervik & I. Martinson (Eds.), *Women in stress: A nursing perspective* (pp. 171–183). New York: Appleton-Century-Crofts.

McElmurry, B. J. (1986). Health appraisal of low-income women. In D. Kjervik & I. Martinson (Eds.), *Women in health and illness* (pp. 116–125). Philadelphia: W.B. Saunders Co.

McElmurry, B. J., Buseh, A., & Dublin, M. (1999). Health education program to control asthma in multi-ethnic, low income urban communities: The Chicago Health Corps Asthma Program. *Chest, 116*(Suppl. 4), 198–199.

McElmurry, B. J., & Huddleston, D. S. (1991a). The perimenopausal woman. In D. Taylor, & N. Woods (Eds.), *Sexuality and the menstrual cycle* (Chapter 18, pp. 213–223). New York: Hemisphere.

McElmurry, B. J., & Huddleston, D. S. (1991b). Self-care and menopause: Critical review of research. *Health Care for Women International, 12*(1), 15–26.

McElmurry, B. J., & Keeney, G. (1998). Primary health care. In J. Fitzpatrick (Ed.), *Encyclopedia of Nursing Research* (pp. 457–458). New York: Springer.

McElmurry, B. J., & Keeney, G. (1999). Primary health care. In J. Fitzpatrick (Ed.), *Annual Review of Nursing Research* (pp. 241–268). New York: Springer.

McElmurry, B. J., & Keeney, G. (2006). Primary health care. In J. Fitzpatrick (Ed.), *Encyclopedia of Nursing Research* (pp. 488–490). New York: Springer.

McElmurry, B. J., Kim, S., & Al Gasseer, N. (2000). Global nursing leadership: A professional imperative. *Seminars for Nurse Managers, 8*(4), 232–238.

McElmurry, B. J., Krueger, J. C., & Parsons, L. C. (1982). Resources for graduate education: Report of a survey of 40 states in the Midwest, West, and Southern regions. *Nursing Research, 31*(1), 5–10.

McElmurry, B. J., & LiBrizzi, S. J. (1986). The health of older women. *Nursing Clinics of North America, 21*(1), 161–171.

McElmurry, B. J., Marks, B., & Cianelli, R. (2002). Primary health care in the Americas: Conceptual framework, experiences, challenges and perspectives. http://www.paho.org/English/HSP/HSO/HSO07/primaryhealthcare.htm

McElmurry, B. J., McCreary, L., Park, C. G., Ramos, L., Martinez, E., Parikh, R., et al. 2008 (in press). Successes and challenges in institutional collaboration to address diabetes care disparities in U.S. urban Latino populations. *Health Promotion Practice.*

McElmurry, B. J., & Misner, S. M. (1996). The minority international research training program. In N. Jeffries (Ed.), *Converging educational perspectives* (pp. 294–297). New York: National League for Nursing.

McElmurry, B. J., Misner, S. J., & Buseh, A. G. (2003). Minority international research training program: Global collaboration in nursing research. *Journal of Professional Nursing, 19*(1), 22–31.

McElmurry, B. J., Misner, S. J., Dresden, E., McCreary, L. M., Popovich, J., & Savage, T. (2003). Nurse researchers implement a curriculum in international ethics in Swaziland. *MNRS Connections, 18*(4), np.

McElmurry, B. J., & Newcomb, B. J. (1980). Midwest Directory of Resources for Graduate Education in Nursing. Evanston, IL: Committee on Institutional Cooperation.

McElmurry, B. J., & Newcomb, B. J. (1995). Graduate nursing concentration in women's health at the University of Illinois at Chicago. *Health Care for Women International, 16*(6), 491–500.

McElmurry, B. J., Newcomb, B. J., Barnfather, J., & Lynch, M. (1981). The manuscript review process in nursing journals. In J. McCloskey & H. K. Grace (Eds.), *Current issues in nursing* (pp. 129–143). Boston: Blackwell.

McElmurry, B. J., Norr, K. F., & Parker, R. S. (Eds.). (1993). *Women's health and development: A global challenge.* Boston: Jones & Bartlett.

McElmurry, B. J., Park, C. G., & Buseh, A. (2003). The nurse-community health advocate team for urban immigrant primary healthcare. *Journal of Nursing Scholarship, 35*(3), 275–281.

McElmurry, B. J., & Parker, R. S. (Eds.). (1993). *Annual review of women's health* (Vol. I). New York: National League for Nursing.

McElmurry, B. J., & Parker, R. S. (Eds.). (1995). *Annual review of women's health* (Vol. II). New York: National League for Nursing.

McElmurry, B. J., & Parker, R. S. (Eds.). (1996). *Annual review of women's health* (Vol. III). New York: National League for Nursing.

McElmurry, B. J., Solheim, K., Kishi, R., Coffia, M. A., Worth, W., & Janepanish, P. (2006). Ethical concerns in nurse migration. *Journal of Professional Nursing, 22*(4), 226–235.

McElmurry, B. J., Swider, S. M., Bless, C., Murphy, D., Montgomery, A., Norr, K., Irvin, Y., Gantes, M., & Fisher, M. (1990). Community health advocacy: Primary health care nurse advocate teams in urban communities. In National League for Nursing, *Perspectives in nursing 1989–1991* (pp.117–131). New York: Author. (No. 41-2281).

McElmurry, B. J., Swider, S. M., & Norr, K. (1991). A community-based primary health care program for integration of research, practice, and education. In National League for Nursing, *Curriculum revolution: Community building and activism* (pp. 77–90). New York: Author.

McElmurry, B. J., Swider, S. M., & Watanakij, P. (1992). Primary health care. In J. Lancaster, & M. Stanhope (Eds.), *Community health nursing: Process and practice for promoting health* (3rd ed. pp. 34–44). St. Louis, MO: Mosby.

McElmurry, B. J., Tyska, C., Gugenheim, A. M., Misner, S., & Poslusny, S. (1995). Leadership for primary health care. *N&HC: Perspectives on Community, 16*(4), 229–233.

McElmurry, B. J., Tyska, C., & Parker, R. S. (Eds.). (1999). *Primary health care in urban communities.* Sudbury, MA: Jones & Bartlett.

McElmurry, B. J., Wansley, R., Gugenheim, A. D., Gombe, S., & Dublin, P. (1997). The Chicago Health Corps: Strengthening communities through structured volunteer service. *Advanced Practice Nursing Quarterly, 2*(4), 59–66.

McElmurry, B. J., & Zabrocki, E. (1989). Ethical concerns in caring for older women in the community. *Nursing Clinics of North America, 24*(4), 1041–1050.

Norr, K. F., McElmurry, B. J., Moeti, M., & Tlou, S. (1992). AIDS prevention for women: A community-based approach. *Nursing Outlook. 40*(6), 250–256.

Norr, K. F., McElmurry, B. J., Moeti, M., & Tlou, S. (1994). AIDS prevention for women: A community-based approach. In S. J. Overberg (Ed.), *AIDS, ethics and religion: Embracing a world of suffering* (pp. 189–199). Maryknoll, NY: Orbis Books.

Norr, K. F., McElmurry, B. M., Slutas, F. M., Christiansen, C. D., Marks, B. A., & Misner, S. J. (2001). Mobilizing Lithuanian health professionals as community peer leaders for AIDS prevention: An international primary health care collaboration. *Nursing and Health Care Perspectives, 22*(3), 140–145.

Norr, K. F., Norr, J. I., Tlou, S., McElmurry, B. J., & Moeti, M. R. (2004). Impact of peer group education on HIV prevention for women in Botswana. *Health Care for Women International, 25*(3), 210–226.

Norr, K. F., Tlou, S. D., & McElmurry, B. J. (1996). AIDS awareness and knowledge among Botswana women: Implications for prevention programs. *Health Care for Women International, 17*(2), 133–148.

Swider, S. M., & McElmurry, B. J. (with Norr, K., & Gantes, M.). (1990). A woman's health perspective in primary health care: A nursing and community health worker demonstration project in urban USA. *Journal of Family & Community Health, 13*(3), 1–17.

Swider, S. M., McElmurry, B. J., & Yarling, R. R. (1985). Ethical decision making in a bureaucratic context by senior nursing students. *Nursing Research, 34*(2), 108–112.

Thongpriwan, V., & McElmurry, B. M. (2006). Comparisons between Thai adolescent voices and Thai adolescent health literature. *Journal of School Health, 76*(2), 47–51.

Watanakij, P., & McElmurry, B. J. (1995). Measuring quality of life in Thai and U.S. communities. *International Nursing Review, 42*(4), 121–123.

Webster, D., Leslie, L., McElmurry, B. J., Dan, A., Biordi, D., Boyer, D., Swider, S., Lipetz, M., & Newcomb, J. (1986a). Re: nursing practice in women's health—A concept paper. In Letters to the Editor. *JOGNN, 15*(3), 273.

Webster, D., Leslie, L., McElmurry, B. J., Dan, A., Biordi, D., Boyer, D., Swider, S., Lipetz, M., & Newcomb, J. (1986b). Re: nursing practice in women's health—A concept paper. In Letters to the Editor. *Nursing Research, 35*(3), 143.

Yang, K., McElmurry, B. J., & Park, C. G. (2006). Decreased bone mineral density and fractures in low-income Korean women. *Health Care for Women International, 27*(3), 254–267.

Yarling, R. R., & McElmurry, B. J. (1983). Rethinking the nurse's role in "do not resuscitate" orders: A clinical policy proposal in nursing ethics. *Advances in Nursing Science, 5*(4), 1–12.

Yarling, R. R., & McElmurry, B. J. (1986). Rethinking the nurse's role in "do not resuscitate" orders: A clinical policy proposal in nursing ethics. In P.L. Chinn (Ed.), *Ethical issues in nursing* (pp.123–134). Rockville, MD: Aspen Systems Corp.

Zabrocki, E., & McElmurry, B. J. (1989). The health of older women. In C. Leppa, & C. Miller (Eds.), *Women's health perspectives: An annual review* (Vol. 2, pp. 143–174). Phoenix, AZ: Oryx Press.

Zabrocki, B. C., & McElmurry, B. J. (1990). Omega women: The health of older women. In C. Leppa (Ed.), *Women's health perspectives: An annual review.* (Vol. 3, pp. 229–260). Phoenix, AZ: Oryx Press.

Beverly J. McElmurry is Professor, Public Health Nursing, and Associate Dean, Global Leadership, University of Illinois at Chicago. She is a graduate of the University of Minnesota at Minneapolis (BS, MEd) and Northern Illinois University (EdD). Women's health, nursing ethics, and community-based primary health care have been enduring areas of interest throughout her academic career. As a long term Director of the UIC WHO Collaborating Center for International Nursing Development of Primary Health Care, she has had extensive opportunities to work with international colleagues and students to strengthen nursing's contribution to global health and development.

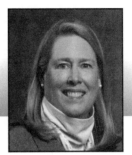

M. Colleen Scanlon

CHAPTER 12

Advocacy in Action: Building the Health of Individuals, Communities, and Society

Ihave never viewed myself as a nurse scholar in ethics or any other area. So I begin this writing with hesitancy and humility, though I am truly honored to be among such distinguished colleagues and friends in this project.

Framing the Issue/Theme

My perspective on ethics and advocacy has been evolutionary. It is not clear to me if this evolution tracked with my professional career, or vice versa. My early understanding of ethics and advocacy was framed almost exclusively within my clinical, patient-centered experience. I became interested in the potential ethical concerns of patients and families, and my advocacy focused on strengthening and supporting their voices. My perspective has grown to encompass a broader, multidimensional view of ethics and advocacy. I am convinced that the knowledge, skills, experience, and commitment nurses possess can transform not only individual encounters, but organizations, communities, government, and even society.

Throughout the decades, *Code of Ethics for Nurses with Interpretive Statements* (Code for Nurses) has been central to the profession, providing ethical grounding, direction, and support (Scanlon & Glover, 1995). The profession's code, as in Provision 9, directs nurses "to engage in political action to bring about social change…" (American Nurses Association [ANA], 2001, p. 25). The ethical values that undergird the profession compel nurses, individually and collectively, to act with and on behalf of others—individuals, communities, and society. Ethics and advocacy have been and are inextricably linked in my mind. One without the other is incomplete.

The Journey

My professional journey has been somewhat nontraditional, and so far I would describe the outcome as eclectic. Actually, I had never considered becoming a nurse, and I did not know any nurses or other health professionals. I initially attended Georgetown University Business School to follow in the footsteps of the men in my family, who for generations had become stockbrokers—that I was destined to go to Wall Street seemed clear. A combination of being on the Jesuit campus dedicated to social justice and service, and living with nurses gradually converted me. Early in my nursing career, I took a course taught by Dr. Mary Trainor. I was wowed by her and the embodiment of humanity, conviction, and compassion. I became convinced that nursing was the profession that would fit me. Looking back, I was very naïve when I began this journey. In that Georgetown environment, I was first exposed to the disciplines of ethics and advocacy and their relevance to the nursing profession.

My true interest and involvement in ethics and advocacy took root with my clinical career. Experiences as a new nurse brought great rewards, but also frustration, confusion, and many questions. On a cancer research unit in Manhattan, I witnessed and participated in many troubling ethical situations and was hesitant to use my voice. In the "do everything, beat disease and death scenario," the patient as a person frequently disappeared while the battle with the body raged. Cure of disease was ultimate—a reality that left patients, families, and staff feeling bewildered and abandoned. I knew of no ethics rounds, committees, or consultants. What existed were "psych" or "clinical" rounds, yet the predominant questions and issues were of an "ethical" nature.

Several years later, another professional opportunity presented itself at Calvary Hospital in the Bronx, NY, which is the only Joint Commission on Accreditation of Healthcare Organizations (JCAHO) accredited acute care hospital in the United States that cares exclusively for advanced cancer patients. I had the privilege of first working as a Staff Development Instructor and later as a Psychiatric Nurse Clinician over my 10 years there. In that environment, my first public speaking and writing occurred (D'Agostino, Gray, & Scanlon, 1990; Fleming, Scanlon, & D'Agostino, 1987).

During these initial years of my professional career, I was also a member of a congregation of women religious, the Ursulines. As I grew in congregational life, I took courses and read in the areas of moral theology, philosophy, religion, and social justice. The interface of these experiences had deep personal and professional impact— being a nurse and a nun was my identity and treasure. Faith helps frame my understanding of nursing—who I am as a nurse is a reflection of who I seek to be in the eyes of God. Faith provides meaning, grounding, and hopefully prevents me from getting too far adrift (Scanlon, 2000).

I viewed the profession as grounded in an ideal of service and saw myself in service of others, a sense of service which required competence and compassion. My ideal of service was not subservience or servitude, but recognition of nurses as learned, independent professionals who strive to benefit others because of their inherent dignity and worth. Encounters with patients, families, and staff were powerful and transforming.

During my years at Calvary, my oldest brother was struggling with a gravely serious cancer diagnosis that led to an array of interventions, including chemotherapy, radiation, surgery, and a bone marrow transplant. No words can describe the impact of that experience—it was transformative in all domains of my life—it is woven throughout.

This was an era of enormous strides in all aspects of cancer care. Yet, despite advances, cancer remained a disease that inevitably progressed and resulted in death for many. Attention began to focus on the needs of patients for whom cure was no longer possible (Scanlon, 1989). There was growing attention to the ethical dimensions of the patient's experience, the nurse's experience, and even the organization's experience. Calvary had a multidisciplinary ethics committee with nursing representation, yet over time this vehicle was not sufficient to address the many ethical issues that nurses faced on a daily basis. Under the leadership of the Director of Nursing Cornelia Fleming, increased attention focused on the ethical concerns of nurses and various forums, resources, and educational tools were provided.

A turning point in my career occurred in the late 1980s, when I decided to pursue a law degree. I had considered advanced education in ethics, but chose not to go that route. I had become aware that legal questions and concerns were frequently present in ethical dialogues and discernment. Physicians, and at times nurses, seemed more concerned about the "legal" ramifications of their decisions than the "moral" ones. Rightly or wrongly, it appeared to me that the law had clouded the world of ethics. I have found that my legal education with a concentration in health policy serves me well and provides more credibility to my voice and activism. The integration of the principled nature of ethics, the analytical foundation of law, and the humanity of nursing has been extremely valuable.

In 1992, I was offered the opportunity to become the second Director of the ANA Center for Ethics and Human Rights (Center). While I recognized how fortunate I was to have such an option, leaving clinical practice was difficult. I tried to view it as an opportunity to bring the richness of my clinical learning to a different point of influence and impact on a national level. The work of the Center created a forum for the natural and needed interface of ethics and advocacy. At the same time I was given an appointment as a consultant for the Center for Clinical Bioethics at Georgetown University Medical Center, which kept me in touch with the clinical world.

Working at ANA was rewarding, challenging, and eye-opening. I had become quite familiar with the politics of the hospital world, yet had not anticipated similar dynamics in a professional association. There was an inherent tension (mostly positive) between the membership and the association's staff in terms of direction, responsibilities, and accountabilities—a balance that was in constant flux. The ANA was not always an easy place to work, but I learned to navigate the rough terrain, build productive relationships, and advance the work of the Center (see Center information at ANA web site, http://nursing world.org).

The Center was steadfast in its efforts to improve the quality of end-of-life care. Throughout the 1990s end-of-life care issues were increasingly predominant. Nurses and the nursing community had a unique opportunity to contribute to future directions in end-of-life care. Examples of influencing efforts by the Center include:

- Creation of a task force on the Nurse's Role in End-of-Life Decisions to examine a broad spectrum of end-of-life issues and develop resources to provide guidance to nurses (ANA, 1992).

- Participation on the Advisory Committee of the American Society of Law, Medicine, and Ethics project on legal barriers to the adequate relief of pain, resulting in a model statute.

- Participation in the Coordinating Council of the National Center for State Courts Project on Care of the Dying: Managing the End-of-Life Decision-Making Process, resulting in the publication of guidelines.

- Collaboration on the development of an educational video and accompanying education monograph on end-of-life care (Marsden, Penticuff, Rushton, Scanlon, & Schwarz, 1995; Sherman, 1995).

- Collaboration with the American Association of Retired Persons on Advance Directives.

- Participation in Choice in Dying's National Outreach Campaign, which produced a public television documentary.

- Testimony before the Institute of Medicine on Care at the End-of-Life, which sponsored an effort to study and make recommendations for improving end-of-life care (Field & Cassel, 1997) and before the Subcommittee on the Constitution of the U.S. House of Representatives Judiciary Committee, "Oversight Hearing on Assisted Suicide in the United States."

- Coalition for Quality End-of-Life Care, in which the ANA joined with the American Medical Association and other professional organizations to advance an agenda focused on improving the quality of care rendered to patients and families at the end of life.

- ANA joined with many other groups in the submission of an amicus curiae ("friend of the court") brief opposing the legalization of physician-assisted suicide (Vacco v. Quill, 1997).

Undoubtedly, one of the most challenging issues that arose at the Center was physician-assisted suicide and the era of Dr. Jack Kevorkian. The increased tolerance of a precipitated death led to my own personal and professional discernment on the issue. Assisted suicide and euthanasia became a focal area for some thinking, writing, and speaking (Portneory, et al., 1997; Scanlon, 1998a, 1998b, 1998c; Scanlon & Rushton, 1996). Shortly before I left the ANA, the findings of a research study dominated the media headlines of the nation (Asch, 1996). Most nursing professionals were critical of the research, but it catalyzed the profession into collective action, focusing needed attention on quality of end-of-life care (Scanlon, 1996).

In 1997, the ANA and the Center initiated a formal process to review, analyze, and revise the Code for Nurses. This daunting undertaking was led by a task force chaired by Dr. Barbara Daly and coordinated by the Center. I vividly remember one of the first meetings when we were discussing the scope of the project, including both provisions and accompanying interpretive statements of the Code. Recommendations for changes to the provisions required formal acceptance by the ANA House of Delegates, whereas changes to the interpretive statements were under the authority of the ANA Board of Directors.

At this preliminary meeting, Dr. Marsha Fowler offered a provocative comparison to the two different procedural options. She compared it to cleaning out a sock drawer—you could open the drawer and rearrange the socks, or you could pull the drawer out, empty it on the floor, and start from scratch. She believed the latter option was warranted. This was a courageous position to take. Listening I felt my panic level rise—I had been at the ANA long enough to appreciate the challenges associated with the ANA House of Delegates approval process. Yet, we embarked on this path, and later I felt significant pride and gratitude, particularly to Barb Daly for her leadership and commitment to the project.

For the past 10 years, I have served as the Senior Vice President, Advocacy at Catholic Health Initiatives (CHI) in Denver, and many new horizons have been opened to me. I was offered this opportunity by Patricia Cahill, JD, Chief Executive Officer (CEO) and President of CHI, who had been the CEO of Calvary Hospital in my early years, my continual role model, mentor, and friend. CHI was and continues to be a bold endeavor that brings together the faith-based ministries of over a dozen sponsoring congregations of women religious. These courageous women, reading the signs of the times, conceived a new model of a lay-religious partnership in Catholic health care. They believed the formation of CHI offered a future for their health ministries which had served this country for well over 100 years (Cahill & Coyle, 2006). CHI has varied health care ministries in 20 states, with over 65,000 employees. Its mission and vision is to nurture the healing ministry of the Church and transform health care delivery—advocacy is central to fulfilling this. The interface of my nursing, ethics, and legal background provides a rich grounding and context for my role.

Early on, I had opportunities to talk with CHI's Board members, representatives of the religious congregations, and senior leadership to understand their views on advocacy. There was consistency in their themes, that advocacy was more than just public policy and government relations; CHI's commitment to advocacy was framed by the social teachings of the Church (Pontifical Council for Justice and Peace, 2005); our primary concern should be directed to those persons who are most vulnerable; and CHI as an organization had internal advocacy obligations as well. This was a call to transform social realities and to consider health broadly for individuals, communities, and society—a call to civic, political, and organizational activism viewed through the lens of faith. CHI, as one of the largest nonprofit health systems in the country, has a unique opportunity to leverage its size, diversity, geographic coverage, and resources to act on behalf of the most vulnerable and achieve its vision of building healthy communities.

There was no roadmap or instructions—just a vision and a challenge to create it. I was simultaneously inspired and terrified. Developing an image or visualization that attempts to depict a particular effort has always been helpful to me. An image can also be valuable when explaining a concept that is dynamic and multidimensional to others. CHI's advocacy model (Figure 12.1, below) has existed for almost a decade, though the approaches and strategies continue to unfold and change.

Within the domain of "individual/community advocacy," there is a commitment to work in partnership within all the urban and rural communities CHI serves across the country. There is a commitment to understand the unique assets, concerns, and needs of each of the communities and to actively address them through collaborative activism. As is known, an alarming number of people go without health insurance coverage and lack access to health care in this country. Barriers such as lack of transportation, language differences, and illiteracy may also impact health care access. Several years ago, every health care ministry within CHI made a commitment to improve access to health care in every community where we are located (waiting for public policy changes was not acceptable). Focus groups, surveys, research data, and meetings with local constituencies (consumers, business leaders, clinicians, spiritual leaders, for example) helped to better understand each communal reality. Subsequently, each community worked to build consensus on the development of a community-based plan to address health care access, including a method for measuring success, and began implementation.

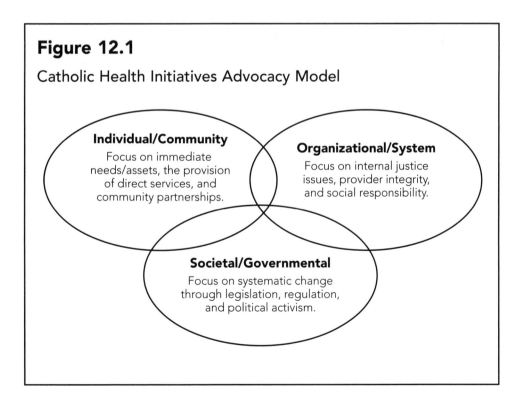

Figure 12.1

Catholic Health Initiatives Advocacy Model

Individual/Community
Focus on immediate needs/assets, the provision of direct services, and community partnerships.

Organizational/System
Focus on internal justice issues, provider integrity, and social responsibility.

Societal/Governmental
Focus on systematic change through legislation, regulation, and political activism.

"Organizational/system advocacy" challenges CHI as a social enterprise to build congruence between what is espoused externally and how we live internally. Corporate activism and accountability such as socially responsible investing, protection of the environment, and codes of conduct can benefit society. Central to corporate social responsibility is good citizenship (Porter & Kramer, 2006). I have often described this area of work as holding "a mirror up to oneself" to force awareness and honesty so as to live and to act with integrity. Being values-driven, rooted in nonnegotiable beliefs, and yet responsive to change makes leading organizations (Lowney, 2003).

Two main areas of activity in this domain are environmental responsibility and socially responsible investing. CHI's environmental efforts continue to expand and include energy efficiency, mercury elimination, waste minimization, toxicity reduction programs, and environmentally preferable purchasing. CHI is a founding member of the Catholic Partnership on Environmental Responsibility. Being a socially responsible steward and conscientious investor of financial resources involves voting of proxies, filing shareholder resolutions, community investment programs, and portfolio screening. Merging social values and investment decisions provides an opportunity—to use shareholder status as an advocate in the investment world. The "best return" is viewed more broadly than profitability. Shareholder activism is a type of political activism that encourages companies to work toward a double bottom line—profit and social good (Brill, Brill, & Feigenbaum, 1999; Price, 2006).

The last, but certainly not the least, important domain is "societal/governmental advocacy"—the area that is most commonly thought of when discussing advocacy which encompasses a range of public policy efforts from evaluating legislative, regulatory, and administrative proposals to political activism. CHI's public policy agenda includes traditional health policy issues as well as nontraditional concerns; for example, affordable housing, gun control, and immigration. By embracing a breadth of health and social policy issues, CHI recognizes that building healthy communities is much more than the provision of medical care services. CHI's concern also extends to the global community.

As a faith-based organization CHI is nonpartisan, yet that does not impede our responsibility to educate legislators, regulators, and other policy-makers. In 2004 the "My Voice, My Vote" campaign was launched to motivate employees, physicians, boards, and volunteers to use their voice and exercise their right to vote. Grassroots advocacy is a vitally important strategic tool. There is a call for faithful citizenship that is more than ideological politics and partisanship, but brings choices grounded in values and seen through the lens of faith (U.S. Conference of Catholic Bishops, 2003). Many—if not all—policy issues have a moral dimension that should be considered.

What has it Meant?

This is an extremely difficult question to answer and probably better answered by others. I suppose one could begin to evaluate the significance of the work quantitatively by counting the number of publications written, presentations given, or awards received. Yet, that seems quite superficial and unsatisfactory. Though it is much harder to assess the quality of the work, the influence it has had, and its continuing relevance, that seems to be a much more important pursuit. Maybe most important of all is the personal impact on one's relationships with patients, families, students, and colleagues. If my thinking and work have had an impact, I do not think it has been in dramatic and obvious ways, but possibly in subtle, hard-to-measure ways.

A recent article highlighting advocacy leaders, including myself, has a poignant introduction: "They fight for those who have no strength. They speak for those who have no voice. They protect those who have no defense. They are advocates, who, like Rosa Parks, champion the battles for human rights and social reform..." (Villaverde, 2006, p. 10). I would be proud to have that as my true legacy!

References

American Nurses Association. (1992). *Compendium of position statements on the nurse's role in end-of-life decisions.* Washington, DC: Author.

American Nurses Association. (2001). *Code of ethics for nurses with interpretive statements.* Washington, DC: Author.

Asch, D. (1996). The role of critical care nurses in euthanasia and assisted suicide. *New England Journal of Medicine, 334*(21), 1374–1379.

Brill, H., Brill, J., & Feigenbaum, C. (1999). *Investing with your values: Making money and making a difference.* Princeton, NJ: Bloomberg Press.

Cahill, P., & Coyle, M. (2006). *Catholic health initiatives: A spirit of innovation, a legacy of care.* Denver, CO: Catholic Health Initiatives.

D'Agostino, N., Gray, G., & Scanlon, C. (1990). Cancer in the older adult: Understanding age-related changes. *Journal of Gerontological Nursing, 16*(6), 12–15, 31–32.

Field, M., & Cassel, C. (Eds.). (1997). *Approaching death: Improving care at the end of life.* Washington, DC: National Academy Press.

Fleming, C., Scanlon, C., & D'Agostino, N. (1987). Study of the comfort needs of patients with advanced cancer. *Cancer Nursing, 10*(5), 237–243.

Lowney, C. (2003). *Heroic leadership: Best practices from a 450-year-old company that changed the world*. Chicago: Loyola Press.

Marsden, C., Penticuff, J., Rushton, C., Scanlon, C., & Schwarz, J. (1995). *End-of-life care: Ethical dimensions* [Monograph]. Glaxo Continuing Nursing Education. Research Triangle Park, NC: Glaxo Inc.

Pontifical Council for Justice and Peace. (2005). *Compendium of the social doctrine of the Church*. Washington, DC: United States Conference of Catholic Bishops.

Porter, M., & Kramer, M. (2006). Strategy and society: The link between competitive advantage and corporate social responsibility. *Harvard Business Review*, December, 78–79.

Portneory, R., Coyle, N., Kash, K., Brescia, F., Scanlon, C., O'Hare, D., et al. (1997). Determinants of the willingness to endorse assisted suicide: A survey of physicians, nurses, and social workers. *Psychomatics, 38*(3), 227–287.

Price, T. (2006). *Activists in the boardroom: How advocacy groups seek to shape corporate behavior*. Washington, DC: Foundation for Public Affairs.

Rockfield, G. (2006). Champions of human rights and social reform. *The College of New Rochelle Alumnae Magazine, 77*(4), 10–17.

Scanlon, C. (1989). Creating a vision of hope: The challenges of palliative care. *Oncology Nursing Forum, 16*(4), 491–496.

Scanlon, C. (1996). Nursing practice and euthanasia: Right question, wrong answer. *New England Journal of Medicine, 334*(21), 1401–1402.

Scanlon, C. (1998a). A road map for navigating end-of-life care. *Medical Surgical Nursing, 7*(1), 57–59.

Scanlon, C. (1998b). Assisted suicide: How should nurses respond. *International Nursing Review, 45*(5), 152.

Scanlon, C. (1998c). Unraveling ethical issues in palliative care. *Seminars in Oncology Nursing, 14*(2), 1–9.

Scanlon, C. (2000, May). "Live the legacy: Forge the future." Commencement Address. Georgetown University School of Nursing.

Scanlon, C., & Glover, J. (1995). A professional code of ethics: Providing a moral compass for turbulent times. *Oncology Nursing Forum, 22*(10), 1515–1521.

Scanlon, C., & Rushton, C. (1996). Assisted suicide: Clinical realities and ethical challenges. *American Journal of Critical Care, 5*(6), 397–403.

Sherman, S. (Producer-Director). (1995). *End of life care: Ethical dimensions* [Video]. Glaxo Continuing Nursing Education. Research Triangle Park, NC: Glaxo Inc.

United States Conference of Catholic Bishops. (2003). *Faithful citizenship: A Catholic call to political responsibility.* Washington, DC: Author.

Vacco v. Quill, 521 U.S. 793 (United States Supreme Court, 1997), No. 95-1858. Amicus brief of American Medical Association, American Nurses Association, American Psychiatric Association, et al., in support of petitioners, 1996.

Villaverde, I. (2006). Introduction to G. Rockfield. Champions of human rights and social reform. *The College of New Rochelle Alumnae Magazine, 77*(4), 10–17.

M. Colleen Scanlon, RN, JD is Senior Vice President, Advocacy at Catholic Health Initiatives in Denver, Colorado. In this role, she has the responsibility for directing the development and integration of a comprehensive advocacy program within one of the largest Catholic health care systems in the country. Prior to this, she was the Director of the American Nurses Association Center for Ethics and Human Rights in Washington, DC and served as a Clinical Scholar in the Center for Clinical Bioethics at Georgetown University Medical Center. Colleen received her BSN from Georgetown University, an MS in Gerontology from the College of New Rochelle and a JD with a health law and policy certificate from Pace University School of Law. Special interests include palliative care ethics, advocacy on behalf of vulnerable persons, and professional and organizational integrity.

✎ SECTION IV ✎
CRITICAL THINKING ACTIVITIES

Perspectives on Advocacy

✦ Compare and contrast the essays in this section on advocacy. What are commonalities among the writers' works and how do they differ?

✦ Thompson stated at the Legacy Seminar, "Advocacy is the central moral concept to my work." Find an example of advocacy from Thompson's essay. Does advocacy truly serve as the central moral concept?

✦ How did Thompson's early work as a nurse midwife in Chile lead to her focus on advocacy?

✦ McElmurry has focused a great deal of time and energy during her career on training primary health providers on a community level. Explain how this work is an example of advocacy.

✦ McElmurry described advocacy at the Legacy seminar as "minimizing or mitigating inequities in power; getting others to speak for themselves; and finding ways to mobilize." Is this a sufficient description? Why or why not? Are nurses adequately prepared to act as advocates given this description? Explain.

✦ Scanlon implies that there is insufficient will for health care reform. Respond and provide examples to support your argument.

SECTION V

Relationship Issues

Connections or involvement between and among health professionals and patients are the foci. The context of action includes the broader community and society as a whole.

To the Mother of the Burned Children

Cortney Davis

When you ask, when your voice
is your own again, and you know
you're not waking from sleep
or a vision of kids napping,
the power gone, candles
shaking light across their faces,
I'll give it to you straight:
Your children are dead.

You can cry one long sound
and we'll let the bed quake,
the burned flesh fall away.
I could bring shots to lull you,
pills to stay your mourning,
but instead I'll tell you:
Walk the fire in your mind.
Carry them out, one by one,
through rooms thick with smoke.
Carry your children, then put them down
safe outside the ring of heat.

Call them by name:
Ramon. Priss. Jamal.

Tell them *Wait.*
Wait here. Wait

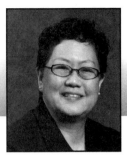

CHAPTER 13

Ethics: The Fabric of Life

I "discovered" ethics by accident and my life was changed, both professionally and personally, in ways I could never have imagined. My relationship with ethics has influenced my interactions with people, provided new perspectives on seemingly mundane everyday situations, and suggested different approaches to the more challenging, often troublesome issues of daily living.

Previously, I never had the inclination to conduct a "life review." Reflection about the beginning of my professional interest in ethics, my current ethics projects, and the legacy that I hope to leave has provided an opportunity to reassess personal and professional goals. I wondered whether my involvement in the study of ethics was a "life plan" or simply coincidence, but from my first formal study of ethics a new career path was born. The relationship between my mentor and me provided venues for growth. In some sense, I feel that I have come "full circle," as I now advise graduate students in their research about ethical issues.

I realize that my path in nursing ethics is analogous to a fine quilt. Personal and professional experiences are the various pieces, each representing a major marker in my career. Splashes of color accent the fabric; the colors represent the many individuals who have influenced my professional being, including my graduate students. These pieces may be sewn together to make a quilt, representing my contributions to nursing and the discipline of ethics. The last pieces are yet to be sewn.

The Context

My discovery and exploration of ethics began several years after acquiring a master's degree in nursing. I was ready for a new challenge. At the same time there was a national effort to prepare more nursing faculty at the doctoral level, so I began pursuing my doctoral degree. Online courses were not available in the 1980s, so commuting between the University of Nebraska Medical Center (UNMC) campus in Omaha to the University of Nebraska campus in Lincoln became a way of life. Life was regimented between full-time teaching responsibilities and life as a student. After three years of this routine, I was exhausted and actually dropped one course in the doctoral program; I registered instead for an independent study that could be arranged on my home campus. At that time I had no idea how this decision would affect my life.

After serious contemplation I concluded that my doctoral education in postsecondary educational administration needed to be more rounded. Discussing the art of academic administration, and faculty, legal, financial, and business management issues, was prescribed, important, but inadequate. I thought actions should be guided by more than administrative concepts and theories. Certainly, there was another framework which could provide a basis for decision-making in administration, as well as in personal matters.

Upon reflection I determined that ethics could provide such a framework for decision-making, not only in health care but for postsecondary educational administrative issues and personal matters as well. I had only dabbled in the field, never having had formal coursework in philosophy or ethics. Therefore I sought out the only faculty member on the UNMC campus who specifically "taught ethics," Dr. Ruth Purtilo. I asked if she would work with me in an independent study course. Gracious as always, Ruth took me on. Later, Ruth encouraged me to apply for a National Endowment for the Humanities Institute in 1983. Invigorated by the Institute, I attended a program at the Hastings Center in 1984, and in 1986 attended the Twelfth Annual Intensive Bioethics Institute and the Kennedy Institute of Ethics at Georgetown University. These experiences were of seminal importance in developing a network of ethics colleagues.

I joined the Society for Health and Human Values (SHHV) in 1983, an interdisciplinary organization addressing humanities education within the health care field, where I was active in the Nursing and Humanities Interest Group. Later I served on the council, and as the Society merged into a new society, the American Society for Bioethics and Humanities (ASBH), I continued on the board and remained in a leadership role in the Nursing Affinity Group. In special recognition of my work in SHHV, I received the 1995 Service Award.

In 1987, under the auspices of the Nebraska Nurses Association (NNA), a colleague and I investigated establishing a nursing ethics committee at the state level (Pinch & Miya, 1989). An ethics committee for educational and consultation purposes was subsequently formed. A number of publications ensued (Boardman & Miya, 1990; Boardman, Miya, & Pinch, 1993; Boardman, Miya, Pinch, & Andrews, 1994; Pinch, Boardman, Miya, & Andrews, 1990; Pinch, Miya, Boardman, Andrews, & Barr, 1995).

Involvement in a Transplant Ethics Study Group in which UNMC and Dartmouth College exchanged scholarly ideas and dialogue (1990–1993) allowed me to network with philosophers, social workers, physicians, and others about issues in organ transplantation. Additionally, as a bioethics consultant for the Visiting Nurse Association, Omaha, Nebraska (1995–1998), the staff and I were able to address increasing violence, end-of-life issues, limited health care resources, and risk management factors, just a few of many issues potentially leading to ethical concerns (Miya & Tully, 1997).

Upon reflection, however, I am most proud of my appointment as chair (2006–2008) of the Advisory Board for the Center for Ethics and Human Rights of the American Nurses Association (ANA), after serving 2 years as a member of the Board. I characterize this opportunity as the pinnacle of my career. The work is challenging, stimulating, and gratifying. The Board has focused primarily on the revision of ANA's position statements, my assignment including those statements on privacy and confidentiality, risk and responsibility, and capital punishment. Through the work of the Board, I now have experienced, and can more fully appreciate, the work of the professional organization and its impact on nursing practice.

Through all of the experiences above, as well as others, I have met many individuals that expanded my view of the world and the many ethical concerns, both of the present and the future. I find it stimulating to assist students in discovering the "grayness" of ethics in both undergraduate teaching and through continuing education programs. Graduate enterprises have centered around my supervision and participation in data analysis of master's research projects. The results of these studies will now, in part, be shared here. In particular, the studies included ethical issues involving relationships between nurses and other individuals, institutions, and the profession, as well as intrapersonal relationships and powerlessness.

Early in my exploration of ethical issues, I was interested in identifying the types of ethical issues facing nursing in neonatal intensive care (NICU) (Miya, Boardman, Harr, & Keene, 1991). Categories of treatment, interpersonal and intrapersonal conflict, and communication were most often described as ethical issues. The dimensions of autonomy, beneficence, nonmaleficence, justice, rights of infants, families, and health care professionals were also identified. Since this initial study, graduate students have replicated the study primarily in the arenas of acute and/or critical care. Two studies, in addition to the one mentioned above, have been conducted in the NICU (Ferris, Grimm, & Hoy, 2002; Sutfin, 1993), three in adult intensive care (AICU) (Biehl, 2007; Camden, Duin, & Sennett, 2007; Liske, 1998), two in emergency departments (EDs) (Danahay & Houlihan, 2005; Haack & Stofferahn, 1997; Miya, Stofferahn, & Haack, 2003), and one in a pediatric intensive care unit (PICU) (Martinez & Murphy, 1995). Other sites have included three in oncology (Kapacee, 2002; Lovejoy, 2000; Reid, 2004) and one in maternity care (Miller, 2007). Non-hospital sites have included hospice (Pepin, 1999), with an additional study exploring ethical issues facing nurse practitioners in Nebraska (Sincebaugh, 1996).

Nursing Research Related to Ethics

Documentation of the ethical issues described by nurses in all of the research studies referenced above included, among others, those involving interpersonal or intrapersonal conflict and powerlessness. Ethical issues were not mutually exclusive to one clinical area or another. In all studies, data was collected using Fry's (1987) Demographic Data Form (DDF) and Moral Conflict Questionnaire (MCQ), modified with permission.

Interpersonal conflict is defined as "those that occurred between two or more individuals related to differences in values, beliefs, and/or behaviors" (Miya, et al., 1991, p. 254). In most instances, nurses experienced conflict with physicians and other nurses. However, nurses also identified situations in which they experienced conflict with families and, rarely, patients. Perceived conflicts with the health care institution in which they were employed were also identified.

Interpersonal conflicts were identified by nurses in all of the research sites, including the NICU, adult intensive care, and the emergency room (ER). However, ER nurse narratives carried with them an even greater sense of urgency. The nature of critical care, with its urgent, high acuity, multifaceted, and multidisciplinary care, is particularly disposed to interdisciplinary conflict. Similar conflicts were found without regard for the demographic variables of age, gender, ethnicity, nursing education, years of nursing practice, clinical specialty, or the hours of work. Some narratives were fairly clinical in nature and most were emotion-laden.

"Intrapersonal conflicts are those in which there was incongruence among a person's own values, beliefs, or behaviors" (Miya et al., 1991, p. 254). Nurses identified situations in which they struggled with their own values and sometimes with the values of the nursing profession. Nurses often expressed guilt over their own inaction. These intrapersonal conflicts are cause for introspection, even years later.

Powerlessness is defined as an individual or group's inability to effect change, which may lead to a feeling of helplessness. Nurses frequently identified feelings of frustration and powerlessness. In many narratives, nurses wrote that the ethical issue they described had been "resolved" because of the patients' death, resulting in the disappearance of the situation. In truth, this is not a true resolution but an ethical challenge that will continue to occur, but with different players. In many situations nurses felt powerless to effect change. There are also narratives from nurses who "took action," but still felt powerless. Sometimes nurses, in retrospect, wish they had taken action but did not because of intrapersonal conflicts.

Dierckx de Casterle (1998) states that powerlessness is common in nursing because nurses have limited authority in ethical choices; organizational, societal, and educational conventions predominate. According to Erlen and Frost (1991), power and powerlessness "can only be seen in terms of relationships," and "the degree of power one has over another is dependent on the extent of imbalance in the relationship" (p. 398). Many times I have heard nurses say, "Oh, but I'm just a nurse." Nurses have a perception of powerlessness when there is physician dominance and a lack of knowledge about alternative choices (Erlen & Frost).

Impact on Health Care Ethics

Based on the research of my students and myself, descriptive documentation of ethical issues confronting nurses in a variety of clinical settings indicates that nurses, over a period of years (1991–2007), continue to experience similar ethical issues over both setting and time. Troublesome ethical issues occur in daily practice despite the inclusion of ethics content in the nursing curriculum, the existence of ethics committees, and/or ethics consultation services in health care institutions. Coupled with the current nursing shortage and resultant increase in workload, as well as perceived powerlessness, ethical issues assume an even greater role in nurses' perception of stress, job satisfaction, and retention of nurses.

Aiken et al.'s (2001) research indicated that nurses experience job stress and dissatisfaction, burnout, and have intentions of leaving the nursing profession due to decreasing quality of patient care, among other factors. This is supported, in part, by a report about the nursing workforce from the General Accounting Office (GAO,

2001), and Cox's (2003) research on intrapersonal conflict. All troublesome ethical issues that have been documented in this paper, as well as the many other equally or perhaps even more troubling issues that are not documented here, in some way affect the quality of patient care, satisfaction, and outcome.

In addition to the ethical issues identified by nurses, the studies cited in this paper also included questions about what resources would have helped them, as nurses, deal with ethical issues both prior to and during the ethical events. Nurses also identified actions, processes, or interventions which would be helpful in similar but future situations. In part, nurses desired more open communication with nurse managers, autonomy in initiating an ethics consultation (i.e., rather than waiting for a physician's request), knowledge of ethics resources available (e.g., especially the night shift), a unit-based ethics resource person, family conferences with staff, inservice training by social workers about guardianship, availability of organ retrieval personnel to answer questions, updates on current laws and practices related to medical treatment or its withdrawal, resources to assist the health care team with assessing quality of life, greater teamwork with physicians, more open communication with physicians, and accountability of physicians for their practices.

Broader Significance beyond Nursing

In today's quickly and ever-changing world, that speed plays a large role in our daily functioning is increasingly apparent. Messages are expected to be communicated quickly and responses transmitted with equal speed. Because of these societal expectations, there is often no time for thoughtful, critical consideration about the communication or its response. There are faxes, e-mail, cell phones, and text messaging. Gratification, sometimes immediate, and/or praise are expected outcomes of individual action. Regardless of the "rightness" or "wrongness" of their action, individuals expect their action to be met with enthusiasm and/or praise for their efforts. This thinking is carried over into clinical settings and situations. Nothing in ethics is clearly a black and white issue. The fabric of ethics is gray. Ethical situations require thoughtful consideration, careful communication, and cooperative teamwork which, one hopes, will lead to an acceptable resolution of the issue at hand. These situations do not lend themselves to speedy communication and may not provide any immediate gratification or praise.

Perhaps part of the solution is a change in the way health care professionals are educated. Opportunities for interdisciplinary discussion, rounding, goal setting, planning, implementation, and evaluation of care may assist the health care professions' ultimate goal—that of quality patient care. Effective communication, respect for individuals, and appreciation of each profession's contributions to patient care could be nurtured during such interdisciplinary education. Nurses need the support of their colleagues and management in addressing the ethical issues they face in their areas of practice. Nurses must empower themselves to engage in discussion, intervention, and resolution of ethical issues without fear of reprisal.

My work in ethics has been critical in my own development as an individual. The study of ethics and its relationship to the arts and humanities has reintroduced me to the fine arts and literature, making my life both richer and satisfying. I have also been provided with opportunities to participate and contribute nationally in my professional organizations. I hope that I have inspired some of my students to continue their exploration of ethics, to provide leadership in their nursing specialties, and to continue to be good stewards of ethics. I end now as I began; the quilt is full of color, the pieces each representing a life experience, and the whole yet to be finished.

References

Aiken, L. H., Clarke, S. P., Sloane, D. M., Sochalski, J. A., Busse, R., Clarke, H., et al. (2001). Nurses' reports on hospital care in five countries: The ways in which nurses' work is structured have left nurses among the least satisfied workers, and the problem is getting worse. *Health Affairs, 20*(3), 43–53.

Biehl, R. R. (2007). [Ethical issues confronting nurses caring for trauma patients in an adult intensive care unit at a level 1 trauma center]. Unpublished raw data.

Boardman, K., & Miya, P. (1990). Withdrawing life support. *Nebraska Nurse, 23*(1), 4–5.

Boardman, K., Miya, P. A., & Pinch, W. J. (1993). A report to the NNA: Implementation of the PSDA in Nebraska hospitals. *Nebraska Nurse, 26*(4), 26.

Boardman, K., Miya, P. A., Pinch, W. J., & Andrews, A. (1994). Health reform: An ethical dilemma for nurses? *Nebraska Nurse, 27*(4), 17.

Camden, C., Duin, P. J., & Sennett, H. (2007). [Ethical issues confronting nursing in critical care]. Unpublished raw data.

Cox, K. B. (2003). The effects of intrapersonal, intragroup, and intergroup conflict on team performance effectiveness and work satisfaction. *Nursing Administration Quarterly, 27*(2), 153–163.

Danahay, J. M., & Houlihan, A. B. (2005). *Ethical issues confronting nurses in emergency departments.* Unpublished master's thesis, University of Nebraska Medical Center, Omaha.

Dierckx de Casterle, B. (1998). Supporting nurses in ethical decision making. *Nursing Clinics of North America, 33*(3), 543–555.

Erlen, J. A., & Frost, B. (1991). Nurses' perceptions of powerlessness in influencing ethical decisions. *Western Journal of Nursing Research, 13*(3), 397–407.

Ferris, B., Grimm, K., & Hoy, S. (2002). *Ethical issues facing neonatal nurses.* Unpublished master's thesis, University of Nebraska Medical Center, Omaha.

Fry, S. T. (1987). *Demographic data form. Moral conflict questionnaire.* Baltimore: University of Maryland.

General Accounting Office. (2001). *Nursing workforce emerging nurse shortages due to multiple factors.* (GAO 01-944). Washington, DC: Author.

Haack, K., & Stofferahn, L. (1997). *Ethical issues confronting nurses in emergency departments.* Unpublished master's thesis, University of Nebraska Medical Center, Omaha.

Kapacee, K. M. T. (2002). *Ethical issues confronting nurses working with hospitalized female patients diagnosed with cancer.* Unpublished master's thesis, University of Nebraska Medical Center, Omaha.

Liske, T. M. (1998). *Ethical issues experienced by intensive care nurses when working with adult patients admitted for cardiac disease.* Unpublished master's thesis, University of Nebraska Medical Center, Omaha.

Lovejoy, B. O. (2000). *Ethical issues confronting nurses in a comprehensive ambulatory oncology treatment center and clinic.* Unpublished master's thesis, University of Nebraska Medical Center, Omaha.

Martinez, K. E., & Murphy, C. A. (1995). *Ethical issues confronting general pediatric and pediatric intensive care nurses.* Unpublished master's thesis, University of Nebraska Medical Center, Omaha.

Miller, C. A. (2007). [Ethical issues confronting maternity nurses in an inpatient hospital setting]. Unpublished raw data.

Miya, P. A., Boardman, K. K., Harr, K. L., & Keene, A. (1991). Ethical issues described by NICU nurses. *The Journal of Clinical Ethics, 2*(4), 253–257.

Miya, P. A., Stofferahn, L., & Haack, K. (2003, October). *Ethical questions confronting nurses in the emergency room.* Paper presented at the meeting of the American Society of Bioethics and Humanities & Canadian Bioethics Society, Montreal, Canada.

Miya, P. A., & Tully, M. E. (1997). Development of a home health agency nursing ethics committee. *HealthCare Ethics Committee Forum, 9*(1), 27–35.

Pepin, K. O. (1999). *Ethical issues confronting hospice nurses.* Unpublished master's thesis, University of Nebraska Medical Center, Omaha.

Pinch, W. J., Boardman, K., Miya, P., & Andrews, A. (1990). Allocation of scarce resources. *Nebraska Nurse, 23*(4), 9, 11.

Pinch, W. J., & Miya, P. A. (1989). Ethics committees in state nurses associations: Report on the national status. *Health Care Ethics Committee Forum, 1*(3), 167–173.

Pinch, W. J., Miya, P. A., Boardman, K. K., Andrews, A., & Barr, P. (1995). Implementation of the Patient Self-Determination Act: A survey of Nebraska hospitals. *Research in Nursing & Health, 18*(1), 59–66.

Reid, C. J. (2004). *Ethical issues confronting oncology nurses.* Unpublished master's thesis, University of Nebraska Medical Center, Omaha.

Sincebaugh, M. T. (1996). *Ethical issues facing nurse practitioners in Nebraska.* Unpublished master's thesis, University of Nebraska Medical Center, Omaha.

Sutfin, A. D. (1993). *Ethical issues confronting NICU nurses: A description.* Unpublished master's thesis, University of Nebraska Medical Center, Omaha.

Pamela A. Miya is Director, Program Services, March of Dimes, Nebraska Chapter. She recently accepted this position after 30 years as a faculty member in the College of Nursing, University of Nebraska Medical Center, where she served as an Associate Professor. Teaching responsibilities included both undergraduate and graduate courses centering on maternal-newborn nursing and women's health. Research interests focused on ethical issues confronting nurses in a variety of clinical settings. She is a graduate of Purdue University (AAS and BSN), Indiana University (MSN), and the University of Nebraska (PhD). She is serving as Chair of the ANA's Advisory Board, Center for Ethics and Human Rights (2006–2008).

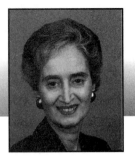

Mary Cipriano Silva

CHAPTER 14

Informed Consent, Administrative Ethics, and Ethical Guidelines: Framework, Journey, Legacy, Impact, and Vision

In this essay, I describe the framework used, the journey taken, the legacy created, the impact felt, and the vision foreseen regarding my ethics scholarship on informed consent, on administrative ethical issues, and on ethical guidelines.

Relationship Issues and Moral Distress

Relationship issues and moral distress implicitly have framed my work in ethics. When I think of a relationship, I think of a connection. A good relationship fosters a caring mutual connection and positive interpersonal practices such as attentive listening, empathic communication, honesty, and empowerment. A troubled relationship fosters a lack of connection and negative interpersonal practices such as avoidance, self-centered communication, deception, and disempowerment. An issue is a point of discussion—one that is often associated with conflict in a relationship.

Also associated with conflict in a relationship is moral distress. According to the American Association of Critical-Care Nurses (AACN) (2006), "Moral distress is a serious problem in nursing. It results in significant physical and emotional stress ...

[and] affects relationships with patients and others and [also] can affect the quality, quantity, and cost of nursing care" (p. 1). Moral distress occurs when one is unable to act ethically.

Journey

My ethics journey has been molded by multiple factors over the past 40 years. However, the most influential factor has been my own desire to explore universal and first-cause issues and themes. This interest led me, while still a teenager, into philosophical and ethical questioning. This interest also accompanied me to Ohio State University (OSU) where, as a nursing major, I elected to take several courses in philosophy.

After obtaining my bachelor's and master's degrees at OSU in 1962 and in 1963, respectively, I took a scholastic hiatus for some teaching experience. That led me to Western Reserve University when Rozella Schlotfeldt was dean. The year was 1964, and the school of nursing was a national leader in nursing and philosophical thought. I was nurtured in this intellectual environment for 5 years.

The next significant part of my ethics journey was my doctoral education. It began in 1972 at the University of Maryland when I was 33 years old. I looked for opportunities to write about philosophical and/or ethical issues and, as a result, had three articles published. The first was a futuristic look at nursing education and included a section on ethical issues (Silva, 1973). The second was a futuristic look at science and ethics and addressed such topics as genetic experimentation, in vitro transplants, and man-machine linkage (Silva, 1974). The third was an analysis of philosophy that also put forth the thesis that research is a moral endeavor (Silva, 1977).

For all of my interest in philosophy and ethics, I did not focus my dissertation on this topic. Why? The decade of the 1970s was the age of empiricism in science. Therefore, I used an experimental design to determine the effects of structured information on spouses' reactions to surgery (Silva, 1979). But all the while, I had developed another interest: the ethics of informed consent.

After receiving my doctorate in 1976, I accepted a position as an Associate Professor of nursing at George Mason University (GMU), where I was to spend the rest of my academic career. My interest in the ethics of informed consent continued during my years at GMU (e.g., Silva, 1985) and was enhanced by three learning opportunities. First, I received a National Endowment for the Humanities Award for June of 1981 to study health care ethics at the Kennedy Institute of Ethics, Washington,

DC. This award taught me theoretical perspectives related to ethics. Shortly thereafter, I received a Kennedy Fellowship in Medical Ethics for Nursing Faculty at Georgetown University. My fellowship focused on ethics and persons with mental retardation and took me into their world. I visited them at their jobs, at their homes, and at state institutions. I also wrote about them in relation to competency and informed consent (Silva, 1984). Finally, in 1987, I became a Visiting Scholar at the Hastings Center for a brief stay. While there, I focused on a review of empirical research about comprehension of information for informed consent and later coauthored an article on this topic (Silva & Sorrell, 1988).

Successful grant writing also fostered my ethics journey. Soon after I arrived at GMU, my dean discovered that I could write, and I was put to the task. My early writings focused on Division of Nursing Advanced Nurse Training and Renewal Grants that were indirectly related to ethics. Then, in 1983, I was asked to write a Division of Nursing Special Project Grant. But about what? After much pondering, I settled on ethical decision-making for nurse executives, because little information existed on this important topic at that time. I reasoned that nurse executives could not help other nurses who were facing ethical dilemmas if they did not understand ethics. The grant was funded from 1984 through 1989. I later coauthored two other ethics grants that were indirectly related to administrative ethics and were funded through the Consortium of Universities of the Washington Metropolitan Area.

The next factors that influenced my ethics journey were the three faculty study leaves that I obtained while at GMU. During these study leaves, I wrote a book on administrative ethics (Silva, 1990) and two monographs on ethical guidelines in nursing research (Silva, 1995a, 1995b). I also conducted research on ethics and managed care (Silva & Williams, 2006).

A final factor that influenced my ethics journey occurred in 1996. I was asked by the American Nurses Association (ANA) to serve as a member of the ANA Code of Ethics Project Task Force that authored the 2001 ANA *Code of Ethics for Nurses with Interpretive Statements*.

Legacy and Impact

By legacy I mean my body of work discussed herein. By impact I mean positive changes to persons or professions as a result of the legacy. One legacy of my ethics writings was to make health care professionals think futuristically and out of the box. That I did achieve some impact was reflected in citations to and commentaries on this body of work.

The continued legacy and impact of my work in ethics was manifested in the 5-year Special Project Grant noted previously. The specific goal of this project was to prepare nurse executives for ethical decision-making. One impact of the project was that nurse executives increased their knowledge about ethics and ethical decision-making, increased their self-confidence in coping with ethical issues, and decreased their moral distress. Other impacts of this project included (a) networking with scholars from the Kennedy Institute of Ethics and with nurse leaders from the community; (b) initiating and distributing an ethics newsletter for the past 20 years; (c) writing a script for an ethics videocassette series that was distributed nationally and internationally; (d) establishing one of the first centers for nursing ethics in the United States on October 10, 1986; and (e) developing ethics content and courses for the undergraduate and graduate nursing programs at GMU.

Finally, perhaps the most enduring legacy of my work was serving on the ANA Code of Ethics Project Task Force that authored the 2001 *Code of Ethics for Nurses with Interpretive Statements*. The impact of this code was and is to offer nurses ethical guidelines for their practice that are nonnegotiable.

Vision

I believe that the three dominant areas I have focused on in my ethics journey will continue to be timely and important in the future. Here is my vision for them:

- Regarding informed consent, it will become more difficult to attain because of the influx of non-English-speaking immigrants to the United States, and because of the increased complexity of medical science and of nursing science, both of which require a sophisticated vocabulary.

- Regarding administrative ethical issues, they will become more stressful and complicated in the future as business environments overtake the management of health care.

- Regarding ethical guidelines, they will remain relatively stable but nevertheless need periodic evaluation to ensure that they are current and continue to set the highest ethical standards to accommodate changes in science and technology and in nursing practice and research (Silva, 1995a, 1995b).

Underlying all three of the preceding areas is the implicit framework of relationship issues and moral distress. Not only will this framework always be with us, but it also will demand more of us in the future as ethical issues become more complex and emotionally taxing.

In summary, I have presented the framework used, the journey taken, the legacy created, the impact felt, and the vision foreseen regarding my ethics scholarship on informed consent, on administrative ethical issues, and on ethical guidelines. However, the four decades of my ethics journey would have been diminished greatly without the help of devoted teachers, caring colleagues, inquiring students, and supporting friends. To each of them I express my deepest gratitude for entrusting a part of health care ethics to me.

References

American Association of Critical-Care Nurses. (2006). *Moral distress position paper.* Washington, DC: Author.

American Nurses Association. (2001). *Code of ethics for nurses with interpretive statements.* Washington, DC: Author.

Silva, M. C. (1973). Nursing education in the computer age. *Nursing Outlook, 21*(2), 94–98.

Silva, M. C. (1974). Science, ethics, and nursing. *American Journal of Nursing, 74,* 2004–2007.

Silva, M. C. (1977). Philosophy, science, theory: Interrelationships and implications for nursing research. *Image, 9,* 59–63.

Silva, M. C. (1979). Effects of orientation information on spouses' anxieties and attitudes toward hospitalization and surgery. *Research in Nursing & Health, 2,* 127–136.

Silva, M. C. (1984). Assessing competency for informed consent with mentally retarded minors. *Pediatric Nursing, 10,* 261–265, 306.

Silva, M. C. (1985). Comprehension of information for informed consent by spouses of surgical patients. *Research in Nursing & Health, 8,* 117–124.

Silva, M. C. (1990). *Ethical decision making in nursing administration.* Norwalk, CT: Appleton & Lange.

Silva, M. (1995a). *Ethical guidelines in the conduct, dissemination and implementation of nursing research.* Washington, DC: American Nurses Publishing.

Silva, M. (1995b). *Annotated bibliography for ethical guidelines in the conduct, dissemination, and implementation of nursing research.* Washington, DC: American Nurses Publishing.

Silva, M. C., & Sorrell, J. M. (1988). Enhancing comprehension of information for informed consent: A review of empirical research. *IRB: A review of human subjects research, 10*(1), 1–5.

Silva, M. C., & Williams, K. (2006). Managed care and the violation of ethical principles: Research vignettes. In P. S. Cowen & S. Moorhead (Eds.), *Current issues in nursing* (7th ed., chap. 73). St. Louis, MO: Elsevier.

Mary Cipriano Silva received her BSN and MS from Ohio State University and her PhD from the University of Maryland. Her interest in bioethics spans several decades, and her scholarship on ethics focuses on informed consent, administrative ethics, and ethical guidelines. She is a Professor Emerita in nursing from George Mason University, Fairfax, Virginia.

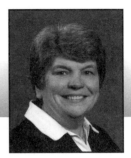

Carol Rae Taylor

CHAPTER 15

Right Relationships: Foundation for Health Care Ethics

In 1983, I was happily teaching in a baccalaureate nursing program when a colleague in philosophy invited me to apply for a grant from the National Endowment for the Humanities to study nursing ethics at Tufts University. The grant aimed to bring teams of philosophers and nurses from different universities to study philosophy and nursing, and to return to our home universities prepared to teach a new course in nursing ethics. Already sensitive to issues in health care decision-making because of my passion for oncology and gerontology, I was bitten by the "bioethics bug" and have not been the same since! In 1987, with the most basic of undergraduate philosophy courses to my credit and a master's degree in medical-surgical nursing, I swallowed my trepidation and enrolled in Georgetown University's doctoral program in philosophy with a concentration in bioethics. My goal was to learn enough philosophy and bioethics to be able to use these disciplines to help make health care effective for those who need it—with special emphasis on the most vulnerable members of society. In 1990, my dissertation director, Dr. Edmund Pellegrino, invited me to help found the Center for Clinical Bioethics at Georgetown University Medical Center, and as they say, "The rest is history."

Originally, in describing my scholarly work and its potential for influencing health care in the future, I would not have chosen relationships to categorize my work. But after a bit of reflection I realized that this was a wise choice. My master's thesis, *Meaning in Suffering and Illness and Its Relationship to Self-Actualization and Despairful "Not-Caring"* (Taylor, 1979), used the work of Victor Frankl and nurse theorists

Travelbee, Pateson, and Zderad as its framework. When I read Paterson and Zderad's (1976) definition of nursing and goal of humanistic nursing, I newly appreciated nursing's potential to effect human flourishing and knew I had a mission.

At heart, I am a "people person," and my scholarly research and service focuses on engaging all of us in the design, delivery, reception, and evaluation of health care in moral reflection and discourse about how to improve the experience of health care and promote better health outcomes. Health care is essentially relational, and good health care depends upon right relationships. In health care, right relationships demand of professionals a clear understanding and acceptance of the power centered in the healing encounter. I absolutely reject the reduction of professional healers to technicians. Right relationships with patients and families, with business partners, and with the public are equally important for institutions and systems committed to healing.

Right relationships are a function of health professionals, and I use this term broadly to include health care executives and managers being trustworthy; that is, not only competent in their role responsibilities, but committed to securing the interests of those entrusted to their care, even when this entails self-sacrifice. Trustworthiness, then, is essential to right relationships.

Ethics Education

Recently I was asked what I do, and to my surprise I said I was a teacher. Reflecting on how and why teacher popped out of my brain/mouth instead of ethicist or nurse or something else . . . I realized how central education is to my identity, and the affirmation and joy I experience when teaching well. My efforts are aimed to educate competent, responsible, and compassionate health professionals.

There are many definitions of ethics. One of the definitions I often use with students and audiences is, "Ethics is the formal study of who we ought to be in light of our identity." For example, nursing ethics is the formal study of who nurses ought to be—how they should make decisions, act, and behave, in light of their identity as professional caregivers committed to patient health and well-being. Using this definition requires one to "unpack" the notion of identity and to raise the question of relativism. Can I (and everyone else!) "invent" my identity as a nurse or a human being, or is there a certain "given-ness" to select identities? My doctoral dissertation, *The Morality Internal to the Practice of Nursing* (Taylor, 1997b), proposes and defends the thesis that there is morality internal to the practice of nursing from which the moral obligations of nurses can be derived. Thus, one of my most important activities as a nurse ethicist is to continually create the moral space for health care professionals to step out of the busyness of their every day to reflect on their personal and professional identities and what these demand.

Ethics then raises questions of truth as well as goodness. Is my personal and professional life faithful to what it means to be human, spouse, parent, Roman Catholic, nurse, ethicist, Georgetown University employee?

Central to these questions for health professionals is the notion of ethical competence. Early in my career I identified the following elements of ethical competence for health care professionals: clinical competence and the ability to be trusted to act in ways that advance the best interests of the patients; to hold themselves and their colleagues accountable for their practice; to work collaboratively to advocate for patients, families, and communities; to recognize and mediate ethical conflict among the patient, significant others, the health care team, and other interested parties; to recognize the ethical dimensions of practice, and identify and respond to ethical problems; and to critique new health care technologies and changes in the way we define, administer, deliver, and finance health care in light of their potential to influence human well-being (Taylor, 1997a). Once we have a robust notion of ethical competence, the challenge lies in communicating it as a core competence that is a requirement for hiring, practice, and promotion, including position descriptions. Many of us fail to be reflective about the efforts needed to develop and maintain the ethical competence needed to practice well.

In 1989 I published the first edition of a fundamentals of nursing text (Taylor, Lillis, LeMone, & Lynn, 2008). As its principal author, I promoted a framework which we now refer to simply as "blended skills." The message to beginning students is that intellectual, technical, interpersonal, and ethical/legal competencies are "all" essential to every clinical encounter. No matter that their early years of study are filled with cramming knowledge into their heads and mastering techniques and procedures, they need to be as intentional and responsible for developing interpersonal and ethical/legal competence as they are for intellectual and technical competence (Taylor, 1995). Because of the value I attach to reflective practice, I have made such exercises a constant in my nursing classes and in this text.

In 1998, Georgetown's Schools of Medicine and Nursing launched the development and implementation of a four-part interdisciplinary curriculum in health care ethics grounded in a robust concept of moral agency. Essential elements of moral agency are freedom, character, valuing, sensibility, responsiveness, accountability, reasoning and discernment, motivation, and advocacy and leadership. The ultimate aim of the curriculum is to foster the cultivation of these capacities in future advanced practice nurses and physicians. "Moral agency" is the capacity to habitually act in an ethical manner, to be able to be counted on to do the right thing for the right reasons. It is unrealistic to assume that the simple desire to be a nurse or physician is accompanied by the natural ability to behave in an ethical way. This ability, moral agency, must be cultivated in the same way that nurses cultivate the ability to do the scientifically right thing in response to a physiologic alteration.

Research/Scholarship

The second edition of the American Nurses Association's (ANA's) *Nursing's Social Policy Statement* (2003) identifies one of the six essential features of professional nursing as the provision of a caring relationship that facilitates health and healing. Given that human caring is essential to nursing, I elected in my doctoral dissertation and subsequent research to describe better both the characteristics of care as a moral orientation and a model of professional caregiving.

According to Rollo May (1969), care must be at the root of ethics, for the good life comes from what we care about. Based upon my own experiences as both a nurse and health care ethicist I would like to suggest that clinicians, who operate from an ethic of care, care about people, relationships, human dignity, responsiveness and responsibility, particulars, and contextual factors.

I believe that every human interaction delivers one of three messages within minutes: "Drop dead, get out of my face," "You are a job to be done, you mean nothing to me," or "You are a person of worth and I care about you." While we go through life receiving these messages at home, school, work, and play, a healthy self-image can go a long way to countering negative messages. Unfortunately, an experience of vulnerability can leave us prey to negative societal messages. Because health care professionals encounter people during moments of exquisite vulnerability and share physically and mentally intimate moments, the messages they communicate can matter dramatically. A friend who was diagnosed with advanced ovarian cancer at the age of 39 and suffered two of the hardest years of dying I have ever witnessed shared the following words with me.

> Carol, please tell your students that when I first got sick it didn't matter how people treated me because I knew who I was...now I become whoever people make me. And if a nurse or doctor walks into my room and treats me like meat, I BECOME MEAT.

I or a member of my profession had the power to take a woman like this and reduce her to MEAT by virtue of what I said or did not say, how I looked, touched, interacted. I believe we need a renewed emphasis on the art of therapeutic or healing presence.

Most clinicians and certainly the public place a high value on professional caring, but find it difficult to describe the nature of professional caring (how it differs from more generic types of caring) and its related moral obligations. Unless we understand what professional care is and can measure it, it will be difficult to hold health care professionals accountable to care. The model of professional caring which I developed is described in an article in the *Kennedy Institute of Ethics Journal* (Taylor, 1998). This model has six necessary and sufficient elements, each with related virtues and moral obligations: affection, cognition, volition, imagination, motivation, and expressiveness. As the one example of an element below illustrates, one strength of the model is that each element can be assessed along a continuum identifying problematic deficiencies and excesses (see Figure 15.1).

- *Affection:* Feeling of positive regard which is experienced as a response to the presence or thought of the one cared for; feelings may range from a simple regard of kinship which acknowledges another human in need, to feelings of loving and tender regard.

- *Continuum:* Simple regard to tender solicitude

- *Deficiency and Excess:* Too little feeling for another can result in the one cared for feeling objectified and depersonalized; too much feeling may overwhelm the recipient of care, incapacitate the caregiver, and make needed therapeutic intervention impossible.

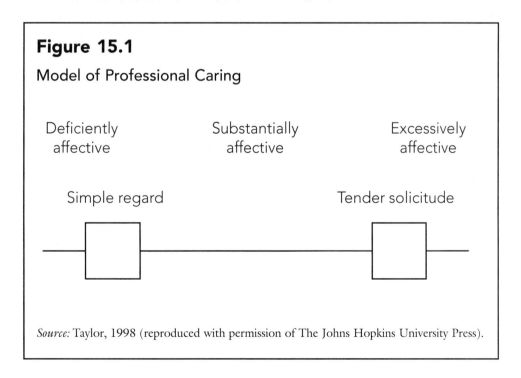

Figure 15.1

Model of Professional Caring

Deficiently affective Substantially affective Excessively affective

Simple regard   Tender solicitude

Source: Taylor, 1998 (reproduced with permission of The Johns Hopkins University Press).

- *Virtues:* Respect (regard), compassion, therapeutic attentiveness

- *Related Moral Obligation:* To practice in a manner that leaves one open to be moved by the experiences of patients and their significant others.

Meaning of this Work for the Future

In an address to Japanese nurse educators at their annual conference on the theme of ethical challenges in nursing education, research, and practice, I cited the following (Taylor, 2004):

- There is currently an acute shortage of professional nurses and nursing assistants which at least in part is linked to nursing's continuing negative image. Nursing is still predominantly a female profession, and women today have numerous career options and are increasingly reluctant to do the "hard work" of nursing. Society continues to devalue and to privatize human caring. This is especially the case with our most vulnerable: the poor, the chronically ill, and the frail elderly.

- Every day we show up for work, we literally hold in our hands the power to influence how people are born, live, suffer, and die. What greater work! When we fail to appreciate our ability to affirm, heal, bruise, or violate humanity, it is time to change careers.

- The steadily increasing costs of health care, coupled with increased competition for limited health care dollars in the United States, have resulted in workplace environments that many nurses find unacceptable. When standards of care drop below an acceptable level of safety and quality, patient safety, health, and well-being are threatened and the integrity of nurses and other health care professionals is compromised. Nurses are leaving active practice for this reason and transitioning to careers in business, law, and sales, for example. Some nurses now report changing their notion of what it means to be a "good" nurse from "making a critical difference in patients' lives," to "giving an honest day's labor for a day's pay," a change that does not bode well for the public! In our research on ethical climate, ethics stress, and the job satisfaction of nurses and social workers in the United States, we suggest strategies to reduce ethics stress and improve the ethical climate of the workplace (Ulrich et al. 2007).

- There have been unprecedented scientific advances in the last 20 years and more are promised daily. The public is being educated to believe that genomic medicine will fulfill all their dreams for a better life. Many, "but by no means all," of these advances will benefit patients. Certain scientific and technologic advances may actually threaten basic human health and dignity. Helping patients to be discriminating and to make wise choices has never been more challenging or more important. It remains true that nurses are often the bridge between exquisite human vulnerability and a dizzying array of therapeutic—and sometimes questionably so—options. While nursing has historically claimed advocacy as central to its role, fewer and fewer nurses find themselves practicing in work environments which support their being skilled advocates. In fact, many practice environments are hostile to nurse-initiated advocacy efforts. Promoting my description of ethical competence and efforts to mandate ethical competence as a core and monitored competence has the potential to redress this deficiency.

■ Paternalistic decision-making (clinician decides what is in the best interests of the patient) has been largely replaced by a model of patient sovereignty exacerbated by consumerism. Many patients and families now believe they can enter a health care system and order up, cafeteria-style, whatever they like: repeat coronary bypass please, hemodialysis if my kidneys fail, treat my sepsis, and on and on. Health Care professionals now find themselves "taking," not "giving," orders and "the model of shared decision-making remains an elusive goal." Some health professionals have responded by reducing respect for the patient's right to be self-determining to a noninterference model which reduces the clinician's obligation to not interfering with the patient's preferences—a far cry from providing the information and support patients need to make scientifically right and humanly good decisions. Sadly, Sally Gadow's rich notion of existential advocacy remains an elusive ideal.

> The ideal which existential advocacy expresses is this: that individuals be assisted by nursing to authentically exercise their freedom of self-determination. By authentic is meant a way of reaching decisions which are truly one's own—decisions that express all that one believes important about oneself and the world, the entire complexity of one's values. Individuals can express their wholeness and uniqueness as valuing beings only if their full complexity of values—including contradictions and conflicts—is clearly in mind, having been reexamined and clarified in the new context (1980, p. 85).

How many nurses today know their patients well enough to facilitate authentic autonomy? And how many nurses value existential advocacy such that they are willing to fight for institutional cultures which demand nothing less. I hope to remain relentless in challenging nurses and other caregivers to make advocacy central to their professional responsibilities.

■ The disparities in health services available to the rich and the poor continue to grow, and never has there been a greater need for advocates for vulnerable populations. Well-documented disparities exist on the basis of factors such as financial resources, race/ethnicity, gender, nature of illness, age, and body size. When the ANA's *Code for Nurses* was revised in 2001, it retained as its first principle:

"The nurse, in all professional relationships, practices with compassion and respect for the inherent dignity, worth, and uniqueness of every individual, unrestricted by considerations of social or economic status, personal attributes, or the nature of health problems" (p. 7). Too often nurses forget the power we have to affirm threatened dignity, worth, and uniqueness by exercising that most basic of our skills, therapeutic presence.

■ Conflicts of interest abound in research and practice sites, and it is not unusual for researchers, health care providers, and health businesses to use the pain and suffering of vulnerable patients to profit financially or otherwise. All of which creates more and more of a demand for strong advocacy on the part of nurses.

■ Finally, love, a sincere commitment to meet human vulnerability with exquisite human caring, seems to be in short supply and can no longer be presumed to be the primary motivation for nursing or for health care in general.

While this quick snapshot may paint a bleaker picture than we would like, it most certainly fails to capture the extraordinary efforts of many nurses to make health care work for those in need. To the extent that this picture is accurate, it dramatically makes the case for work in ethics. I remain committed to this work and grateful for the opportunities it gives me to help make health care work for those who need it.

References

American Nurses Association. (2001). *Code of ethics for nurses with interpretive statements*. Washington, DC: Nursebooks.org.

American Nurses Association. (2003). *Nursing's social policy statement* (2nd ed.). Silver Spring, MD: Nursebooks.org.

Gadow, S. (1980). Existential advocacy: Philosophical foundation of nursing. In S. F. Spicker & S. Gadow (Eds.), *Nursing, images and ideals: Opening dialogue with the humanities* (pp. 79–101). New York: Springer.

May, R. (1969). *Love and will*. New York: Norton.

Paterson, J., & Zderad, L. (1976). *Humanistic nursing*. New York: John Wiley & Sons.

Spicker, S. F. & Gadow, S. (Eds.) (1980). *Nursing, images and ideals: Opening dialogue with the humanities* (pp. 79–101). New York: Springer.

Taylor, C. (1979). *Meaning in suffering and illness and its relationship to self-actualization and despairful "not-caring" in selected hospitalized persons with metastatic carcinoma*. Unpublished master's thesis. The Catholic University of America, School of Nursing, Washington, DC.

Taylor, C. (1995). Rethinking nursing's basic competencies. *Journal of Nursing Care Quality, 9*(4), 1–13.

Taylor, C. (1997a). Ethical issues in case management. In E. Cohen & T. Cesta, (Eds.), *Nursing case management: From concept to evaluation* (pp. 314–334). St. Louis, MO: Mosby.

Taylor, C. (1997b). *The morality internal to the practice of nursing.* Unpublished doctoral dissertation. Georgetown University, Graduate School of Philosophy, Washington, DC.

Taylor, C. (1998). Reflections on nursing considered as a moral practice. *Kennedy Institute of Ethics Journal, 8*(1), 71–82.

Taylor, C. (2004). Meeting the ethical challenges in nursing education, research, and practice. Same commitment to patients but new responsibilities. *Journal of Japan Academy of Nursing Education, 14*(2), 37–55.

Taylor, C., Lillis, C., LeMone, P., & Lynn, P. (2008). *Fundamentals of nursing: The art and science of nursing care* (6th ed.). Philadelphia: Lippincott, Williams & Wilkins.

Ulrich, C. M., O'Donnell, P., Taylor, C., Farrar, A., Danis, M., & Grady, C. (2007). Ethical climate, ethics stress, and the job satisfaction of nurses and social workers in the United States. *Social Science & Medicine, 65*(8), 1708–1719.

Carol Rae Taylor is a faculty member of the Georgetown University School of Nursing and Health Studies and Director of the Georgetown University Center for Clinical Bioethics. She is a graduate of Holy Family University (BSN), the Catholic University of America (MSN), and Georgetown University (PhD in Philosophy with a concentration in bioethics). Bioethics has been a focus of her teaching and research since 1980 linked to her passion to "make health care work" for those who need it. Special interests include health care decision-making and professional ethics.

⁀ SECTION V ⁀
CRITICAL THINKING ACTIVITIES

Relationship Issues

✦ In the poem that introduces this section on relationships, the nurse chooses not to delay patient mourning through administration of drugs. What does this say about the relationship between this nurse and the mother?

✦ You have been appointed to the hospital's ethics committee where you work. Based on the issues raised in Miya's essay on the ethical issues encountered by nurses in clinical settings and your own experience, describe the content of an orientation program for new members of the ethics committee. In other words, what would you need to know to be an effective committee member?

✦ Silva predicts that administrative ethical issues will become more problematic in the future as business environments overtake the management of health care and as the nursing population ages. Propose two or three strategic measures that nurse administrators should take to address these related problems.

✦ Taylor cites Sally Gadow's classic work on existential advocacy (Existential advocacy: philosophical foundation of nursing practice. In S. Spicker & S. Gadow, 1980 [pp. 79–101]). How would you respond to Taylor's question that she draws from Gadow's work: How many nurses today know their patients well enough to facilitate authentic autonomy?

✦ Taylor proposes core competencies in ethics similar to other competencies in nursing such as technical competencies. Make a list of core competencies in ethics that all nurses should possess. How would you measure mastery of the competencies you have identified

SECTION VI

Concerns Related to Vulnerability

Ethical issues related to the situation of or treatment of social groups who are at risk for various untoward actions because of the characteristics of that group (for example: gender, ethnicity, disability, etc.). Particular treatments include disenfranchisement, stigmatization, discrimination, and/or marginalization.

Nunca Tu Alma

Cortney Davis

I turn my eyes from the girls' thin bodies
in Sarajevo and from corpses that float down river
like matchsticks, but here in the clinic
I sit with Maya—a twelve-year-old, raped
by her sister's friend—who asks me *Am I still a virgin?*
I examine her crimson vagina. Three
delicate tears lace her perineum, as if Maya
has had a rough delivery.
I culture for GC, chlamydia, draw blood
for pregnancy, HIV.
Am I still a virgin? she asks, her voice disembodied
above her knees, bent and open,
her hips narrow as a boy's beneath the sheet.
I struggle with mechanical *vs.* emotional, consider
the penis as metaphor. When we're finished,
Maya and I lean close, face to face.
Virginity is a matter of love, I say, when you give yourself
out of joy. Rape takes only your body, never your soul.
Maya nods, repeats this in Spanish
to her mother and sister, three dark women
singing like birds. Maya imitates me, her fist
strikes her palm: *Nunca, nunca tu alma.*
Her tests are negative.
Maya's more like thirty than twelve,
the nurse whispers, and I agree.
I crumple the sheet and dump the bloods swabs.
Shove the metal stirrups into the table, out of sight.

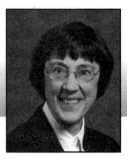

Judith A. Erlen

CHAPTER 16

Ethics and Vulnerable Populations: My Passion for the Underdog

The Context

During my formative years I developed a set of values that continue to guide my life, in general, and my role as a professional nurse, in particular. My parents led by example, encouraging me always to do what was right and make good choices. The values that I acquired because of my parents' perspective and my religious upbringing, as well as through my participation in the scouting movement and other organizations, served as guides for making good decisions. I learned that critically important decisions were not made haphazardly, but rather were made after some thought; making the right choices and acting on those choices were emphasized.

When I was 15 years old, I visited my grandfather, who at the time was a resident in a long-term care facility. I remember spontaneously reaching out and touching a young lad who could not raise his head from his pillow. I neither knew his name nor anything about his health problem; I later learned that he had hydrocephaly. I remember my father commenting to me about how my small act of caring brought a smile to this boy's face. My father noted that I had not stared at or pitied him; instead, I had made a difference for at least a few moments because I saw him as someone in need of a smile and a touch of a hand.

Selecting nursing as a career fit with the values that I was developing. There were many instances during my baccalaureate and master's programs, and my early days as a staff nurse, where I had the opportunity to attempt to make a difference in the way that patients were being treated. For example, there was a large ward for "clinic" patients on the maternity unit where I worked. I remember that some of the staff made disparaging remarks about these women because of their frequent pregnancies. To me, these new mothers were women who needed the same teaching and support as other maternity patients. I offered what I could to try to help them. The staff would say to me, "Why are you wasting your time? They will only be back next year."

Because I, as one individual, was unable to make lasting changes that I believed were important when caring for maternity patients, I focused on becoming a nurse educator in order to develop an "army" of nurses who could go out and "do battle" with the health care system and help to transform the way that patients were sometimes treated. I felt that becoming an educator might be an effective strategy to make this change, as I would be able to influence how young nurses should treat patients and enable them to have more control over their personal health needs. My guiding principle was that one should care for a patient as one would want someone to care for one's family member.

As I look back, there were some other life events which clearly demonstrated to me the extreme vulnerability of patients. One example occurred during a visit with a great-uncle who was a resident in a skilled nursing facility. He had been a Lutheran minister for much of his working life, but this aspect of his life seemed to go unnoticed by the staff. During my visit a staff member came over to see if my uncle needed anything. She called him "Pops." I was appalled by her use of this term. Where was respect for persons? Why was it necessary to use such "shorthand" rather than a person's name?

In numerous other situations, patients were described in rather disparaging ways. Yet, in no instance in my experience did I hear the patient or any accompanying family member make a comment to the health care provider. Quite possibly, if the patients had known what was being said, they may have tried to change the situation or they may have just said, "That's just the way it is. I can't do anything to change this." Family members may have thought that it is important that my loved one receive care; saying something may lead to an unpleasant scene and possible negative consequences.

Some time later, I read *The House of God* by Samuel Shem (1988) and realized that sometimes health care providers create a set of shorthand terms to describe particular groups of patients, such as "GOMER" or "GORK." The author, a physician, had vividly pointed out how we, as health care providers, can easily fall prey to engaging in this same practice. The result is that when patients are labeled, they take on the characteristics of the term that has been applied. This use of disparaging terms may label and stigmatize patients, making them even more vulnerable and powerless. One question that will continue to need to be addressed is why no one challenges the use of terms of endearment such as "dearie," "honey," or "pops," or the use of acronyms such as "GOMER," or the use of the common vernacular such as "roadkill" or "frequent flyer" to describe patients. Is it that this is such a common practice that nurses, other health care providers, and patients and their families have just gotten used to such terms?

My passion for ethics, however, did not actually awaken until I was engaged in doctoral study. Taking advantage of several learning opportunities during that program and becoming acquainted with the work of ethicists in the Dallas, Texas area and the work of my mentor and dissertation chair, Dr. Barbara Carper, helped to provide me with a stronger foundation in ethics and challenge my thinking. Subsequently, I had two additional postgraduate learning experiences: one focused on nursing ethics and the other centered on literature and medicine, which helped to strengthen my knowledge and understanding of ethics and the role of the humanities in health care.

Having knowledge and understanding of ethics gave me the basis for teaching courses in nursing ethics to both undergraduate and graduate students, as well as students from the various schools of the health sciences. Co-taught by my husband, an expert in the history of medicine and health care, and me, we were able to show how ethical issues and practices have changed as health care has changed.

Upon reflection, I realize that these opportunities have shaped my career in nursing ethics and the focus of my work on the concept of respect for persons, particularly as related to vulnerable populations. Thus, this essay traces my work spanning nearly 40 years that describes personal and professional encounters with patients and families, as well as research with nurses, patients with HIV infection, and patients with Alzheimer's disease and their informal caregivers.

Framing the Theme

Vulnerable populations are those individuals who lack control over at least some portion of their lives; they are often characterized as being powerless. They may be immobilized or seem helpless in regard to trying to change their situation. Their sense of powerlessness may occur because of their physical or mental impairments or their lack of knowledge and understanding. Because others are seemingly in control, vulnerable populations are unable to assert themselves in order to make their needs known and have their needs met. Their knowledge and understanding of the health care situation is elusive; they are unable to make well-informed decisions. Their ability to access health care services, or even to participate in the available services, may be limited at best. They may lack advocates to assist them to meet their needs and decrease their sense of powerlessness. They may not have advocates who can bring about changes within society that will reduce the negative responses that they encounter. As I have thought about the role of nursing, I realize that nurses need to be there to enable and to possibly empower these individuals; nurses need to recognize their advocacy role in regard to people who are vulnerable and seize the opportunity to make a difference.

Vulnerable populations may experience discrimination and stigmatization; as noted earlier, they may be discredited, devalued, and labeled negatively by others within the society because of particular discrediting attributes that they possess. Goffman (1963) has poignantly described this phenomenon of stigmatization; individuals are shunned by society because they are different in some way. Their identity becomes "spoiled." Others' opinions about these individuals are slanted or biased and may lead to avoidance behaviors (Erlen & Jones, 1999). The result is that such patient populations, for example patients with HIV/AIDS, feel controlled rather than in control. They feel disempowered; they may be unaware of how to affect any type of change.

The research that I conducted with patients with AIDS during the late 1980s through the mid-1990s clearly demonstrated how the homophobic attitudes of others left their mark on these individuals. At that time, patients with AIDS were very sick; they were living with a life-threatening illness. Many were shunned by both friends and family. Their vulnerability increased because many of these patients engaged in behaviors such as homosexuality and illicit drug use that society did not condone or felt were wrong. Some led two lives; they closeted those behaviors that were not approved of by society.

However, patients are not the only vulnerable group within our society. Given some of the findings from my early research (Erlen & Frost, 1991), I would classify nurses as another vulnerable group. They, too, may feel that they lack autonomy and are not respected despite their education and experience. The voice of nurses is not always heard when patient care decisions are made, even though nurses may have important, relevant knowledge about the patient and family that others may not have. Nurses and their work seem almost invisible (Wolf, 1989).

Thus, the ethical issues that arise with vulnerable populations are decreased respect, an increased risk of harm and suffering, and the potential for injustices to occur. Lack of respect can lead to limited decision-making on the part of the individual. There is the possibility that the person may be treated differently.

Impact on Health Care Ethics

The qualitative study that I conducted with a small group of nurses working in a critical care environment provided an opportunity for nurses to describe one or more "troubling" stories that had left a lasting impression on them (Erlen & Frost, 1991). One of the first things that I noticed was that even though these patient situations may have occurred some time ago, the nurses talked about them as if they had happened only yesterday. This storytelling seemed to provide a kind of catharsis for some of them. The themes that were identified focused on powerlessness and the nurses' inability to affect patients' and families' abilities to make decisions. When discussing their interactions with physicians, the nurses expressed that they felt blocked from taking any action.

This work set the stage for me to do some writing on the concept of moral distress. Now, as I reflect back, the nurses in this qualitative study were describing instances of moral distress in their practice (Erlen, 2001). They were distressed because they remembered experiencing indecision about the action to take, powerlessness to implement what they believed to be the right action, and a lack of support from peers or supervisory personnel.

More recently, my research has focused on vulnerable populations such as patients with HIV/AIDS and Alzheimer's disease. Each of these patient populations experiences different, yet common, characteristics, predisposing them to being even more vulnerable than other groups of patients.

My entrée into research with HIV/AIDS patients focused on whether or not there was a difference in the quality of care that this patient population received when compared with general medical-surgical patients cared for by the same nurse (Erlen, 1992–1996). Our research team found that the quality of care did not differ significantly between the two groups of patients. Both groups received the expected standard of care, placing the quality of care at a mid-range level. Because researchers, based on findings in the literature, suggested that patients with a diagnosis of AIDS might be shunned, we examined the idea of avoidance, using the field notes that had been kept by the research nurses as they made their observations of nurse-patient behavior. Contrary to what we expected, nurses did not avoid patients with HIV/AIDS. The nurses had more positive verbal behaviors, made more eye contact, and touched patients with AIDS more often than general medical-surgical patients (Siminoff, Erlen, & Sereika, 1998). Quite possibly the age of the patient may have been a factor accounting for this nursing behavior, or nurses may have become less fearful of contracting AIDS because of their increased knowledge and understanding of AIDS.

I followed this quality of care study with one in which I used a life review intervention with patients with AIDS to examine whether life review helped them to make sense of this "off-time" event (earlier death), and reflect on and identify meaningful events in their lives, and thereby increase their quality of life. Following the use of the life review intervention, we found trends showing that the treatment group had fewer depressive symptoms and exhibited increased purpose in life, quality of life, and self-esteem (Erlen, Mellors, Sereika, & Cook, 2001). Upon reflection, life review might be used as an intervention to help patients see that, although their illness and its burden may contribute to their sense of powerlessness, other aspects of their lives have afforded opportunities to help them have a meaningful life and to seek reconciliation with estranged family members.

The advent of protease inhibitors in the mid-1990s changed the management of patients with HIV/AIDS. I put together a team of researchers to test the efficacy of a nurse-delivered telephone intervention to help patients adhere to a complex medication regimen (Erlen, 2003–present). As part of the preparatory work for this longitudinal study, we conducted interviews with five patients in order to understand the experience of taking a complex antiretroviral regimen. We found that patients discussed the "blessings" and the "burdens" of taking these regimens (Erlen & Mellors, 1999). In effect, they were describing a sense of powerlessness. Some of them lacked information about their illness and its management, which limited their understanding and increased their vulnerability.

When patients complete our longitudinal study, we ask them to participate in an exit interview. One comment that my staff often hears is, "You care about me. I matter." Something happens between my staff and the patients with HIV, who are the participants in the study, through the multiple contacts they have with each other over a period of 18–24 months. These patients are important; their contributions as volunteers in our study are helping to advance the science of adherence. Also, those who are in the intervention arm are learning ways to better manage their medications through habit formation and problem solving, giving them greater control over their lives.

As part of this study we have also followed patients with HIV who are deemed to be 100% adherent at baseline. We have interviewed these individuals and characterized their medication-taking experience (Lewis, Colbert, Erlen, & Meyers, 2006). These informants have described both facilitators and barriers to being adherent to their regimen.

My other research, funded by the Alzheimer's Association, has focused on another vulnerable patient population, individuals with dementia. Our findings suggest that, while patients are vulnerable because of their decreased cognitive ability, the informal family caregivers are also expressing a sense of powerlessness and vulnerability related to the difficulties of obtaining information or accessing health care services.

Influence of My Work on Ethics

My work has helped to inform the ways in which health care professionals and patients interact with and treat each other and make decisions regarding issues that affect their lives. As I have explored the relationships that are constituted when individuals with different levels of power, control, and authority communicate with each other, I have learned that mutual respect and appreciating differences in people are critically important considerations.

I have no doubt that vulnerable populations will continue to exist within our society. The work that I have done provides a framework for continuing to ask the questions and frame the issues. Although my work has been primarily published in nursing journals, numerous individuals from other disciplines have contacted me when they want information about a particular paper that I have published. When I conduct ethics seminars with third-year medical students during one of their clerkships, I often have the opportunity to discuss the meaning of patient and professional vulnerability and lack of control with these students. They have said that they are the "low persons on the totem pole." They may observe patient situations and yet not be able to do anything about what they see. While they can tell nurses or physicians what patients have said or requested, medical students say that they have no authority to act in such situations. They fear that if they do something without permission, such as answering a patient's questions, they will experience some repercussions during their evaluations at the end of the rotation. Similar to the other groups I have described, the medical students are saying that they also are in a vulnerable position because the evaluator has the power to "make or break" them.

As I reflect on my scholarly focus in ethics, I realize that my work has certainly given me increasing insight into nurses and patients as vulnerable populations, as well as benefited others. Staff nurses and students from across the health science disciplines have been exposed to my teaching and have had the opportunity to delve into the literature, examine selected ethical questions, and consider how the situation might unfold in the real world. In the long run, I hope that my work has actually benefited patients and their families. Certainly, the perspective that I have been using in my current research with patients with HIV who are taking antiretroviral therapy suggests that involving patients and engaging them in shared decision-making about issues regarding medication taking has afforded them more power, so they can question their health care provider. These patients are feeling more in control of their lives. Because of the changes in therapy, they look to fulfilling their hopes and dreams. Would that this outlook were true for all patients with HIV and with Alzheimer's disease. There are many patients who continue to be shunned and disregarded. Likewise, nurses continue to express an inability to exert influence when ethical situations arise; they feel as if their perspective is often ignored.

Over the years, I have called for conversations surrounding these issues and the use of peer support and advocates to help empower vulnerable populations. As I come to the end of this essay, I realize that this message needs to be underscored. I challenge nurses and other health care professionals to continue to fulfill their advocacy role, empower patients, give them control, treat them with respect, enable them to access needed health care services, and thereby reduce their vulnerabilities.

References

Erlen, J. A. (1992–1996). AIDS and the quality of nursing care. National Institute of Nursing Research, National Institutes of Health, Bethesda, MD (RO1 NR02664).

Erlen, J. A. (2001). Moral distress: A pervasive problem. *Orthopaedic Nursing, 20*(2), 76–80.

Erlen, J. A. (PI). (2003–present). Improving adherence to protease inhibitors. National Institute of Nursing Research, National Institutes of Health, Bethesda, MD (RO1 NR04749).

Erlen, J. A., & Frost, B. (1991). Nurses' perceptions of powerlessness in influencing ethical decisions. *Western Journal of Nursing Research, 13*(3), 397–407.

Erlen, J. A., & Jones, M. (1999). The patient no one liked. *Orthopaedic Nursing, 18*(4), 76–79.

Erlen, J. A., & Mellors, M. P. (1999). Adherence to combination therapy in persons living with HIV: Balancing the hardships and the blessings. *Journal of the Association of Nurses in AIDS Care, 10*(4), 75–84.

Erlen, J. A., Mellors, M. P., Sereika, S. M., & Cook, C. (2001). The use of life review to enhance quality of life of people living with AIDS: A feasibility study. *Quality of Life Research, 10*(5), 453–464.

Goffman, E. (1963). *Stigma: Notes on the management of spoiled identity.* Englewood Cliffs, NJ: Prentice-Hall.

Lewis, M. P., Colbert, A., Erlen, J. A., & Meyers, M. (2006). A qualitative study of persons who are 100% adherent to antiretroviral therapy. *AIDS Care, 18*(2), 140–148.

Shem, S. (1988). *The house of God.* New York: Dell Publishing.

Siminoff, L. A., Erlen, J. A., & Sereika, S. M. (1998). Do nurses avoid AIDS patients? Avoidance behaviours and the quality of care of hospitalized AIDS patients. *AIDS Care, 10*(2), 147–163.

Wolf, Z. R. (1989). Uncovering the hidden work of nursing. *Nursing & Health Care, 10*(8), 463–467.

Judith A. Erlen, Professor and PhD Program Coordinator, School of Nursing, also holds a secondary appointment in the Center for Bioethics and Health Law at the University of Pittsburgh, Pittsburgh, PA. She is the Associate Director of the Center for Research in Chronic Disorders in the School of Nursing, as well as the Director of the Center's Research Development Core. She received a Bachelor of Science in Nursing from the University of Pittsburgh, a Master of Science in Nursing from Wayne State University, and a PhD in Nursing from the Texas Women's University. Ethics in nursing and health care has been a focus of her research and teaching since the late 1970s. Her work centers on powerlessness in relation to the nurse's role in affecting ethical decisions, respect for persons and its relationship to vulnerable populations, and quality of life.

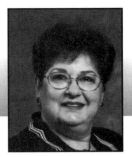

Shaké Ketefian

CHAPTER 17

Research in Nursing Ethics: A Journey

One typically does not sit down and take stock of the corpus of one's work and the journey one has taken over so many years, with its twists and turns. So I feel both honored and humbled to be included in this project to dialogue and share with so many wonderful colleagues, providing me with yet one more opportunity to learn and be instructed by such accomplished friends and colleagues.

The Beginnings: Nursing Science

During graduate school at Teachers College, Columbia University, I came upon the idea that, while nursing research in a variety of areas was increasing, there was no evidence that the findings were being used by anyone in a serious way. At the time, late 1960s and early 1970s, while research in nursing science was new, there existed a body of research, so I decided to study the extent to which scientific knowledge (read research) was being used in designing nursing curricula around the country. I selected five schools from a broad survey of schools where curricular innovations based on scholarly works were taking place. I did this through a case study approach. The available literature, mostly from social scientists, viewed application of scientific, research-based knowledge into practice (in any form) through the prism of change and the change process and adoption of innovation, while my concern was whether nursing, and eventually nursing practice and patients, were benefiting from the research being produced by nurses and others. With hindsight, this issue ultimately is an ethical one.

As I joined the faculty of New York University, I stayed with the same area of research as the dissertation for a while and designed a study to find out the extent to which a specific practice, temperature determination, on which there was much research and replication (this was before electronic thermometers) was being applied and used in practice settings (Ketefian, 1975). I found that the research finding was not being used. The lesson was that if we want to see new knowledge move to the practice arena, systematic methods and approaches needed to be developed to bring the new science and ideas to the nurse at the bedside, and that it cannot happen by itself. This concept is now referred to as evidence-based practice, with its concomitant requirement to develop and conduct translational research to help move research closer to a form that is ready for application. This is a salutary and welcome development for the discipline and for patients.

Around the time the above paper was published, I was asked to be on the first ethics committee of the New York State Nurses Association; the charge was to find ways in which the association could publicize the American Nurses Association's (ANA) *Code for Nurses with Interpretive Statements* (1968) among its members and determine how violations could be monitored. At the same time, I was invited to serve on the ANA committee to revise the Code, out of which came the 1976 revision. These two experiences stimulated me to read extensively on ethics and to consider ways in which one could study matters of ethics empirically rather than philosophically, as I did not have in-depth background in philosophy. Further, there was nothing in the literature at that time using empirical methods to study ethics questions. Then I heard Catherine Murphy's presentation of her research, in which she described her study on the moral development of nurses, and I became familiar with the work of Laurence Kohlberg and his colleagues. This was the stimulus to begin serious empirical work in addressing ethical questions. I met with Professor James Rest, who developed the "Defining Issues Test," a paper-and-pencil test for measuring moral reasoning and an alternative to Kohlberg's Moral Judgment Interview (1979). I designed several descriptive studies of nurses and nursing students, looking at the relationship between cognitive development and moral development to see if the tenets of Kohlberg's theory hold in these populations. They did (Ketefian, 1981a, 1981b).

The next and crucial question was what difference does it make if someone has high moral reasoning/cognitive levels with regard to decisions/judgments in real-life ethical conflicts? To address this type of question it was necessary to have a tool that would measure the person's ethical judgments and decisions. Since this cannot be accomplished by observation, I began the arduous task of developing an instrument, which eventually was titled "Judgments about Nursing Decisions" (JAND). Thus, the JAND makes it possible to see to what extent nurses are aware of the correct action in an ethical dilemma (see Table 1; read what the Code would have them do, column A), and compare this to the extent to which nurses are likely to act in the way respondents identified as the correct action (column B). Several findings from these studies are instructive. First, that nurses know what the right/appropriate action is almost universal; second, despite knowledge of the right action, in many cases they indicated the nurses on their unit would not act in accordance with the right action; third, the relationship between moral reasoning and the extent to which respondents would choose the right action in practice was positive, but with a very low correlation magnitude and statistically not significant (Ketefian, 1989). Many investigators used the JAND, both in the United States and abroad. Later I worked with one of my doctoral students to launch a major revision to give the scenarios a more contemporary flavor.

It is often said that research ends up raising more questions than it answers. This definitely was so in the case of these studies. Thus, the need to explain the major and consistent discrepancy noted between what the nurse should/should not do, on the one hand, and what colleagues would or would not do in a given case in practice became an issue of concern and focus for the next steps. This question took me back to the literature and a series of informal discussions with some of my study subjects and colleagues to pin down the reasons for this discrepancy. I hypothesized that there were elements in work environments that might account for this discrepancy. But what were they?

The Role of Autonomy

Further readings on these matters, especially some of the writing by Curtin, Aroskar and Davis, Murphy, and McElmurry, provided some direction for next steps. I identified several variables that intersect individual and organizational features, to find out if they influenced the way nurses make ethical judgments (using the JAND). Toward this end I developed another instrument, which I called "Perceived Job Characteristics," to measure nurses' perceptions of autonomy, standardization, and work stress. In addition, I chose the construct Nursing Role Conceptions; this was developed by a sociologist in the 1960s and modified in the 1970s by a nurse (Pieta, 1976). These reflect value orientations and reveal which of three role expectations nurses have internalized: professional role conception, bureaucratic role conception, and service role conception. Other variables included were moral reasoning and ethical decision-making (Ketefian, 1985; Kim & Ketefian, 1993).

Table 17.1

Judgments about Nursing Decisions
Sample Story: Story One

Rebecca and Nancy, good friends, were working on a pediatric unit. Matthew, a 1-year-old patient, went into heart failure and was transferred to the PICU. Immediately after transfer Rebecca told Nancy that she (Rebecca) had made a medication error and had given Matthew a larger dose of the digoxin than was prescribed. She said that she had not reported the error and did not intend to report it. Rebecca pleaded with Nancy not to say anything to anyone.

For each action below indicate your level of agreement with the nursing action to be taken by Nancy (Column A) and nurses on your unit (Column B), by placing a number in the appropriate box according to the following scale:

5 = strongly agree   4 = agree   3 = neutral   2 = disagree   1 = strongly disagree

NURSING ACTIONS	Column A Nancy should:	Column B In my unit nurses are realistically likely to:
Overlook this one error because Rebecca is basically a competent nurse.		
Discuss the meaning of professional responsibility and accountability with Rebecca, and suggest that she immediately report the error to the PICU staff and Matthew's physician.		
Call the PICU anonymously, tell of the overdose, and hang up.		
Discuss the matter with the charge nurse and seek advice as to what she should do.		
Explain to Rebecca that information on a drug overdose cannot be considered confidential when patient safety is compromised.		
Tell Rebecca that it is difficult to acknowledge a medication error, but that she will support her during the process of reporting the error.		
Volunteer to present an education program to the pediatric unit staff about ethical responsibilities in reporting medication errors.		
Comments:		

A few of the most notable findings are (also see Figure 17.1):

■ Autonomy had a negative relationship with work stress;

■ Autonomy influenced ethical decision-making through its strong relationship to both professional and service role conceptions, which then strongly influenced ethical decision-making;

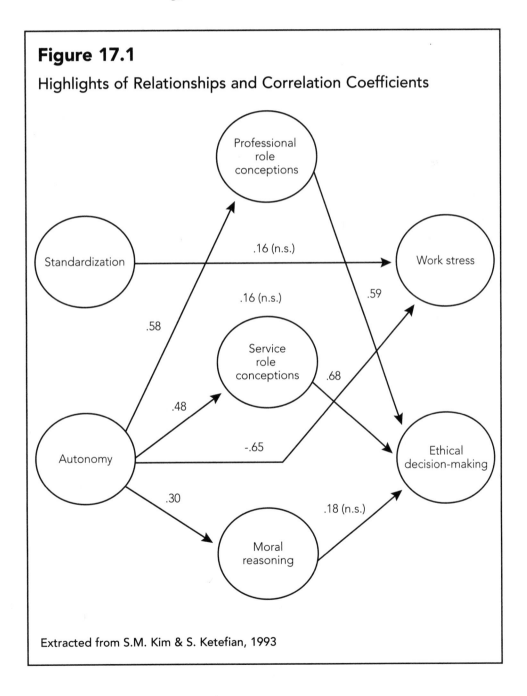

Figure 17.1

Highlights of Relationships and Correlation Coefficients

Extracted from S.M. Kim & S. Ketefian, 1993

- Autonomy is significantly related to moral reasoning;

- Moral reasoning and ethical decision-making were not related (negative but not significant) (for possible explanations of this finding, see Rest, 1979).

Scientific Integrity

In the mid-90s I was asked to co-organize a survey and report on nursing doctoral program directors' views of scientific integrity (read research ethics). We found that these individuals had a very narrow view of scientific integrity and understood it to refer to protection of human subjects in research, in a legalistic sense (Lenz & Ketefian, 1995; Ketefian & Lenz, 1995). This was shocking to me as a director of a doctoral program at the time and an eye-opener.

As an outcome of this survey two important initiatives resulted, from my perspective. One was the development of a University-wide course at Michigan on scientific integrity. The University eventually converted this to a required online course a few years ago. The second initiative occurred through the Midwest Nursing Research Society (MNRS), whereby the Board appointed a committee to develop scientific integrity guidelines, and I served as chair of the committee. This resulted in the first document that provided scientific integrity guidance to nurse scientists. We now have the second edition of the guidelines (MNRS, 2002). The guidelines were subsequently translated into Spanish and Chinese.

Meta-analytic Studies of Moral Reasoning and Ethical Practice

Nursing research was making great strides in generating new knowledge in nursing ethics, although the research was moving in many different directions. I felt that it was important to take stock periodically and examine the overall knowledge yield. So it was that in the late 1980s I spent 2 years doing an integrative review of research on moral reasoning and ethical practice, however defined, accepting a variety of definitions by investigators so that relevant studies would not be excluded (Ketefian, 1988, 1989). Overall, despite the dramatic increase in research, there was little evidence that research was cumulative. Due to serious limitations, little meaningful knowledge yield resulted from the studies reviewed.

Ten years later, in the late 1990s, I worked with the ethics research section of Midwest Nursing Research Society to do a formal meta-analysis of the relationship of education and moral reasoning to ethical practice. We reviewed only quantitative studies conducted since the previous integrative review 10 years earlier, dealing with two of the same variables (Ketefian, 2001).

Like the earlier integrative review, the findings indicate that the work being done is neither cumulative nor programmatic. None of these quantitative studies included variables within practice environments and institutional settings that might better explain the quality of ethical decisions. On the whole, I have noted too much focus on the individual nurse and her/his qualities, and not enough on the environmental and institutional realities (or the interplay between individual and organizational factors) that might hinder or facilitate high-quality, ethical practice (Ketefian, 2001).

International Endeavors

In the late 1990s, an opportunity presented itself to form an international organization on doctoral education to enable doctoral educators and students around the world to network together and benefit from one another and improve the quality of doctoral education worldwide. The outcome of this effort was the formation of the International Network for Doctoral Education in Nursing (INDEN: www.umich.edu/~inden/). As founding president, I have had quite a ride, but it also dovetailed with my appointment as the director of a new office of international affairs. Overseeing international visiting has expanded my understanding of international issues, especially those regarding doctoral education in other countries. My work on INDEN has broadened my view through visiting many countries, to speak and do workshops for faculty and students on ethics and doctoral education alike. Many of my writings and presentations during this period focus on doctoral education globally (Ketefian & McKenna, 2005; Ketefian, Phancharoenworakul, & Yunibhand, 2001).

An issue of great concern to me has been the relevance of nursing science (or lack of it) produced in the United States to other countries and settings. Our science is imbued with our Western values, implicitly or explicitly, reflecting our assumptions, norms, and values. Nurses in many parts of the world look to our research for guidance, without recognizing that these are not always appropriate for their settings. Therefore, it behooves us to work with our international colleagues and assist them to design their own studies in their own settings and contexts, so they can generate relevant and usable research. Related to this concern is the fact that we do not do enough work with our own international students to help them make the assessment and evaluation of what they learn in the United States to determine to what extent they are applicable in their own countries, and whether any "translation" is indicated before U.S.-based knowledge can be usefully applied to their countries.

Given the above point, the question has been raised about the extent to which the JAND is applicable/valid for use in other countries. For example, while patient autonomy is an important value in the United States, it is not a major value in some cultures, since families are crucially important. Thus, in many instances patients cede their decision-making to their families and accept the decisions of the family unit. This type of examination needs to be done for each nursing action, to determine validity to different countries. Therefore, the values embedded in the JAND are not universal, and may or may not apply in different countries.

My work and interest in ethics have been anchors in my various activities, and I find that ethics is relevant in so many different domains, such as in interactions with students, teaching, research, and in educational administration. My roles as editor, associate editor, and columnist over the years have given me a unique perch from which to address ethical concerns, especially in scientific integrity/research ethics.

Impact

I find it hard to discuss the impact of this body of work, much of it interconnected over a career, in ways that make sense to me but are difficult to communicate. In addition, without a measure or yardstick, this difficulty is compounded. From my perspective, a few thoughts suggest themselves.

My early work and interest in the use of scientific knowledge to improve practice and education have become a major concern in the field today, represented as evidence-based practice in the literature, which is now having a major, positive effect on nursing practice. In this regard, nursing is now developing models to translate research to practice and is beginning to address research methodologies to bring research to the practicing nurses and to the bedside. Various methods are now proposed to enable this type of translation of scientific knowledge. One of these methods is meta-analysis; I used this technique to evaluate and summarize ethics research on two occasions, 10 years apart, in collaboration with others (Ketefian, 1988, 2001). These enabled me to combine my early interest in knowledge use (with the recognition that any single study could not, indeed should not, be applied to practice without replications or without the evaluation of a larger body of work to seek confirmation of given findings), with my interest in ethics research and the directions it was taking. This enabled me to assess the state of research in nursing ethics and to set forth recommendations for future directions.

In launching my empirical work in nursing ethics several decades ago, I was among a very small group of people dealing with nursing ethics in this manner; it had been previously thought that one cannot do empirical research in ethics, as it was all about values. However, it was possible to show that while research could not tell people what values they should hold, it could bring forth the value orientations nurses were using in making judgments about ethical issues they faced, along with their actual decisions. This was accomplished through the development of the first instrument to measure ethical practice; its foundation was the Code for Nurses (1976) of the American Nurses Association, which set forth the values of the profession.

When I began my research in ethical practice, I mainly thought of its determinants in terms of personal characteristics and qualities of the individual nurse. A major evaluation of the research occurred with the insight that, as important as the personal qualities of individuals may be, the variables and factors in work environments and organizations are more powerful in shaping behavior, in facilitating or hindering ethical practice. Therefore, I consider the current and ongoing nursing administration research on work environments a wonderful development; while the intent of such research is not expressly to facilitate ethical practice, my research suggests that as work environments for nursing practice improve, become more collegial, as policies are put in place that empower nurses, all of these will be supportive of nurses, and will encourage them to make ethically sound judgments, for ethical practice is ultimately an integral part of nursing practice, rather than something that exists apart from it.

In the area of scientific integrity, my work has served to raise awareness of this area in the field and created the recognition that there are many issues that require attention, by scientists and educators alike. The *Guidelines for Scientific Integrity* (MNRS, 2002), the development of which I led through two editions, has been an important development in the life of that Society (MNRS). It is extensively used by researchers and faculties to guide both their research/scholarly activities and in their teaching/mentoring of graduate students. This is a work in progress. As new concerns emerge with new technologies and societal developments, the guidelines need to be revised periodically in order to serve the field well. The integrity of research is crucially connected to the credibility of the science produced.

One hopes that one has made a difference to one's students' lives of the mind, that one's writings have invited readers to think in different and more creative and productive ways on the issues at hand, and most important, to make connections across boundaries of knowledge. I have found that sometimes impact occurs slowly, incrementally, without one realizing, and over many years. I hope this is the case here.

References

American Nurses Association. (1968). *Code for nurses with interpretive statements.* Kansas City, MO: American Nurses Publishing.

American Nurses Association. (1976). *Code for nurses with interpretive statements.* Kansas City, MO: American Nurses Publishing.

Ketefian, S. (1975). Application of selected nursing research findings into nursing practice: A pilot study. *Nursing Research, 24*(2), 89–92.

Ketefian, S. (1981a). Critical thinking, educational preparation, and development of moral judgment among selected groups of practicing nurses. *Nursing Research, 30*(2), 98–103.

Ketefian, S. (1981b). Moral reasoning and moral behavior among selected groups of practicing nurses. *Nursing Research, 30*(3), 171–176.

Ketefian, S. (1985). Professional and bureaucratic role conceptions and moral behavior among nurses. *Nursing Research, 34*(4), 248–253.

Ketefian, S. (with Ormond, I.). (1988). *Moral reasoning and ethical practice in nursing: An integrative review.* New York: National League for Nursing.

Ketefian, S. (1989). Moral reasoning and ethical practice in nursing. In Fitzpatrick, J. J., and Taunton, R. L. (Eds.), *Annual Review of Nursing Research, 7,* 173–195.

Ketefian, S. (2001). The relationship of education and moral reasoning to ethical practice: A meta-analysis of quantitative studies. *Scholarly Inquiry for Nursing Practice, 15*(1), 3–18.

Ketefian, S., & Lenz, E. R. (1995). Promoting scientific integrity in nursing research, Part II: Strategies. *Journal of Professional Nursing,* 11(5), 263–269.

Ketefian, S., & McKenna, H. P. (Eds.). (2005). *Doctoral education in nursing: International perspectives.* London: Routledge.

Ketefian, S., Phancharoenworakul, K., & Yunibhand, J. (2001). Research priorities in nursing ethics for Thailand. *Thai Journal of Nursing Research, 5*(2), 111–118.

Kim, S. M., & Ketefian, S. (1993). Effects of environmental factors and individual traits on work stress and ethical decision making. *The Journal of Nurses Academic Society, 23*(3), 417–430. [This is the official journal of the Korean Nurses Academic Society.]

Lenz, E. R., & Ketefian, S. (1995). Promoting scientific integrity in nursing research, Part I: Current approaches in doctoral programs. *Journal of Professional Nursing, 11*(4), 213–219.

Midwest Nursing Research Society. (2002). *Guidelines for scientific integrity* (2nd ed.). Wheat Ridge, CO: Author.

Pieta, B. A. (1976). *A comparison of role conceptions among nursing students and faculty from associate degree, baccalaureate degree, and diploma nursing programs and head nurses.* Unpublished doctoral dissertation, State University of New York at Albany.

Rest, J. R. (1979). *Development in judging moral issues.* Minneapolis: The University of Minnesota Press.

Shaké Ketefian is Professor of Nursing at the University of Michigan School of Nursing. She is a graduate of the American University of Beirut (BS), and Teachers College, Columbia University (MEd, EdD). Her areas of teaching have been research in nursing ethics, research methods, and scientific integrity. Her scholarship has dealt with international doctoral education, international nursing, ethical decision-making, and scientific integrity. She has conducted several meta-analytic studies of research within nursing ethics.

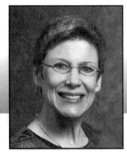

Joan Liaschenko

CHAPTER 18

"...to take one's place... and the right to have one's part matter"

The Question

A retrospective account of one's scholarship cannot be a precise representation. Rather, it is a hybrid of the extant work, the memory of the history of one's ideas, and what one has learned since then. It is the outcome of a dialectical relationship between the ways in which one's earlier work informed what subsequently called out for explanation and how those explanations, in turn, generated new questions. There is a question that has come to occupy me over the past few years, one that I will use to bridge the task of linking legacy and vision within my work. It is a question to which the title of this essay (adapted from Heilbrun, 1988) is an abbreviated answer. But first, the context of the question. I have been exceedingly fortunate in that my teaching and scholarship blend in ways not always possible for many who teach ethics in schools of nursing. And for this, I owe much to Dr. Mila Aroskar, who was instrumental in recruiting me to the University of Minnesota where she was a key figure in initiating, developing, and sustaining ethics education.

Since January of 2001, I have taught nursing ethics to students in the master's degree program three times a year, and to doctoral students every other year. The content and method of my teaching in the master's degree program follows directly from my dissertation, that is, I start where students are. The students are given the assignment on the first day to write a narrative from their practice about which they were ethically concerned. The instructions are to include as much detail as possible about the key persons involved, but with all identifying information removed. These narratives are subsequently discussed throughout the duration of the course. Over the years, two observations have remained astonishingly consistent. The first is that the day-to-day experience of working nurses has changed little since I started school in 1967. I say this from a perspective of first-person knowledge, since I worked continuously from 1970 through mid-1996. The second is that the moral concerns of students' collective experience are overwhelmingly one of conflict between themselves and others involved in the care of a patient.

These observations are not unrelated in that their concerns are linked to the history of modern, professional nursing, gendered labor, class, and the economic independence of women. Nurses' moral concerns reflect conflict with others regarding the moral understandings of a particular situation. The conflicts typically involve competing aims and epistemologies that are most commonly formed along disciplinary boundaries. The majority of their moral concerns involved either end-of-life situations or instances in which a patient was "going bad," and the nurse's concerns and/or recommendations were not taken seriously, were ignored, or dismissed. The narratives describe the nurses' generally unsuccessful attempts to make their case to the relevant people. What captured my attention (and continues to do so) was that students frequently wrote that they should have known more, the implication being that if they did, they would have been able to convince the physician to alter the course of clinical actions. The knowledge they feel they should have known was always scientific. Particularly noteworthy is that this was the case for new nurses and nurses who had been reassigned to areas outside of their practice specialty. Invariably, others dismissed nurses as noncredible knowers and, not surprisingly, "not knowing enough" figured centrally in their moral evaluations of themselves.

On one hand, this is understandable. People generally wish they had been able to do something to prevent or reverse harm, and this is especially the case when a person has special knowledge of some kind. This explanation was not entirely satisfactory to me. I could understand their "desire" to know more, but not the implied assumption underlying the desire that if they did know more, they would have been heard. Likewise, I wondered why they thought they "should" have known more and, if they did, what difference did they think that would make.

Over the years, I became increasingly cognizant that students actually believe that having such knowledge would, indeed, make a difference. They believe they will be "empowered" and finally regarded as equal in value and social status to physicians, at which point their concerns will be taken seriously and not dismissed, ignored, sentimentalized, or trivialized. I found their naïveté shocking. Here were nurses writing in significant detail about issues they identified as moral concerns, e.g., issues of physical and psychological harm to patients and families, and issues that affected their identities as nurses, their moral understandings of responsibilities, relationships, and values. Arresting by their absence were any evaluations of the others they were trying to convince. The language they used was remarkably devoid of moral language. I am not referring to the language of rule-based ethics, care ethics, or religious ethics. Rather, I am referring to language that calls for recognition of moral practices and moral identities, a language capable of reflecting social positionality, work, knowledge, and concerns, a language calling for and expressing the moral understandings of those involved in a given situation. Something like the following: "I am holding you morally accountable to take my concerns seriously because my part in the care of this patient is just as important as your part."

Never, not once, did any student say something like this. Why is this? Why have I never encountered this type of response? This is the question I pursue in this essay.

My Answer

At the most general level, my answer is that nurses do not say something like this because they do not experience the freedom to speak and act in ways that other occupational groups in health care do. "I am holding you morally accountable..." is a communicative act of assertion that does three things: claims a legitimacy to speak; makes the claim of being a credible knower; and demands accountability within a set of social relationships in which power, privilege, and cognitive authority are not equal. As such, it is an assertion of power but not power over, or the power to force. Rather, this power is the "ability to take one's place in whatever discourse is necessary to action and the right to have one's part matter" (Heilbrun, 1988, p. 18). As a group, nurses occupy a social space that privileges others to name what counts as knowledge, moral or otherwise, to label what counts as an ethical problem, and what ways are appropriate to respond.

The social space that nurses occupy in patient care is a space of gendered labor. For most of human history, care of the sick, the dying, and the dead has been done by women. Nursing is part of a long history of gendered labor associated with the body. Such work has been devalued as manual work and shunned as dirty. This is still the case, at least in the experience of my students over the past six and a half years, and in my recent research, just as it was in my earliest experiences.

Hierarchies of privilege, social prestige, and authority abound within groups as well as between them. Those between nursing and medicine receive much press, but there are hierarchies among nurses that are sustained and reproduced through institutional structures. To some, discussions of these issues might seem quaint and unnecessary, but my students show me they are not. I want to be clear here. I am not suggesting that nurses are passive victims to deliberately orchestrated domination by physicians and/or administrators. I am saying social organization is ongoing and accomplished through social actors in real space and time in which identities, responsibilities, relationships, and values are reproduced. This is one side of the issue—the "way the world is" side. The other side is how this is reinforced through language and various social practices by nursing academia, nursing management, and professional nursing organizations.

Nurses' moral concerns are best understood by these two interactive and mutually reinforcing social processes which construct the social identity of nurses as nurses. On one side is the objectified knowledge of bioethical theory and organized medicine, routinely backed by the hierarchical, social order of institutions in which the unequal distribution of power is normalized and reproduced, and which denies nurses' knowledge as knowledge (Ceci, 2004). On the other side is nursing's response. That is, nurses believe that if they had more scientific knowledge or case knowledge (Liaschenko & Fisher, 1999), they would be seen as credible knowers. Nurses fail to claim credit for their nonscientific knowledge that is absolutely necessary for patient care. Following from this, both physicians and nurses fail to see that the knowledge nurses have and the work they do actively contributes to the production of the facts on which the supposedly scientific knowledge depends (Stein-Parbury & Liaschenko, 2007).

Moral concerns are not generic but arise from the organization of social life (Chambliss, 1996). Disciplines, occupational groups, and professions are one way of organizing social life. Central to such organization is the distribution of knowledge and responsibilities among groups. For the purposes of this discussion, I am using "knowledge" to mean a warrant to believe "x" and, therefore, a rationale for acting in a specified way. For example, a nurse can be said to "know" the side effects of "x" drug if she believes certain things. The link between knowledge and action has a special status in the professions. The health care professions are not theoretical disciplines but practical disciplines, that is, knowledge is important not for its own sake but because it enables us to do something to and for patients. In nursing, the link between knowledge and action involves speaking and acting for others (Liaschenko, 1995b). I believe Virginia Henderson said it best: nursing is helping the patient to do what he would do for himself if he had the capability, knowledge, and will (Henderson, 1966). That this definition of nursing is accurate seems obvious. But nurses also speak and act for physicians and particular institutions as well as for other social bodies such as insurers and the state, which is less obvious (Liaschenko, 1994, 1995a, 1998, 2001, 2002).

Furthermore, the concerns are not about issues over which the nurse has sole control, such as whether the patient prefers to have a pillow or a rolled towel supporting her neck and head—and this is not a trivial matter if you are the patient. In this case, the nurse has the cognitive authority to act; there is no need to seek approval from another, demanding that one's concerns be taken seriously. Rather, the concerns reflect issues about which the nurse bears witness but lacks the cognitive authority to act on her own accord. Keeping all of this in mind, the following are factors that influence the mutually reinforcing processes that construct the social identity of nurses as nurses and help to explain the question, at least for me.

In my view, the "way the world is" side includes the following issues:

- Bioethical theory silences nurses by "epistemic rigging" and "conceptual imperialism."

- The privilege and cognitive authority of medicine as an institution powerfully sustains the supposedly objective stance of bioethics.

- Although care ethics was proposed largely as an alternative to rule-based ethics, there are significant limitations to its standing as a robust alternative at the present time. Even feminist bioethicists shun interprofessional relationships, preferring to focus solely on issues directly affecting women as receivers of care, or on the provider-patient relationship.

In my view, the "way nursing is" side includes the following issues:

- Although nursing academia generally believes that the socialization, knowledge, and status of nursing have changed with the move to the university, I do not share this view. In contrast, I think we moved the diploma schools into the university and took the culture of conformity, the commitment to institutional hierarchy, and the belief in the early ideas of a nurse as a proper, middle-class woman, while simultaneously leaving behind what was valuable—skills that students mastered and remembered in their bodies.

- The discourses of nursing and the cultural ethos of both nursing education and nursing administration in health care institutions support and nurture the message that nurses have to be better and do things better than anyone else in health care.

- Within academia, there is a tension between both the meaning and value of "holistic care" and "scientific knowledge," which is rarely acknowledged or meaningfully discussed.

■ Nursing academia, like the culture at large, has a profound ambivalence about care work, and especially, body work, that leads directly to a disdain for staff nurses.

Legitimacy to Speak

"An assertion is a speech act in which something is claimed to hold" (Pagin, 2007). What holds is the identity of the nurse to speak as a nurse and to demand that accountability be mutual and not unidirectional; the right to be seen as a credible knower; and the right to have her part matter. The most striking aspect of the assertion is the use of first person pronouns, "I" and "my." In using these, the nurse takes direct ownership of the words and the meaning she intends and is willing to risk the consequences of their effect on the hearer. There can be no mistake that the listener will fail to note this. There is directness with neither hesitancy nor doubt regarding the legitimacy to speak. Consider much of the communication in busy health care today—it is factual, e.g., the hemoglobin is 16 gm/ml. Using "I" disrupts the statement of facts by stopping action and it is precisely the human embodied person that is put back in. Not using "I" obscures the role of human judgment from embodied persons. As if facts are just out there to be reported but not weighed and sifted through the sieve of embodied judgment within a community, discourse, and network of practices that define what comes to count as a "fact" (Ceci 2004; Code 1991).

In speaking the assertion, the nurse makes the claim that she is a credible knower. She is claiming her ability to take her place in the discourse necessary to action. She is acknowledging that her work is necessary to make the "facts" appear in the first place (Stein-Parbury & Liaschenko, 2007). The right to have her part matter is her acting assumption. There is neither doubt nor inferiority that infects this belief. Thus, the nurse does three things. She changes the terms of the conversation from a merely scientific one to a moral one and she puts the "I," that is, her agency, into that discourse. The "I" is not the generic self of moral theories but a situated "I," the "I" of a particular nurse, right here, right now. And very importantly, it is an "I" that recognizes the interdependence of nurses and physicians to the well-being of patients. In making this assertion, the nurse is saying that accountability goes in both directions.

What I Make of This

Envisioning a nursing ethics for the future is not something that I can readily do. Perhaps it is because I am too rooted in the here and now and, perhaps, because I am in an existential crisis regarding nursing. I no longer know what nursing academia is doing—the logic escapes me. I wonder what identities are being produced and against which nurses will evaluate themselves. What moral resources is nursing academia providing?

It saddens me deeply that nursing increasingly devalues the manual, the bodywork of care work. In this, it is in keeping with a very long history in Western thought. Nursing has made a false god of scientific knowledge—believing it the panacea to its "damaged identities" (Nelson, 2001). As an academic discipline, we try to fix our damaged identities by copying much of what medicine does, even as we vehemently maintain that we are different. I do believe that the devaluation of care work and, by extension, those who do it, is a serious problem. Perhaps, rather than nurses trying to make their cases on the basis of scientific knowledge, those of us in nursing ethics should give Walker's model, that is in contrast to the dominant model of morality as a kind of formal knowledge, a try (Walker, 1998). It would not be easy. Epistemic rigging, privilege, the distribution of responsibilities, moral costs, and those who bear them would be made transparent; some practices will not survive the scrutiny. On the other hand, if our moral understandings do survive the transparency, health care labor would be markedly less hierarchical. Nurses could count on physicians to join them at the bedside (Peter & Liaschenko, 2004), to not abandon nurses there (Stein-Parbury & Liaschenko, 2007), and nurses could help to support physicians in their management of uncertainty. In this model, power is not distributed merely on the basis of group membership. Rather, "power is the ability to take one's place in whatever discourse is necessary to action and the right to have one's part matter" (Heilbrun, 1988, p. 18)—and it is for everyone.

References

Ceci, C. (2004). Nursing, knowledge and power: A case analysis. *Social Science & Medicine, 59*(9), 1879–1889.

Chambliss, D. (1996). *Beyond caring: Hospitals, nurses, and the social organization of ethics.* Chicago: University of Chicago Press.

Code, L. (1991). *What can she know? Feminist theory and the construction of knowledge.* Ithaca, NY: Cornell University Press.

Heilbrun, C. (1988). *Writing a woman's life*. New York: Ballantine Books.

Henderson, V. (1966). *The nature of nursing: A definition and its implications for practice, research, and education*. New York: Macmillan.

Liaschenko, J. (1994). The moral geography of home care. *Advances in Nursing Science, 17*(2), 16–26.

Liaschenko, J. (1995a). Artificial personhood: Nursing ethics in a medical world. *Nursing Ethics, 2*(3), 185–196.

Liaschenko, J. (1995b). Ethics in the work of acting for patients. *Advances in Nursing Science, 18*(2), 1–12.

Liaschenko, J. (1997). Ethics and the geography of the nurse-patient relationship: Spatial vulnerabilities and gendered space. *Scholarly Inquiry for Nursing Practice, 11*(1), 45–59.

Liaschenko, J. (1998). The shift from the closed to the open body—Ramifications for nursing testimony. In S. D. Edwards (Ed.), *Philosophical issues in nursing* (pp. 1–16). Houndsmill, Basingstoke: Macmillan.

Liaschenko, J. (2002). Health promotion, moral harm, and the moral aims of nursing. In L. Young & V. Hayes (Eds.), *Transforming health promotion practice: Concepts, issues, and applications* (pp. 136–147). Philadelphia: F.A. Davis.

Liaschenko, J., & Fisher, A. (1999). Theorizing the knowledge nurses use in the conduct of their work. *Scholarly Inquiry for Nursing Practice, 13*(1), 29–41.

Nelson, H. L. (2001). *Damaged identities: Narrative repair*. Ithaca, NY: Cornell University Press.

Pagin, P. (2007). Assertion. In E. N. Zalta (Ed.), *The Stanford encyclopedia of philosophy*. Retrieved November 27, 2007, from http://plato.stanford.edu/archives/ spr2007/entries/assertion/

Peter, E., & Liaschenko, J. (2004). Perils of proximity: A spatio-temporal analysis of moral distress and moral ambiguity. *Nursing Inquiry, 11*(4), 218–225.

Stein-Parbury, J., & Liaschenko, J. (2007). Understanding collaboration between nurses and physicians as knowledge at work. *American Journal of Critical Care, 16*(5), 470–477.

Walker, M.U. (1998). *Moral understandings: A feminist study in ethics*. New York: Routledge.

Joan Liaschenko, MA, MS, RN, PhD, FAAN, is originally from Philadelphia where she completed basic nursing studies and obtained a BS from Hahnemann University and an MA from Bryn Mawr College. She migrated west where she obtained an MS, PhD, and completed a postdoctoral fellowship at the University of California, San Francisco. She joined the University of Minnesota Faculty in January of 2001 where she is jointly appointed in the Center for Bioethics and the School of Nursing. Both her research and teaching are largely informed by feminist scholarship. She teaches masters and doctoral students in the School of Nursing, which is noteworthy for their commitment to ethics education, requiring ethics at all educational levels: baccalaureate, masters, and doctoral. Through the Center for Bioethics, she has taught courses on 'The Social Construction of Health and Illness' and 'Stories of Illness,' a course that relies primarily on the writings of ill people. Her major research interest is the morality of nursing work, specifically, the ways in which the context of the work shapes nurses' moral concerns, the language they use to articulate them, and how they seek to resolve them. She has studied home care, intensive care units, and psychiatric nurses as well as nurses who run biomedical clinical trials. She has published widely and has been a visiting scholar in Australia, Canada, Germany, Japan, Turkey, and upcoming, New Zealand. She holds adjunct faculty appointments at the Universities of Toronto and Calgary.

⤳ SECTION VI ⤳
CRITICAL THINKING ACTIVITIES

Concerns Related to Vulnerability

✦ Select any essay and tell/create a patient story that represents the author's perspective on the theme of the section. Describe the ethical dilemma it creates and how one might problem solve in that situation.

✦ What are the barriers to and facilitators of nurses acting on what they believe to be the morally correct action?

✦ Erlen raises concerns about derogatory labels of vulnerable patients. What types of patients are particularly vulnerable to this kind of stereotyping? How do you and coworkers respond when a patient is labeled in a demeaning manner? What does labeling do to those who label?

✦ Ketefian asks, "What difference does it make to have high moral reasoning? Will it be translated into practice?" Review Ketefian's chapter and respond to her questions.

✦ Power and powerlessness are central concerns of Liaschenko's essay. What are the tools of power that nurses lack? What are the tools of power nurses possess? Do nurses take advantage of the power they do have to effect change? Are the tools of ethics (principles, theories, concepts) a source of power for nurses?

SECTION VII

Caring and Care in Nursing

These are central concepts for the provision of professional nursing services, especially when integrating an ethical dimension. Care/caring has been variously described as a theory, way of knowing, behavior, and principle, for example.

I Want to Work in a Hospital

Cortney Davis

where it's okay
to climb into bed with patients
and hold them—
pre-op, before they lose
their legs or breasts, or after,
to tell them
they are still whole.

Or post-partum,
when they have just returned
from that strange garden,
or when they are dying,
as if somehow because I stay
they are free to go,
taking with them
the color of my eyes.

I want the daylight
I walk out into
to become the flashlight they carry,
waving it
so God might find them
as we go together
into their long night.

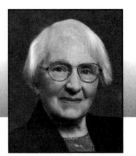

Marie Simone Roach

CHAPTER 19

A New Awakening in the Call to Care

This paper represents the unfolding of my thinking, over 40 years, with highlights of writings and presentations essentially exploring the meaning of human care and its foundation for ethics. The convergence of spirituality and human caring seemed a natural progression of my thought, and global concerns raised a new consciousness of our place in the universe. Issues involving human ecology and our stewardship of the planet Earth, our habitat, are staggering and present new challenges for the moral life.

I became Chair of the Nursing Department, St. Francis Xavier University, Antigonish, Nova Scotia, in 1970, and for a variety of reasons became preoccupied with a need to understand more fully the nature of human caring. I gave the first public lecture, *Care and Caring: The Center and Foundation for Nursing Ethics,* as the Nettie Douglas Fildler Lecture, University of Toronto, in 1979 (unpublished). This was followed by a presentation of the same lecture, sponsored by the School of Nursing, McMaster University, Hamilton, Ontario. In 1979, I was appointed by the Canadian Nurses Association to direct a project on the development of a new code of ethics.

Research on caring proceeded with an inquiry into the question: What is a nurse doing when he or she is caring? The response covered all activities of the nurse, with a list of such a high degree of specificity that appropriate categories had to be developed. These categories known as the five "Cs"—compassion, competence, confidence, conscience, and commitment—became the focus for further writing and numerous presentations to nursing groups. A sixth "C," comportment, was subsequently added. At the request of the Faculty of Nursing, University of Toronto, I prepared the first of their *Caring Monograph Series* (Roach, 1984).

The "Six Cs" provided a practical context for observation and assessment of caring performance in nursing. After using the model of the "Six Cs" for some time, I had a strong intuition that the model, by itself, was not sufficient since it did not address a fundamental question in my inquiry on human caring. This question, "What is caring in itself?" was raised by reflections in my doctoral studies in philosophy of value, a work that subsequently influenced my research and writing. A postdoctoral year as a Scholar in Ethics at Harvard Divinity School provided rich resources and, along with a World Health Fellowship Grant from the Canadian Government, supported my research. This grant enabled me to travel and consult with Richard McCormick, S.J., Georgetown University; Paul Ramsey, Princeton University; James Gustafson, University of Chicago; and many others. While this exploration expanded my thinking and was a most positive experience, the philosophical-theological project itself did not materialize.

Over time I acquired an insight that served as the ground for caring ontology, "caring, the human mode of being." Enlightened by the breadth of research of other scholars, I arrived at meaningful categories from which questions about human caring could be raised—the ontological, anthropological, ontical, epistemological, and pedagogical. My work focused on ontology; caring, the human mode of being; and the ontical category appropriate for reflections on the Six Cs.

From 1986 to 1990, I was a Project Advisor to Jan Dyck, Vice President Nursing, St. Boniface General Hospital, Winnipeg, Manitoba. During this time I taught ethics in the School of Nursing, and in a planning workshop with faculty, revised the method of teaching ethics, identifying ethics content for each level of the program.

The monograph published by the University of Toronto was further expanded into a book, *The Human Act of Caring: A Blueprint for the Health Professions* (Roach, 1987, 1992). The book was also published in Japan. On request of the author, the publisher retrieved the original title of the manuscript, *Caring, The Human Mode of Being: A Blueprint for the Health Professions,* for the 2002 revised edition. This change in title was significant since it more accurately described the intent of my research. Membership and involvement in the International Association of Human Caring greatly influenced the success of my work, promoting global interest, travel, and presentations in many countries.

As I continued my research on caring, I became attracted to the relationship of caring as the human mode of being, and spirituality, later more clearly understood to be a characteristic of being human (Rolheiser, 1999). After 2 years of reading and auditing courses at Regis College in Toronto, I edited a book with 12 contributors (Roach, 1997).

A Seismic Shift in Focus

Becoming involved in an environment project of my congregation, the Sisters of St. Martha of Antigonish, I proceeded from a congregational concern for environmental issues to the critical issues concerning the health and survival of our home planet, Earth. This involvement developed my consciousness of an additional moral call for care of our planet and prompted the writing of a paper, *Caring for Self and the Universe*, presented in June 1998 at a Nursing Reflection Conference, Cambridge University, England. This awakening of the moral demands of our time placed a new and urgent emphasis on the meaning of human care and related ethical responsibility.

A Paradigm Shift and the New Universe Story

A paradigm shift, altering our understanding of self, the universe, and the planet on which we live, is both the gift and challenge of this millennium. An enlightened consciousness continues to heighten awareness of relationship with all creation, and the human being as the celebratory manifestation of the universe becomes conscious of itself. The planet Earth, the most glorious of the planets ever known, is our habitat. Its flourishing is dependent upon peoples of the Earth, newcomers on this planet, existing only within 70,000 years of the universe's 15-billion-year history.

At present and in the immediate future, we are faced with ethical challenges of which we are just beginning to become aware. Nonetheless, the ethical issues and problems of the past will continue to demand our attention, and with the ongoing development of science and technology, they are growing beyond expectation. But for me, the critical issue of our time is that we are destroying all life forms and resources at a rate challenging the highest standards of ethical stewardship. Survival of all life on this planet depends upon the choices we make in the immediate future.

Nolan (2006) reflects on the experience of Jesus, who lived in a prescientific, preindustrial age, relating to all of nature as God's creation, seeing the whole universe as alive with divine action and creativity. The universe of Jesus was full of mystery. In his reflections, Nolan includes the experience of the mystics as an experience of oneness with God and with all of nature. St. Francis of Assisi can perhaps be better understood as living within this paradigm of God, nature, and human beings, not separated but joined in an intimate oneness with God and all creation. And Teilhard de Chardin (1960) taught us to see ourselves as part of an evolving universe, not living "in" the universe, but as part of an ongoing process.

While the new science reveals a time-development portrayal of the universe never before known within modern Western culture, something has been lost in the narrative; primarily, a loss of the sacred dimension of all creation. The influences of mechanism, dualism, individualism, the privatization of religion, and the root metaphor of the machine, radically shaped the way of thought and the development of the Western worldview. Reason became supreme; given time, science was to find the solution to all problems. The loss of balance among the scientific, technological, and the spiritual, between technoscience and the humanities, crafted the erosion of the sacred dimension of all creation, leading to a crisis never before experienced by the human community. We now live on a planet where belief in unlimited economic progress, exploitation of air, water, soil, and vegetation has stretched to the limit the basic planetary resources needed for human survival.

At least 30 years ago, Thomas Berry (1978), in a prophetic appeal, urged us to ponder the meaning of the future in light of:

- Energy sources beginning to fail;

- Pollution darkening the sky, poisoning the seas;

- Tensions between nations and within nations intensifying;

- Military methods growing more destructive;

- Multitudes of mankind doubling in numbers (in the year 2000, 300 cities of over a million will exist; early in the 20th century, there were a dozen such cities);

- Swarming of people toward great urban centers (p. 1).

These concerns are those of every member of the human community and, as Berry notes, we meet as absolute equals to face ultimate tasks as human beings within a human order.

Continued enumeration of threats to the planet at this time can easily immobilize to inactivity (nothing can be done), or mobilize the global community to care for "mother earth" and, in doing so, to care for ourselves. Such an effort starts with one person, one group, with people who, as Von Hildebrand (1953) describes as having an attitude of "religio," of reverence for all of creation. Perhaps this begins with an attitude that moves one to mourn; mourn the loss of land, of vegetation, of all living species, of diminishing the resources available to our descendants (see Hessel & Ruether, 2000).

We need a new story—a new celebratory cosmology that encompasses the universe as community in bondedness, not bondage; that celebrates the Earth as subject, not as object to be exploited and consumed. In the great odyssey that is our story, we need to be empowered with a vision of the human person as a participant, not observer, engaged in a web of relationships. We need a new language that replaces the mechanomorphic language of scientific reductionism; a new language about God and about all creation. We need to re-think our understanding of the biblical creation story, to recover the mentality of the image of the human person bonded with the earth as "farmer," to till and cultivate, not to dominate and subdue (see Hiebert, 2000).

The accomplishments made possible through the genius of physicists and the achievements of science and technology have, on the one hand, developed the capacity to destroy the entire planet and, on the other hand, the capability to pierce the veil into outer space, revealing a universe in the process of expansion, inviting us to capture a new vision of ourselves in relationship with an interconnected cosmos. Responsibility lies in the choice we have in a limited period of time, to opt for planetary annihilation or the ecstasy of greater discovery; to lose or save the most magnificent of all planets, the only one we know to date that is capable of sustaining human life. Caring, as the human mode of being, calls all professional groups to flesh out a timely response. "For what is at stake—is not simply an economic resource, it is the meaning of existence itself. Ultimately it is the survival of the world of the sacred. Once this is gone, the world of meaning truly dissolves into ashes" (Swimme & Berry, 1993, p. 31).

The implications for ethics are staggering! Garesché (1929), in his work in ethics, uses the phrase "noblesse oblige" that inspires and empowers us by the claim that there is something about nursing itself that is noble, calling all of us to assume our identity as persons for and of care. The desire to care is at the heart of our professional lives whether practitioner, teacher, researcher, or administrator.

Health care is a moral enterprise involving professionals, families, and communities. It is a moral enterprise because it brings persons into unique relationships. Whenever we are in a relationship with another person, we establish bonds, and these bonds grounded in trust entail duties and responsibilities—an ethic of relational responsibility. When we studied ethics in the 1940s, the content, when examined in the context of health care in the 21st century, was relatively simple. Nonetheless, I propose the values subsumed under "noblesse oblige" still hold, if not take on greater significance.

As noted at the beginning of this paper, over the course of many years of reflection and research on human caring, I have noted the many ways that nurses expressed caring as administrators, researchers, and caregivers (the Six Cs) and came to an understanding of caring as the human mode of being. One cares, not because he or she fills a particular role, but because one is a human being. Caring is a fundamental characteristic of being human. Humanity may be shown through love or compassion, sorrow or joy, sadness or solicitude, or bruised to the very core of its being. Caring is the unique manifestation of a person's being-in-the-world (Roach 2002, pp. 29–30). This research focused on the "being" of caring, arriving at a caring ontology that has served as a foundational conceptual basis for study and application.

Caring is expressed in virtuous action and in habits acquired over time, and provides the energy that transforms doing things to and for people into service as ministry. Caring is not an exceptional quality, nor the response of an exceptional few. Caring may be expressed with special grace and a unique quality by a special person or, indeed, may not be manifested or expressed at all. Nonetheless, caring is the most common, authentic criterion of humanness. Caring is humankind at home, not through dominating or controlling, but by being who we really are, being real, being true to self (Roach 2002, p. 28). It is human caring that evokes a sense of urgency for the preservation of every species on planet earth, that commits a person more fully to a call to life-giving, life-enhancing, life-protection of human and other kind (see Roach 2002, p. 13).

The Ultimate Moral/Ethical Challenge

Do we have a context that fits the moral mandate of our time, the essential moral foundation stones for ethical reflection? I suggest the following as the basic premises underlying broader parameters for moral discernment.

- The Earth with all its life forms is the primary referent for moral thought and action.

- We live in a relationship with planet Earth, called to a new consciousness of being engaged in an ongoing process within a self-expanding universe.

- Human beings live in a global community where ethnic/religious and national divisions are but arbitrary boundaries separating peoples from each other; the aspiration for all humanity is ultimately the "omega point" (Teilhard de Chardin, 1960).

- Our most fundamental moral attitude is that of reverence, "religio" (Von Hildebrand, 1953).

- Caring is the human mode of being (Roach, 2002).

- The responsibility of stewardship of the Earth is that of each individual living at this time on our planet.

As human persons, we are called to witness by our lives to the virtue of caring. As human persons with a spirituality that is an essential characteristic of our humanness (Rolheiser, 1999), we unfold its potential through the desires and focus of who we want to be (O'Connell, 1998). Herein lies the foundation of our moral lives.

References

Berry, T. (1978). *The ecological age.* Riverdale Papers: Vol 11. Riverdale, NY: Riverdale Center for Religious Research, 1–19.

Garesché, E. F. (1929). *Ethics and the art of conduct for nurses.* Philadelphia: W. B. Saunders.

Hessel, D. T., & Ruether, R. R. (Eds.). (2000). *Christianity and ecology.* Cambridge, MA: Harvard University Press, Harvard Center for the Study of World Religions.

Hiebert, T. (2000). The human vocation: Origins and transformations in Christian traditions. In D. T. Hessel & R. R. Ruether (Eds.), *Christianity and ecology* (pp. 134–154). Cambridge, MA: Harvard University Press, Harvard Center for World Religions.

Nolan, A. (2006). *Jesus today: A spirituality of radical freedom.* Maryknoll, NY: Orbis Books.

O'Connell, T. E. (1998). *Making disciples: A handbook of Christian moral formation.* New York: Crossroad Pub.

Roach, M. S. (1984). Caring, the human mode of being: Implications for nursing. In *Perspectives on caring: Monograph 1 series,* Toronto, Ontario: University of Toronto, Faculty of Nursing.

Roach, M. S. (1987). *The human act of caring: A blueprint for the health professions.* Ottawa, Ontario: Canadian Healthcare Association Press.

Roach, M. S. (1992). *The human act of caring: A blueprint for the health professions.* Ottawa, Ontario: Canadian Healthcare Association Press.

Roach, M. S. (Ed.). (1997). *Caring from the heart: The convergence of caring and spirituality.* New York: Paulist Press.

Roach, M. S. (2002). *Caring, the human mode of being: A blueprint for the health professions* (2nd rev. ed.). Ottawa, Ontario: Canadian Healthcare Association Press.

Rolheiser, R. (1999). *The holy longing: The search for a Christian spirituality*. New York: Double-day Publishing.

Scharper, S. B. (1998). *Redeeming the time: A political theology of the environment*. New York: Continuum Publishers.

Swimme, B., & Berry, T. (1993). The universe story: A new, celebratory cosmology. *The Amices Journal, Winter,* 30–31.

Teilhard de Chardin, P. (1960). *The divine milieu: An essay on the interior life*. New York: Harper & Row.

Von Hildebrand, D. (1953). *Christian ethics*. New York: D. MacKay Co.

Marie Simone Roach, CSM, PhD was born in Scotchtown, on the outskirts of New Waterford, Cape Breton, Nova Scotia. She did primary education there before entering a diploma program in Nursing at St. Joseph's Hospital, Glace Bay, NS, graduating in 1944. She entered the Sisters of St. Martha, Antigonish, NS in 1945. Engaged in health care ministry, she obtained a BSc in Nursing at St. Francis Xavier University, Antigonish; a Masters in Nursing Education Administration at Boston University, and a PhD in Education from The Catholic University of America with a major in Philosophical Foundations. She did further study in ethics in a post-doctoral fellowship at Harvard Divinity School, and a year as Reader at Regis College, Toronto School of Theology for further research and writing on the Ontology of Human Caring, a focus of her professional research and writing. Her studies in ethics were grounded in this research. She is presently engaged in study and writing in the area of Transformative Suffering using the spiritual journey of her own biography as context.

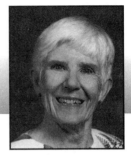

Anne H. Bishop and John (Jack) R. Scudder, Jr.

CHAPTER 20

The Primacy of Caring
Practice in Nursing Ethics

Our interpretation of nursing ethics grew out of our attempt to interpret nursing philosophically. We were interested in the meaning of nursing and, for us, that included its moral dimension. Our first book, *The Practical, Moral, and Personal Sense of Nursing* (Bishop & Scudder, 1990), and our second, *Nursing: The Practice of Caring* (Bishop & Scudder, 1991), both stress the moral sense of nursing. Interpreting nursing as a moral enterprise led us to interpret nursing ethics as integral to nursing practice.

The Context

Our joint work began when Anne accepted the position of founding chair of the nursing department at Lynchburg College where Jack was a well-established professor of philosophy. We soon discovered that we both were interested in the meaning of caring and practice—Jack's particular interest being education and Anne's being nursing. Anne was particularly concerned with whether nursing is a science, an art, or a practical activity. She saw in Jack's phenomenological interpretation of caring and practice a way to "make sense" of nursing. During this period, Anne was awarded a fellowship to a National Endowment for Humanities Seminar, "Ethics in Nursing," at Michigan State University. Upon returning from the seminar, we discussed ethics and how it was being influenced by the stress on technology in health care, especially in medicine. We both concluded that defining ethics as solving problems wrought by technology was a limiting approach to nursing ethics. Nurses treat patients in ongoing caring situations in which the moral and professional are integrally related. In most cases, nurses do not face "once and for all" decisions, such as to treat or not to treat, in the way that physicians often do.

Impact of Our Work on Health Care Ethics

One of our first projects was a conference and an edited publication entitled *Caring, Curing, and Coping* (Bishop & Scudder, 1985). The simplistic assumption that physicians cure, nurses care, and patients cope was challenged by all presenters, asserting that our focus should be on our common caring vocation. A vocation that is designated as caring is going to have moral considerations at its heart, not as occasional occurrences that require "outside" expert help.

Our approach to nursing ethics grew out of our interpretation of nursing as a caring practice with practical, moral, and personal senses. Fry (2001) and Zaner (2001) affirm that our integral approach has contributed to nursing ethics. By practice, we mean a sociocultural way of being developed over time that seeks to foster a good (for those interested, see Gadamer [1976/1981] and MacIntyre [1984]). A practice includes practical methods, science, applied science, personal relationships, moral imperatives, and much more. Rather than being neutral like a science or applied science, nursing practice is designed to achieve human good.

The primary way of being in nursing is caring. The way Nel Noddings (1984) describes caring makes its moral sense evident. The primary moves in a caring relationship are "'engrossment and motivational displacement' on the part of the one caring, and a form of 'responsiveness or reciprocity' on the part of the cared-for" (p. 150). Engrossment means being concerned for the well-being of another and, as much as possible, seeing through their eyes. Motivational shift refers to replacing concern for one's own well-being with that of the well-being of another in a particular situation.

Nursing is learned by engaging in a practice that is inhabited with caring presence. Caring practices are given to the uninitiated through human habitation. Those who fail to appropriate that caring presence often become nurses who think of nursing as a set of fixed skills. When nursing students become interns or engage in clinical experience, they learn more than skills by appropriating the caring presence that originally brought the practice into being. An appropriated caring sense is flexible and open in that it reaches out to different persons in different circumstances.

Zaner (1981) stresses availability and empowerment in caring relationships. Many patients are unable to accomplish thinking and actions without the help of others. When nurses help these people to care for themselves, they are empowering them. However, some patients will never be able to care for themselves adequately. They are empowered by learning how to cooperate with others in order to accomplish certain things. Through disclosing their availability, nurses help patients realize that they are agents of empowerment.

In past years, being a good nurse meant following the rules, "cooperating," and following principles. The stress in our ethics is on "being" a good nurse. Being a good nurse requires, at least, attentive, efficient, and effective nursing practice and the sentiment to care for the well-being of others through that practice.

Good nurses focus on caring relationships with patients, but their concern goes beyond that in seeking the improvement of the practice of nursing and the context in which the practice takes place. Consequently, rather than seeking to preserve the status quo, those engaged in practice, as we interpret it, continually search for ways of improving it and the context in which it works to achieve its moral end.

The meaning of being a good nurse is given primarily through concrete examples disclosing that meaning. In this work, we will attempt to show what it means to be a morally good nurse with two brief examples.

Margie Smith discloses the meaning of being a morally good nurse by becoming a patient's advocate in a situation that requires challenge to usual hospital practice. Margie Smith cared for Mrs. Cooper, 78 years old, who already had an ill-fitting prosthesis and was admitted for another prosthesis for her recently amputated leg. The physician and physical therapist rejected a prosthesis due to her limited prospects for walking. Margie and the nursing staff observed that Mrs. Cooper had skills and determination that made her a likely candidate. Margie persistently, working over five weeks, developed a team approach that not only gave Mrs. Cooper her new prosthesis but, with additional pressure, a replacement for her old prosthesis. Soon she was walking 300 feet with a walker (Smith, 1993).

Why do we consider Margie Smith a morally good nurse? She is a sound practitioner of nursing—the first requirement of good nursing. Her outstanding qualities concern the personal way she relates to her patient, becomes her advocate in the face of professional opposition, and forms the necessary teamwork to foster her patient's good. From her wealth of experience, Margie knows that positive attributes of Mrs. Cooper make success in recovery likely in spite of some limitations. By communicating with others, Margie found that several of the staff shared her assessments of Mrs.

Cooper's prospects and used this knowledge to get the physician to alter the discharge plans and to secure two new prostheses and therapy.

Ethics articulates moral actions in a way that discloses why they are good. An ill or debilitated person needs an advocate most when there is inadequate support for her cause. The moral worth of Margie's advocacy is especially evident in her forming a team of advocates and then bringing those in opposition onto that team.

Ethics could contribute to Margie's grasp of the moral significance of her actions by helping her and others to recognize and articulate the moral excellence of what nurses do. She fails to adequately articulate the moral significance of her actions. She regrets that she cannot describe her actions as "positive team-building" as the profession requires. She seems not to recognize the moral significance of her team building to confront the powers that blocked good action. She describes what she did as playing "an instrumental role in improving the quality of life for this patient" (Smith, 1993). In using the word "instrumental," she is employing language associated with technology and usually considered amoral.

She could have articulated how well she fulfills the moral sense of nursing by using the moral and feminist language of Carol Gilligan (1982) to say that she fostered Mrs. Cooper's good by overcoming opposition from those in charge through cooperative action that empowers from the bottom up. She could say that she works as a moral, as well as a professional advocate, to foster Mrs. Cooper's well-being. In nursing language, professional is often used as a substitute for moral, but in actual practice they are integrally related to each other.

Margie's care for Mrs. Cooper is holistic in that she is continually making decisions in which the moral and the personal are integrally related to her care. Margie recognized how Mrs. Cooper's determination was rooted in her desire to live a normal life. In short, Margie did not care for "any" patient but for Mrs. Cooper, this "particular" person assigned to her care.

In our second edition of *Nursing Ethics* (Bishop & Scudder, 2001), we changed the subtitle from *Therapeutic Caring Presence* (Bishop & Scudder, 1996) to *Holistic Caring Practice*. This edition is actually a reinterpretation of our nursing ethics, recognizing that much of nursing ethics involves ongoing relationships between nurse and patient that involve more than therapy. We gave holistic care a more central place in nursing ethics and replaced "in between care" with "wholistic care." By wholistic, we mean bringing the different specialties together in a more unified, integral care, rather than a negative situation in which nurses are caught in between various caregivers. Nursing, by its very nature, places nurses in a setting that requires integrating specialties in order to foster the well-being of their patients. We use the term wholistic to clarify the distinction between holistic care given to a particular person, and the care that brings together the separate specialties in health care such as physician's directives, administrative support, specialty treatment, the patient's aspirations and abilities, the family, and the specialized care unique to nursing. Margie engaged in wholistic care when she secured the physician's reluctant support and set in motion a cooperative effort of various team members that led to Mrs. Cooper's acquiring two new prostheses and learning to walk again. Having to unify these various forms of care can place nurses in a difficult situation, but it also puts them in a position of great power to foster good.

One way in which nurses find the courage to be morally good nurses is by spiritually grasping the moral sense inherent in nursing practice. A nurse in our fulfillment study related a time when she was ready to quit nursing. She said it was killing her. One day she was bringing a very young child back from radiology when the child stopped breathing while they were in an elevator. She responded with mouth-to-mouth resuscitation. The child recovered, and the mother praised her for saving her child. The nurse said that any nurse would have done the same. "But it was you," the mother replied. This recognition led this nurse to see the moral sense of everyday nursing. That event ended her burnout by infusing her being with the caring presence that is inherent in the practice of nursing (Bishop & Scudder, 1990).

There is a difference between caring for "the" patient and caring for "a particular" person who is a patient. The philosopher Martin Buber (1923/1970) articulates this difference by distinguishing between I-It and I-Thou relationships. By "It," he means treating people categorically. In nursing, this means referring to the patient with such-and-such medical or health problem and then relating to them on that basis alone. "I-Thou" means relating to this person as present to you in a given situation and responding to that person personally. Margie obviously responds to Mrs. Cooper in an I-Thou relationship that says to Mrs. Cooper that she is a person of worth, not just a patient. As Buber says, there are many situations in which you have to relate to other people in I-It relationships. The cardiopulmonary resuscitation (CPR) rescue by the nurse of the child in the elevator is an example of an I-It relationship—a procedure that is done to any patient for a specific purpose. The mother, however, converts that relationship to I-Thou when she thanks "her" as a person, not as a nurse, for saving "her" child.

Although hospital procedure inclines nurses to operate on an I-It basis, nurses discover the moral sense of nursing by relating to patients personally. A nurse, Beverly, made this discovery by facing her patient Midori's impending death with her. They sat in silence with tears streaming from their eyes. Midori spoke first by proclaiming that she wanted to die at home without her family knowing of her impending death. She confessed to Beverly that she felt selfish, asking her to share her burden. Beverly responded by affirming her worth and strength. Later in the day, Beverly returned to wash Midori and take her for a walk. As she washed Midori, she could see her reflection in a mirror. Midori looked weak and helpless, her body constantly straining to stay alive. Beverly knew where in the huge sprawling hospital in the middle of the city there was a place of peace and beauty that Midori would appreciate. A large window that overlooked the busy city in the daytime came alive with flickering lights in the twilight. Midori's plight vanished in the beauty of the moment.

Beverly held Midori gently, affirming her love and concern her. Midori, for a moment, forgot her illness, and then thanked Beverly for helping her through this crucial time of deciding how to spend the last few days of her life. Midori had helped Beverly see nursing in a new way. She realized that the tasks of nursing had come to define her practice. Caring for Midori had shown her "what it 'really' meant to be a nurse" (Dyck, 1989).

The I-Thou relationship between Midori and Beverly infuses Beverly's nursing with a new spirit that is so pronounced that Beverly proclaims that she finally knows what it really means to be a nurse. Beverly was called into being a nurse in the full sense by responding to Midori in a way that gives a spiritual meaning to advocacy. She enters into Midori's situation spiritually, discovering how Midori wants to die, and sensitively assists her to carry out her wishes. Beverly's struggle, unlike Margie's, has nothing to do with overcoming opposition from other health care professionals. Her struggle is in caring for someone who is dying that she has come to respect and love. Often novice nurses are warned against personal relationships on the grounds that they might injure the nurse and may inhibit good nursing practice. Beverly's relationship with Midori challenges this impersonal approach to nursing. Even though she will be hurt by Midori's death, it is evident that this relationship has enhanced her spiritually and morally as a nurse and as a person.

New Directions

Often nurses look for spiritual strength to carry out their moral obligations from sources outside of nursing, especially from religion. Usually this means praying, reading the Bible, attending church, and discussing Christian ethics to bolster the nurse's spirit for facing the tasks encountered in practice. We advocate finding spiritual power and enrichment in the practice of nursing. We have come to call the latter "implicit spirituality" and contrast it with the "cloistered spirituality" in formal religious settings. The story of Midori and Beverly is an example of implicit spirituality in that they discovered the spiritual in their relationship as nurse and patient without reference to specific religious commitments or practices.

Their relationship is an example of an ethic of love. An ethic of love, developed in a Christian context, often contrasts personal love with agape love. Personal love is love that grows out of attachment to a particular person. In contrast, agape love is a love given to all persons without considering personal factors. It is obvious that Midori and Beverly love each other personally and that their love is unconditional. A relationship in which personal love and agape love are integrally related to each other is the most desirable relationship for nurse and patient. We recognize that in actual nursing care, limited time often prevents personal love relationships from developing. In addition, some nurses encounter patients who make unreasonable demands that make it impossible to love them personally. Agape love calls us to care for those whom we do not love personally.

Nurses sometimes make the mistake of thinking of love as a principle or moral standard to be used to judge the goodness of nursing care. Instead, we claimed that stories such as the parable of the Good Samaritan call us into being persons who care for others out of love in varied situations and settings (Bishop & Scudder, 1997). We interpreted ethics as being called to care rather than using principles or rules to govern behavior. As the parables of the Bible call us into being good persons, the stories of good nursing call us into being good nurses. But is acting out of love the only definition of being a morally good nurse? All of us have been in situations in which our love was not adequate to do what we ought to do. When that happens, we believe that one way to be a good nurse is to act out of duty, as advocated by Emmanuel Kant and others. This approach has been so ingrained in nursing care that, in the past, to engage in nursing was called "to be on duty." Currently, nurses often refer to acting out of duty as "being professional."

Granting one's right to autonomously decide how one should die can be well supported by a Kantian ethic. Beverly, however, is not affirming one's rights, she is affirming Midori as a person she loves in a relationship of I and Thou. Speaking of one's rights refers to anyone in a given category. An I-Thou relationship refers to this person directly relating to that person. Granting one's right is primarily an intellectual endeavor, whereas affirming another person's being occurs in a direct and open dialogical relationship between two whole persons who come into being together.

We discovered a way of evoking the spirit of love in dialogical relationships by following a procedure that Wayne Teasdale (2002), a monk, used to evoke the spiritual from scripture and other religious writing. We applied his four steps to the story of Beverly and Midori. When we asked what in the story inspired us, we found that it was the quality of their relationship that came from a dialogical relationship of love. Then we allowed that deeper meaning to affect our way of being in the world.

Finally, we gave thanks for the mysterious source of love that so enlivens and enriches our lives. We have found that reading many stories about nurses in caring relationships has, in fact, deepened our own spiritual life. Thus, it becomes a forceful way of enhancing the spirit of caring love in other relationships.

Spiritual empowerment comes into being when we awaken to and avail ourselves of the caring sense that inhabits the practice of nursing. By inhabiting the practice of nursing, nurses can appropriate the sense of caring that leads to being an authentic nurse. Practice of nursing does not primarily refer to a set of skills and understandings but to relationships between persons who are related in ways that foster healing and health. When this is not possible, as for Midori, the caring relationship supports the dying person in as much comfort, awareness, and dignity as possible. Put succinctly, nursing ethics primarily concerns relationships between nurses and patients that foster the good of each by fulfilling the practical, moral, personal, and spiritual senses inherent in the caring practice of nursing.

References

Bishop, A. H., & Scudder, J. R., Jr. (Eds.). (1985). *Caring, curing, coping: Nurse, physician, patient relationships*. University, AL: University of Alabama Press.

Bishop, A. H., & Scudder, J. R., Jr. (1990). *The practical, moral, and personal sense of nursing: A phenomenological philosophy of practice*. Albany, NY: State University of New York Press.

Bishop, A. H., & Scudder, J. R., Jr. (1991). *Nursing: The practice of caring*. New York: National League for Nursing Press.

Bishop, A. H., & Scudder, J. R., Jr. (1996). *Nursing ethics: Therapeutic caring presence*. Boston: Jones and Bartlett.

Bishop, A. H., & Scudder, J. R., Jr. (1997). On being a neighbor: Nursing's moral standard. *Journal of Christian Nursing, 14*(4), 9–12.

Bishop, A. H., & Scudder, J. R., Jr. (2001). *Nursing ethics: Holistic caring practice* (2nd ed.). Boston: Jones and Bartlett.

Buber, M. (1970). *I and thou* (W. Kaufmann, Trans.). New York: Charles Scribner's Sons. (Original work published 1923).

Dyck, B. (1989). The paper crane. *American Journal of Nursing, 89*(6), 824–825.

Fry, S. T. (2001). Foreword. In A. H. Bishop & J. R. Scudder, Jr. *Nursing ethics: Holistic caring practice* (2nd ed.). Boston: Jones and Bartlett.

Gadamer, H. G. (1981). *Reason in the age of science* (F. G. Lawrence, Trans.). Cambridge, MA: MIT Press. (Original work published 1976).

Gilligan, C. (1982). *In a different voice: Psychological theory and women's development.* Cambridge, MA: Harvard University Press.

MacIntyre, A. C. (1984). *After virtue* (2nd ed.). Notre Dame, IN: University of Notre Dame Press.

Noddings, N. (1984). *Caring: A feminine approach to ethics and moral education.* Berkeley: University of California Press.

Smith, M. (1993). Two legs to stand on. *American Journal of Nursing, 93*(12), 42–44.

Teasdale, W. (2002). *A monk in the world.* Novato, CA: New World Library.

Zaner, R. M. (1981). *The context of self: A phenomenological inquiry using medicine as a clue.* Athens, OH: Ohio University Press.

Zaner, R. M. (2001). Foreword. In A. H. Bishop & J. R. Scudder, Jr. *Nursing ethics: Holistic caring practice* (2nd ed.). Boston: Jones and Bartlett.

Anne H. Bishop is Professor of Nursing Emerita, Lynchburg College in Virginia. She is a graduate of the University of Virginia (BSN, MSN, EdD). She has been writing on nursing as practice and nursing ethics since the early 1980s. She has co-authored books, articles, and presentations with John R. Scudder, Jr., Emeritus Professor of Philosophy, Lynchburg College in Virginia.

John (Jack) R. Scudder, Jr. is Professor of Philosophy Emeritus, Lynchburg College in Virginia. He is a graduate of Vanderbilt University (BA), University of Alabama (MA), and Duke University (EdD). At the time he began working with Anne Bishop, he had been interpreting philosophy of education from a phenomenological perspective. Anne recognized possibilities for interpreting nursing phenomenologically. They have been thinking and writing together since the early 1980s.

⤳ SECTION VII ⤳
CRITICAL THINKING ACTIVITIES

Caring and Care in Nursing

✦ Roach states that, "Nursing is the best way to show charity." Think about the various meanings of "nursing" in this sentence, such as professional nursing or the basic act of nursing someone who is sick or injured. Does the meaning of the word "nursing" change your agreement or disagreement with the claim Roach makes? Why or why not?

✦ Bishop emphasizes that caring is not "touchy, feely, fuzzy, or fluffy." If Bishop is correct, what then is caring? How does your definition compare to the descriptions of care in Roach's and Bishop and Scudder's essays?

✦ Barbara Carper's "The Ethics of Care" article in *Advances in Nursing Science (ANS)* (1979), 1(3), 11–19, is extensively cited in the literature when various authors discuss nursing, ethics, and care. Obtain her article and compare/contrast her perspective on care with either Roach's or Bishop and Scudder's viewpoints.

SECTION VIII

Diversity and Disparities Issues

Diversity means varied, and can include any characteristic of the individual or group that is different from the norm generally seen in the population, from local to international. Diversity requires ethical attention when it results in disparity in the treatment of those persons. Diversity factors include geography, history, occupation, and religion, for example.

continued

The Good Nurse

Cortney Davis

A good nurse kisses her patients when she says good night.
Elie Wiesel

Our kiss is in gratitude
for rumpled sheets, the hourly
turning of patients. For pillows
placed between legs,

cotton booties pulled over raw heels,
and in thanksgiving
for the patients' needs:
Their thirst quelled

by our cold glass.
Their pain,
sharp and relentless as a bee
charmed by our fingertips.

The kiss has everything to do
with sons who look at us
and disappear, daughters
who line their eyes with blue

and borrow our too-loud laughter.
We want to bind them
in our arms. Instead we tend
the patient who longs for us.

He knows we will rush to him,
stroking his earlobe, kissing lightly
his eyelid, his cheek—
not for love,

but for what is constant:
the way skin hurries
to bruise, and the last gaze
freezes the mind.

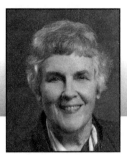

Anne J. Davis

CHAPTER 21

Nursing Ethics and Cultural Diversity: A 32-Year Journey Still in Motion

How It All Began

Thirty-two years ago, in 1975, the Kennedy Foundation opened its postdoctoral fellowship in bioethics to nurse educators for the first time. More than 200 people applied; 12 of us were invited to Washington, DC, for interviews; six of us survived the first interview and had a second; four fellowships were awarded. I received one of these fellowships, and this event changed my career and my life. Without the Kennedy Fellowship, my career would have continued in psychiatric nursing and international health. A year to focus on one discipline without the usual academic demands was as close to my idea of heaven as I may ever get.

While ethics has been in nursing since Nightingale's time with emphasis on the virtuous nurse, bioethics, as an emerging discipline, was fairly new then and greatly influenced by the Beauchamp-Childress book (1979) that focused on ethical principles and rules. I was privileged to be an early participant in what would become a worldwide movement. Mila Aroskar and I met at the Kennedy Summer Institute of Bioethics before arriving at Harvard.

Since our Creighton colleagues asked us to look to the past and the future, this chapter focuses on (a) my early work in nursing ethics, (b) my international professional experiences and how they impacted my work in ethics, and (c) comments about the future of nursing ethics.

Early Work in Nursing Ethics

Early in that glorious New England autumn, Mila and I discussed how we would plan our year and decided to write a textbook which would organize our reading (Davis & Aroskar, 1978). I cannot really remember, but I do not think we had any grand plan that a new nursing ethics book was sorely needed or that it would put us on the national bioethics and nursing ethics maps.

After the fellowship, I returned to the University of California at San Francisco (UCSF) to teach and conduct research, but my focus now had shifted. At UCSF, like other places in those days (and in these) to get promoted, it was necessary to measure and count things in your peer-reviewed publications. While that sort of research is extremely important, less room is left for qualitative research and even less for polemical essays on ethical issues. At the time, we knew little in an organized way of the ethical problems facing clinical nurses, so I decided to embark on a number of "think pieces" (Davis, 1979b, 1981a, 1981b, 1982; Davis & Garrison, 1983), small studies (Davis, 1979a, 1988, 1989, 1991; Davis & Jameton, 1987), and larger studies (Davidson, et al., 1990; Davis, Phillips, et al., 1995; Davis & Slater, 1989) to investigate this aspect of nursing ethics. This approach continued until I went to work in Japan in 1995. Invitations to participate in national and international conferences and to be on national boards kept me busy, along with teaching the Nursing Ethics course twice each academic year at UCSF.

In addition to membership on the UCSF ethics research committee Institutional Review Board (IRB) and the Clinical Ethics Committee (Davis, 1998b; Davis & Kreuger, 1980), a most beneficial aspect of my work was my nonsalaried appointment in Nursing Service at the UCSF Medical Center. I gave nursing service 100 hours of my time annually. I was asked to come to the hospital for an informal ethics round on a unit with the staff about a specific ethical problem they were having. Sometimes it was the entire staff, and other times, the nursing staff. These sessions were not only fascinating, but beneficial to me since this was the clinical front line, with real people grappling with complex ethical issues. I also participated in orientation for new nurses, informing them about the clinical ethics committee.

During this time, IRBs were being established and in places that I visited, the newly formed committee would tell me how they were preparing for this work. As an early member of the IRB at UCSF, I remember my first meeting, when discussion centered on a qualitative research proposal. Questions were asked about the hypothesis, sample size, and control group, for example—all inappropriate for this methodology. After listening, I mentioned the inappropriate nature of these questions and was told by the lawyer member that this IRB would not approve the work of Sigmund Freud or Margaret Mead. My work was cut out for me on this committee.

It was a time that Allison Lurie (1998) might call "the bright full present" in bioethics. Much activity in many directions was afoot. Health care professionals were eager to learn and discuss ethics. Students and clinical nurses arrived at my office for advice, and letters came from all over, telling me about ethical issues. One post marked Budapest sought information about an Ethics Code. And so my days were full of nursing ethics, and time moved on.

In 1989, I received an honorary Doctor of Science degree for my work in Human Rights from Emory University in Atlanta, where I had been a mediocre undergraduate student. Not much had caught my imagination until pubic health nursing and psychiatric nursing courses late in those years. At the same time as this degree, I also received the First American Nurses Association (ANA) Human Rights Award. I had served on, and chaired, the very active ANA Ethics Committee.

My previous international work, coupled with living in large, multiethnic U.S. cities, led me increasingly to focus on cultural diversity in health care ethics. While these remarks reflect my professional life, my interest in international work and questions of morals and ethics began long before the fellowship year. These interests were nurtured around the dinner table with my parents, whom I now thank for their love and guidance. My childhood and early teen years were greatly shaped by World War II, with discussions of the Nazi concentration camps, the U.S. atomic bombs devastating Japan, and later the Nuremberg trials.

When the war was over, with the resulting rebuilding of Europe and Asia, I suddenly saw the world as a place to explore, enjoy, and learn from my adventures. During these postwar years as a psychiatric nurse, I pondered numerous ethical issues long before the bioethics movement began. The foundation for my career shift is easy to see and not limited to the Harvard year.

International Work: Cultural Diversity and Ethics

My work in nursing ethics and diversity can be better understood by looking at my international work from 1962, when I lived in Israel for a year, including time on a kibbutz and later teaching for the Ministry of Health. I taught communication skills to nurses who had immigrated to Israel from many countries, speaking numerous languages and learning Hebrew. The next year I worked in a mental hospital in

Copenhagen. During the 1970s I spent a year on a World Health Organization (WHO) Travel Fellowship in the Sub-Saharan African countries of Ghana and Kenya, with additional months in Nigeria at the University of Ibadan. These countries and those I visited on my way home, Ethiopia, Sudan, and Egypt, left a deep impression about the lives of people, health care, and human rights (Davis, 1964, 1972, 1974, 1984; Davis & Olesen, 1971). My first night back in the United States, I watched television before joining friends for dinner in New York City. One television advertisement informed me that the big breakthrough was new dog food for overweight dogs. Having spent a year in Africa, where about 50-60% of children died before the age of five from preventable causes and recent famines caused deaths from starvation, this, too, left a deep impression.

In the 1980s, a sabbatical in India visiting nursing schools and mental hospitals pushed me to ask many questions about India, but also and importantly, about the United States. With a group of nurse educators, I developed the school of nursing at King Abdul Aziz University in Saudi Arabia, where I graciously refused the first deanship. All of my international experiences, but especially in Africa, India, and the Middle East, led me to write much later:

> This fundamental problem of how to balance the general value of tolerance for cultural differences with the questioning or condemning of cultural practices differing from one's own remains a central issue in discussions of human rights and international ethics, with ramifications for health care and nursing ethics, especially in the international arena. Some years ago, a popular saying was that: "If you don't stand for something, you will fall for anything" (Davis, 2000b, p. 66).

In other words, without some basic global values, anything goes and can be justified as morally permissible, if not actually moral (Davis, 2003). This remains a lifelong question for me.

In addition to my numerous, rich, international professional experiences, involvement in a 1990 WHO-Geneva project on female genital mutilation required that I look more closely and dig more deeply for some answers to questions of cultural diversity, ethics, and human rights (Davis, 1998a). Later, I was involved in another WHO project on long-term care and social justice issues throughout the world and especially in developing countries (WHO, 2002).

But the most profound experiences of cultural diversity and values came from my involvement in Asia. My first visit to Japan for the 1977 International Council of Nurses quadrennial came at the end of the postdoctoral year when Mila and I had just completed the manuscript. For years, UCSF enrolled numerous graduate students from Japan, and I had had the pleasure of working with them. This first visit opened doors for me that later would open more widely and would lead to a wonderful new career when I retired from UCSF after 34 years.

In the 1980s, I began to visit China annually, and together, Lin Ju Ying, then president of the Chinese Nurses Association, and I traveled in much of that large country, meeting nurses and other health professionals. I was invited to lecture, and these were as much a learning experience for me as for them. Because of this close, trusting friendship with Lin, I could question her and she could be frank with me. Her rusty English, gained in her university years, educated me about China and its long traditions and multiple upheavals. With an American and some Chinese colleagues, we conducted two studies in China. One study examined virtue ethics in the first baccalaureate nursing (bachelor of science in nursing–BSN) students (Davis, Ghan, Lin, & Olesen, 1992) in the new China, and the other explored resource allocation for chronically ill children (Davis & Martinson, 1999; Martinson, Armstrong, et al., 1997; Martinson, Davis, et al., 1995), and older people (Davis & Martinson, 1994, 1995, 1998; Davis, Martinson, et al., 1995) being cared for at home.

Two research projects that I conducted while still at UCSF compared and contrasted a variety of cultures. The first project, undertaken in seven countries, Australia, Canada, China, Israel, Sweden, United Kingdom, and the United States examined nurses' attitudes toward physician-assisted suicide and active euthanasia (Davidson, et al., 1990; Davis, Davidson, Hirschfeld, & Lauri, 1993). The other project focused on terminally ill cancer patients and their families from four different ethnic groups: (a) Anglo-Americans, (b) Afro-Americans, (c) Chinese-Americans, and (d) Hispanic-Americans. This federally funded study examined cultural diversity, informed consent, and ethical issues (Barnes, Davis, Moran, Portillo, & Koenig, 1998; Davis, 1996b; Davis & Koenig, 1996; Marshall, Koenig, Barnes, & Davis, 1998; Orona, Koenig, & Davis, 1994).

While still at UCSF and not thinking about retirement, Hiroko Minami, a former doctoral student and today president of the International Council of Nurses, asked me if I would consider teaching in Japan when I retired. In 1995 after all those years at UCSF, I did retire at the age of 62 and fulfilled a prior commitment as a visiting scholar at Ersta Bioethics Institute in Stockholm, and then I joined the Nagano College of Nursing faculty in Honshu, the main island of Japan. I lived in Komagane, population 30,000, located in a lovely valley between the southern Japanese Alps and the central Japanese Alps almost five hours away from Tokyo and another world. My initial two-year contract became six and a half years of living and working in another culture very different from my own, learning much about them and me, and making many good friends.

Japan, Another World View:
International Cultural Diversity

Japan, an ancient culture influenced by China, was isolated (1639–1853) from most of the world during the formative era of modern philosophy and the rise of modern science that laid the foundation of liberal humanism and rationalism in the West. Essentially, Japan remained a feudal society, almost totally untouched by Christian missionaries, until the Meiji Restoration began in 1868 when the United States was engaged in civil war over the moral question of slavery. Emiko Konishi and other Japanese colleagues and I published papers examining the Japanese nursing ethics scene. Among these, we wrote the following comments about Japanese culture depicting the differences found there when compared with the West:

> Ethical traditions are born out of the ethos and mores that have been uniquely nurtured and accumulated in the long histories and cultures in the east and west. Ethics is neither ahistorical nor acontextual. The Japanese word for "self" (jibun) means the socially embedded self and not the individual self. This definition supports the important cultural concepts of mutual dependency (amae) and a reliance on another to make decisions (omakase) as well as filial piety (oyakoko) The sources of ethics and therefore health care ethics in Japan include: Shinto, Confucianism, Taoism, Buddhism (the Ch'an school of Chinese Buddhism or Zen) and Bushido, the code of the warrior (samurai) (Konishi & Davis, 2006, p. 253).

The clear-cut dualism of good/bad and right/wrong characteristic of unilateral determinism in the West is not congenial to the Japanese sense of morality. Morality is socially relative in that it does not lie within the individual but within relationships. I have come to realize how much my thinking is structured in this Western manner.

Teaching the ethics course in Japan to 95 third-year undergraduate students was the single most difficult responsibility in those years. I spent much time thinking about Western ethics and Japanese culture, and how this was like trying to force my big American foot into a tiny Japanese woman's shoe…it did not fit. While I agree with Ruth Macklin (1999) that there are universals at certain levels of a culture, I would be careful labeling certain behavior in Japan as paternalism because it would be so labeled in this country. The most problematic ethical principle, autonomy, assumes a specific definition of the self and notions of individual rights. Even the principle "do no harm," while used in Japan, may have culturally diverse content. The Japanese cultural value, protective truthfulness, is very strong and permits information to be withheld and untruths to be told.

Research in Japan

During my years in Japan, I wrote on numerous topics that interested me (Davis, 2000b; Davis & Konishi, 2002, 2003, 2007; Davis, Konishi, & Tashiro, 2003), or were central to Japanese nurses' concerns at the time (Barnes, Asahara, Davis, & Konishi, 2002; Davis, 1996c, 1996d, 2001b; Davis, Ota, Suzuki, & Maeda, 1999), and conducted research on end-of-life ethical issues which in the West focuses on the individual competent adult. Individual autonomy has been a problem for the Japanese given the above-mentioned values and cultural norms, since their emphasis is on obligations and not on rights. This research then led us to focus on dying and death ethical questions, when there was much discussion about the definition of death and whether to use "brain dead" or not. Decisions in Japan are usually made collectively and often information, especially about a cancer diagnosis, is not given to patients, so others making decisions for them (omakase) is not uncommon. However, many nurses say that while the patient has not been told, the patient knows and this creates problems for them (Davis, 1994; Davis & Konishi, 2000; Davis, Konishi, & Mitoh, 2000, 2002a, 2002b).

These experiences raised many questions about nursing ethics and bioethics, and I began to examine Western ethics differently (Davis, 1996a, 2000a, 2001a, 2002; Lorensen, Davis, Konishi, & Bunch, 2003). I wondered about universalism and relativism in ethics, as well as the influence of American nursing ethics internationally (Davis, 1999). And I began to see more clearly and then question more deeply my taken-for-granted world that holds my ethics to be reasonable and right.

Because of differences found in the Japanese and other cultures that I have visited but know less well, my concern regarding the influence from American nursing ethics internationally has been voiced in several places. I am delighted to act as an informal consultant to nursing ethics projects undertaken by colleagues in other countries, but it is important that we in the United States and colleagues elsewhere have cultural sensitivity to ethical issues and their solutions, which may differ from our own. I do not subscribe to the concept, cultural competency, and wonder if it is useful. We may be better off realizing that we are not culturally competent, since then we might be more culturally sensitive.

Possible Influence

One never really knows what, if any, influence one has had on others. Perhaps the Davis-Aroskar book, simply because it was among the early ones to extend the field beyond virtue ethics, had some impact. It certainly has been used, and work on the fifth edition is underway.

All the national and international presentations and teaching hopefully at least raised questions in people's minds and moved some to be more ethically sensitive. For me the most fun, and the most educational activity, was working with doctoral students. Most of these students were enrolled in the nursing doctoral programs, but others were in theology, sociology, anthropology, and education. Internationally, it is difficult to gauge the difference that my work has made. It certainly made a difference in me. I would venture a guess that I have had as much influence in nursing ethics to date as any nurse or other colleagues in Japan. How much this extends to international nursing is more difficult to know.

In an article examining the content of the journal of *Nursing Ethics* from its first 11 years of publication, the editor wrote, "This meant that an international editorial board needed to be appointed and in this connection, Professor Anne J. Davis needs to be mentioned as a key person in the first decade. Her many contacts world-wide and her experience of the subject matter were invaluable" (Tschudin, 2006, p. 66).

Since I retired in 2001 and came home from Japan, I have been busy with several projects. One is the book on teaching nursing ethics written for an international audience that I mentioned earlier (Davis, Tschudin, & deRaeve, 2006). Another is a project with 13 colleagues in four countries, Australia, Canada, United Kingdom, and United States, focused on women prisoners' health and human rights (Fisher, Hatton, & Davis, 2008). Last August some nurse educators and social scientists spent time at the Rockefeller Study Center in Bellagio, Italy, working on this book. I had wanted to write more on health policy issues, and the work of two colleagues, former doctoral students, led to this involvement. This book is for health professionals who seem woefully uninformed about this population and the health and ethical issues involved. This book essentially says health and human rights are connected, as I noted in a 1971 article (Davis, 1971).

At present a multinational Asian project is underway focused on cancer patients' perception of the Good Nurse. This is one attempt to see if a more culturally sensitive nursing ethics is necessary in Asia. A so-called "Asian nursing ethics" may have similarities with "Western nursing ethics." I am a consultant to this project, and while in Hong Kong in February 2007 working with PhD students, we planned an August 2007 East-West working conference using these data.

The Future of Nursing Ethics

Few of us can predict the future accurately. We extend the past and present into what seems a logical future, but we rely on certain assumptions and lack knowledge of possible future events. Historians refer to this as the fallacy of uninterrupted trends.

So, rather than engaging in predications, I shall list what I would like to see as the future of nursing ethics.

- More dialogue among nurses in the West about virtue ethics, principle-based ethics, caring ethics, and feminist ethics.

- More thinking, discussing, and writing by Asian nurses focused on nursing ethics and what it means for that part of the world. They cannot simply take what has been developed in the West and use it without thinking about the cultural diversity involved.

- Nursing ethics courses become more central to nursing school curricula. Ethics is at the core of our practice. So why is it often absent or an elective course? What does this say about the nursing profession, other than it may not have enough prepared teachers of nursing ethics? And if this is so, why is it so?

I sometimes wonder if we had a Golden Age of Nursing Ethics in the 1970s–1980s, and today we look back on it and wonder why this did not continue. Or this may only be that I have been away learning about and experiencing cultural diversity even more deeply than before.

I hope that in the future not only is cultural diversity factored into what is now mostly Anglo-American health care ethics, but also that nursing's place in health care ethics grows and influences care delivery. To reach this goal, I believe it is necessary to develop required courses in nursing ethics at the undergraduate and graduate levels that focus on the multiple ways we have to frame and address ethical issues. Focusing only on virtue ethics, or principle-based ethics, or caring ethics, or feminist ethics limits the ways nurses think about ethics and does not provide them with the full range of possibilities for the future.

References

Barnes, D. M., Davis, A. J., Moran, T., Portillo, C. J., & Koenig, B. A. (1998). Informed consent in a multicultural cancer patient population: Implications for nursing practice. *Nursing Ethics, 5*(5), 412–423.

Barnes, L. E., Asahara, K., Davis, A. J., & Konishi, E. (2002). Questions of distributive justice: Public health nurses' perceptions of long-term care insurance for elderly Japanese people. *Nursing Ethics, 9,* 67–79.

Beauchamp, T. L., & Childress, J. F. (1979). *Principles of biomedical ethics.* New York: Oxford University Press.

Davidson, B., Vender Laan, R., Davis, A. J., Hirschfeld, M., Lauri, S., Norberg, A., et al. (1990). Ethical reasoning associated with the feeding of terminally ill elderly cancer patients. *Cancer Nursing, 13*(5), 286–292.

Davis, A. J. (1964). Health problems of life on an Israeli collective. *International Nursing Review, 11*(February), 12–15.

Davis, A. J. (1971). The poor can least afford it: Poverty and health in the United States. *International Nursing Review, 18*, 362–365.

Davis, A. J. (1972). Health problems and nursing practice in Sub-Saharan Africa. *International Journal of Nursing Studies, 12*, 1–4.

Davis, A. J. (1974). Preventive intervention: Healing in West Africa. *Journal of Psychiatric Nursing & Mental Health Services, 1*, 7–9.

Davis, A. J. (1979a). Clinical nurses' ethical decision-making in situations of informed consent. *Advances in Nursing Science, 11*, 63–69.

Davis, A. J. (1979b). Ethics rounds with intensive care nurses. *Nursing Clinics of North America, 14*, 45–56.

Davis, A. J. (1981a). Compassion, suffering, morality: Ethical dilemmas in caring. *Nursing Law and Ethics, 2*, 1–2, 6, 8.

Davis, A. J. (1981b). Ethical considerations in gerontological nursing research. *Geriatric Nursing, 2*, 269–272.

Davis, A. J. (1982). Authority-autonomy, ethical decision making and collective bargaining in hospitals. In C. Murphy & H. Hunter (Eds.), *Ethical problems in the nurse-patient relationship* (pp. 62–76). Boston: Allyn and Bacon.

Davis, A. J. (1984). Ethics and international nursing. In M. M. Andrews & P. A. Ludwig (Eds.), *Nursing practice in a kaleidoscope of cultures* (pp. 134–151). Salt Lake City: University of Utah Press.

Davis, A. J. (1988). The clinical nurse's role in informed consent. *Journal of Professional Nursing, 4*(2), 88–91.

Davis, A. J. (1989). Informed consent process in research protocols: Dilemmas for clinical nurses. *Western Journal of Nursing Research, 11*(4), 448–457.

Davis, A. J. (1991). The sources of a practice code of ethics for nurses. *Journal of Advanced Nursing, 16*, 1358–1262.

Davis, A. J. (1994). Search for meaning in life and death. *Journal of Hospice and Palliative Care in Japan, 4*(5), 368–372.

Davis, A. J. (1996a). A critique: Aspects of moral knowledge in nursing. *Scholarly Inquiry for Nursing Practice, 9*(4), 355–358.

Davis, A. J. (1996b). Ethics and ethnicity: End-of-life decisions in four ethnic groups of cancer patients. *Medicine and Law, 15,* 429–432.

Davis, A. J. (1996c). Nursing ethics in terminal care. *Nursing Education, 37,* 27–31. (In Japanese).

Davis, A. J. (1996d). Some ethical questions about HIV infected blood: The Japan case. *Kango, 12,* 32–38. (In Japanese).

Davis, A. J. (1998a). Female genital mutilation: Some ethical questions. *Medicine and Law, 17,* 6–10.

Davis, A. J. (1998b). A nursing perspective of ethics committees in health care and research: Promises and paradoxes. In K Hoshino (Ed.), *The Memorial International Symposium for Liaison Society of Ethics Committees of Medical Schools in Japan: The role of ethics committees-international comparisons* (pp. 37– 48). Kyoto, Japan: Onbunkaku Shuppan Sha.

Davis, A. J. (1999). Global influence of American nursing: Some ethical issues. *Nursing Ethics, 6,* 118–125.

Davis, A. J. (2000a). The bioethically constructed ideal dying patient in the U.S.A. *Medicine and Law, 19*(1), 161–164.

Davis, A. J. (2000b). Ethics in international nursing: Issues and questions. In N. Chaska (Ed.), *The nursing profession: Tomorrow and beyond* (pp. 65–74). London: Sage Publications.

Davis, A. J. (2001a). Labeled encounters and experiences: Ways of seeing, thinking about, and responding to uniqueness. *Nursing Philosophy, 2*(2), 101–111.

Davis, A. J. (2001b). Trends in the ethics of conducting nursing research with human subjects. *Japanese Journal of Nursing Research, 162,* 3–8.

Davis, A. J. (Ed.). (2002). *Nursing ethics: Theory, practice and research.* Tokyo: Japanese Nursing Association. (In Japanese).

Davis, A. J. (2003). International nursing ethics: Content and concerns. In V. Tschudin (Ed.), *Approaches to ethics: Nursing beyond boundaries* (pp. 95–104). Edinburgh: Butterworth-Heinemann.

Davis, A. J., & Aroskar, M. A. (1978). *Ethical dilemmas and nursing practice.* New York: Appleton-Century-Crofts.

Davis, A. J., Davidson, B., Hirschfeld, M., & Lauri, S. (1993). An international perspective of active euthanasia: Attitudes of nurses in seven countries. *International Journal of Nursing Studies, 30,* 301–310.

Davis, A. J., & Garrison, S. H. (1983). Least restrictive alternative: Ethical considerations. *Journal of Psychosocial Nursing, 21*, 17–23.

Davis, A. J., Ghan, L. C., Lin, J. Y., & Olesen, V. (1992). The young pioneers: First baccalaureate nursing students in the People's Republic of China. *Journal of Advanced Nursing, 17*, 1166–1170.

Davis, A. J., & Jameton, A. (1987). Nursing and medical students' attitudes toward nursing disclosure of information to patients. *Journal of Advanced Nursing, 12*(6), 691–698.

Davis, A. J., & Koenig, E. (1996). A question of policy: Bioethics in a multicultural society. *Nursing Policy Forum, 2*(1), 6–11.

Davis, A. J., & Konishi, E. (2000). End-of-life ethical issues in Japan. *Geriatric Nursing, 21*, 89–91.

Davis, A. J., & Konishi, E. (2002). The ethics of peer review. *Quality Nursing, 8*, 49–56. (In Japanese).

Davis, A. J., & Konishi, E. (2003, October 6). Vulnerable by tradition: Ethics data for advocacy intervention. *Vulnerable groups in society: A nursing issue* [Third European Nursing Congress Proceedings], Amsterdam, Netherlands.

Davis, A. J., & Konishi, E. (2007). Whistle blowing in Japan. *Nursing Ethics, 14*, 194–202.

Davis, A. J., Konishi, E., & Mitoh, T. (2000). Rights and duties to die: Perceptions of nurses in the west and in Japan. *Eubios Journal of Asian and International Bioethics, 10*, 11–13.

Davis, A. J., Konishi, E., & Mitoh, T. (2002a). Framework for information disclosure to the terminally ill in Japan. In A. J. Davis (Ed.), *Kango Renri: Riron, Jissen, Kenkyuu* (pp.213–222), [Nursing ethics: theory, practice and research]. Tokyo: Japanese Nurses Association. (In Japanese).

Davis, A. J., Konishi, E., & Mitoh, T. (2002b). Telling and knowing of dying: The philosophical bases for hospice in Japan. *International Nursing Review, 29*, 226–233.

Davis, A. J., Konishi, E., & Tashiro, M. (2003). A pilot study of selected Japanese nurses' ideas on patient advocacy. *Nursing Ethics, 10*, 404–413.

Davis, A. J., & Kreuger, J. (1980). *Patients, nurses, ethics.* New York: American Nurses Association.

Davis, A. J., & Martinson, I. (1994). The impact of chronic illness on the urban elderly and their caregivers in the PRC. *Chinese Journal of Nursing, 4*, 3–7. (In Chinese).

Davis, A. J., & Martinson, I. (1995). Informal care givers in the Peoples' Republic of China: Caring for the urban chronically ill elderly at home. *Journal of Cross-cultural Gerontology, 2*, 76–81.

Davis, A. J., & Martinson, I. (1998). Informal care givers for urban chronically elderly people at home in the People's Republic of China: A qualitative study. *Health Care in Later Life, 3,* 3–14.

Davis, A. J., & Martinson, I. (1999). Care for chronically ill children and elderly in the People's Republic of China. *Nursing and Health Sciences, 1,* 229–233.

Davis, A. J., Martinson, I., Ghan, L. C., Liang, Y. H., Jin, Q., & Lin, J. Y. (1995). Home care for the urban chronically ill elderly in the People's Republic of China. *International Journal of Aging and Human Development, 41,* 345–358.

Davis, A. J., & Olesen, V. (1971). Communal work and living: Notes on the dynamics of social distance and social space. *Sociology and Social Research, 55*(2), 191–202.

Davis, A. J., Ota, K., Suzuki, M., & Maeda, J. (1999). Nursing students' response to a case study in ethics. *Nursing and Health Science, 1,* 3–6.

Davis, A. J., Phillips, L., Drought, T. S., Sellin, S., Ronsman, K., & Hershberger, A. K. (1995). Nurses' attitudes toward active euthanasia. *Nursing Outlook, 43*(3), 174–179.

Davis, A. J., & Slater, P. V. (1989). U.S. and Australian nurses' attitudes and beliefs about the good death. *Journal of Nursing Scholarship, 21,* 34–39.

Davis, A. J., Tschudin, V., & deRaeve, L. (2006). *Essentials of teaching and learning in nursing ethics: Perspectives and methods.* Edinburgh: Churchill Livingstone/Elsevier.

Fisher, A., Hatton, D. C., & Davis, A. J. (2008). Women prisoners, health, and human rights. In V. Tschudin, & A. J. Davis (Eds.), *Globalization of nursing: Ethical, legal, political issues.* Abingdon, U.K.: Radcliffe Publishing.

Konishi, E., & Davis, A. J. (2006). The teaching of nursing ethics in Japan. In A. J. Davis, V. Tschudin, & L. de Raeve (Eds.), *Essentials of teaching and learning in nursing ethics: Perspectives and methods* (pp. 251–260). Edinburgh: Churchill Livingstone/Elsevier.

Lorensen, M., Davis, A. J., Konishi, E., & Bunch, E. (2003). Ethical issues after the disclosure of a terminal illness: Danish and Norwegian hospice nurses' reflections. *Nursing Ethics, 10,* 175–185.

Lurie, A. (1998). *The last resort.* New York: Henry Holt.

Macklin, R. (1999). *Against relativism: Cultural diversity and the search for ethical universals in medicine.* New York: Oxford University Press.

Marshall, P., Koenig, B. A., Barnes, D. M., & Davis, A. J. (1998). Multiculturalism, bioethics, end-of-life care: Narratives of Latina cancer patients. In D. Thomasma & J. Monagle (Eds.), *Health care ethics: Critical issues for 21st century* (pp. 421–431). Gaithersburg, MD: Aspen Publishers.

Martinson, I., Armstrong, V., Qiao, J., Davis, A., Yi-Hua, L., & Gan, M. (1997). The experiences of the family of children with chronic illness at home in China. *Pediatric Nursing, 23*(4), 371–375.

Martinson, I., Davis, A. J., Liu-Chiang, C. Y., Liang, Y. H., Jin, Q., Ghan, L. C., et al. (1995). Chinese mothers' reactions to their child's chronic illness. *Health Care for Women International, 16*(4), 365–375.

Orona, C. J., Koenig, B. A., & Davis, A. J. (1994). Cultural aspects of nondisclosure. *Cambridge Quarterly of Healthcare Ethics, 3,* 338–346.

Tschudin, V. (2006). How nursing ethics as a subject changes: An analysis of the first 11 years of publication of the journal Nursing Ethics. *Nursing Ethics, 13*(1), 65–75.

World Health Organization. (2002). *Ethical choices in long-term care: What does justice require?* Geneva: Author.

Anne J. Davis is a Professor Emerita, retired, from the University of California, San Francisco. Her career at UCSF spanned 34 years. Beginning in 1962, Dr. Davis's teaching experience took on an international component with appointments in Israel, Japan, Korea, and Taiwan. These rich experiences led to the development of her overriding interest in cultural diversity and nursing ethics. She is a graduate of Emory University, Atlanta (BS, Nursing), Boston University (MS, Psychiatry), and University of California, Berkeley (PhD, Higher Education). Dr. Davis has been the recipient of numerous awards including an honorary Doctor of Science from Emory University and election as a Fellow in the American Academy of Nursing.

Anita J. Tarzian

CHAPTER 22

Exploring Diversity and Disparities: An Evolving Journey

The roots of my interest in ethical concepts have shaped a rather unconventional career thus far. Here I will explore the scope of diversity in health care and describe the conundrum that is presented to the scholar who must choose a focus among a multitude of ethical problems. I call for expanding ethics education in nursing and involving nurses in ethical decision-making, debate, scholarship, and research across academic and health care settings at a global level.

Framing the Issue

End-of-life (EOL) and palliative care, culture, and ethics are umbrella concepts that impact health care across disciplines and subspecialties. Having chosen these areas for my professional focus makes identifying my specific contributions a bit of a challenge. I'm proud that the themes of diversity and disparities emerge from my work, as they are foundational concepts in both nursing and ethics. When we talk about "diversity," many think merely in terms of racial or ethnic differences and the need to be "tolerant," implying that diversity is measured in terms of degree of difference from a dominant group, and should be "put up with" by that group to avoid conflict. Beyond culture, ethnicity, and race, differences exist in terms of gender, age, physical and mental abilities, religion, sexuality, education, family structure, and socioeconomic status. A descriptive approach advocates recognizing that diversity exists; a normative approach advocates promoting diversity in actions that we take.

Unfortunately, these diversity issues often get short shrift in nursing school curricula, despite their ever-presence in clinical care. The trend to integrate them throughout the curriculum, recognizing their wide scope of application, unfortunately increases the chance that they fall through the cracks or are only superficially addressed. I once heard about a Nigerian nursing student taken to the hospital for a presumed psychotic break. Her loud wailing and prostrations, it turned out, followed failing an important exam. Her behavior was thus a culturally acceptable form of response to the shock and despair of academic failure, a source of tremendous shame to her family. I was struck by how often we get the Golden Rule backward and how much we could benefit from learning more about our own and others' cultural beliefs and traditions. For example, cultural norms could affect an understanding of plagiarism. Foreign students from more communitarian cultures could have special needs, where fiercely protecting a single individual's "intellectual property" may not be a shared value. Both nursing students and faculty should be encouraged to examine their own cultural norms, values, and beliefs as the first steps toward "cultural competence."

The term "cultural competence" evolved from Madeleine Leininger's work (1991, 2002), whose goal in her theory of transcultural nursing is to provide "culturally congruent and competent care." The term "cultural competence" has been criticized as overly ambitious, and I tend to agree—it would take years of living in another culture to come close to being able to deliver such care. Superficial approaches to achieve cultural competence may paradoxically lead to stereotyping and do more harm than good. In my opinion, "cultural competence" grows out of cultural self-awareness, and the latter is partly developed by exploring how culture influences one's own and others' values, beliefs, and practices, a process akin to Hunt's (2001) conception of "cultural humility."

Recruiting faculty and clinical staff that represent the student or patient population is important. Cortis (2003) suggests the following to achieve "culturally competent" health care providers: (a) promoting equality, recognizing that "being equal does not necessarily mean being the same" (p. 37), (b) valuing difference, and (c) challenging racism. I would amend the latter to "challenging bigotry" of any kind (e.g., based on religion, gender, culture).

Next, promoting these activities among all nurses could also serve to address the growing disparities in quality and access to needed health care among poor and minority groups, as shown in two major reports (National Academy of Sciences [NAS], 2002; U.S. Department of Health and Human Services, 2003). The Institute of Medicine (IOM) reviewed over 100 studies involving quality of health care for different racial and ethnic minorities, controlling for a number of relevant variables. Of great concern to the study committee was the consistency of research findings, " ...

even among the better-controlled studies, the vast majority indicated that minorities are less likely [than] . . . whites to receive needed services, including clinically necessary procedures, . . . [in] a number of disease areas . . . and [for] a range of procedures. [The committee concluded, although] myriad sources contribute to these disparities, some evidence suggests that bias, prejudice, and stereotyping on the part of health care providers may contribute to differences in care" (NAS, p. 2).

Pivotal Experiences along the Way

Looking back on my experiences, I notice significant contributors to my long-standing interests in race and culture. Early in my nursing career, at a large medical center in inner-city Chicago, I was surrounded by racially diverse coworkers and patients. Chicago has an unfortunate history of racial tension. As a young person, I held idealistic hopes for bridging differences and overcoming disparities. During a year abroad in Barcelona, Spain, as an undergraduate, I learned first-hand how culture influences our values and behaviors. I found a natural progression of my dual interests in race and culture when serving as a Peace Corps volunteer in the Dominican Republic (DR). Dominicans share a distinct Latin-Caribbean culture, but would be considered black by race. Yet, they do not have a word in Spanish for a "black" or "white" person; rather, they have names for various shades of skin tone. Racism is still present there (against darker-skinned people), but begs the question of "what is race?" And how is it influenced by socioeconomic class and politics?

In my first years as a nurse working in a surgical-oncology floor at a large, tertiary-care medical center, I quickly became involved in issues related to end-of-life care and decision-making. This was in the mid-1980s, when hospital ethics committees were just beginning to emerge, and the hospice movement was starting to gain momentum. Yet, "slow codes" were still called, and "do not resuscitate" (DNR) orders were rarely written. My interest in clinical ethics began with my experiences caring for patients who knew they were dying, knew what they wanted, but whose wishes were not followed. Physicians were still functioning within a paternalistic framework where patients were "protected" from the truth. I became involved in studying the issue of DNR orders at that hospital, which had no ethics committee at the time.

The fates converged when I returned from the Peace Corps, as I was accepted as a graduate student at the University of Maryland where I was able to combine my interests in culture (at the master's level) and ethics (at the doctoral level). When working as a hospice nurse during my graduate studies, I noticed that, while a lot of attention had been given to pain management at the end of life, little had been given to other symptoms like shortness of breath. I decided to focus on acute breathlessness or "air hunger" for my dissertation, partly because of my patients' experiences (Tarzian, 2000). Such patients and their caregivers evoked vulnerability at its extreme. Yet, how did I choose the topics of "DNR orders" and "air hunger" as my focus from the many problems I confronted?

Two related memories come to mind. The first is a grand rounds lecture I gave at University of California at Davis in 1998. I spoke about how air hunger in a dying patient should be considered a "palliative care emergency," one that demands a paradoxical combination of rapid response and calming presence. In discussing how palliative care at the end of life differs from the typical high-tech medical care that the hospital staff is used to providing, one physician in attendance raised his hand. He recognized the need to provide a holistic approach to address a dying patient's need for physical, psychological, spiritual, and emotional care that also addressed needs of the family. But how could he possibly meet all of his patient's needs?

His understandable reaction is no stranger to me. I'm thinking of one of the many mornings that I sat in my rocker in the pine-board, tin-roofed, window-slatted room in La Descubierta, D.R., during my stint as a Peace Corps volunteer from 1990–1992. I would ponder what to do that day, whether it would lead to any lasting benefit for anyone. A lot of sickness could be avoided by focusing on basic hygiene and health promotion through education. Health education, that's where I would focus my energy. Yet, would not raising the basic level of education by improving the school system make more sense? Right. What the town's people needed was a better formal educational system. But wait. I saw a lot of children who were clearly undernourished having trouble focusing in school. No one can learn without proper nutrition. One would have to start with access to a balanced diet through sustainable agriculture and livestock projects. But that takes capital. Okay, so microenterprise is the way to start, perhaps small loans to support economic development to provide funding for people to grow and manage their own food supply. But wait. That requires educating people. Back to the beginning: an infinite regress! Where should I start?

Well, first, with a pronoun adjustment. There was little hope that "I," alone, could do much to help the people of La Descubierta. Similarly, the physician querying about meeting all of his patients' many needs must realize that he simply cannot, not by himself. So that's the first lesson. If we focus too much on what "we alone" can do to "fix the world," it can overwhelm us to the point of hopelessness and inaction—we need to look for allies. The second lesson here is this: faced with multiple needs, deciding which should be acted upon is difficult. Sometimes what needs to be done is obvious and we just need to find material resources or courage to act. Other times we are faced with too many choices and we have to pick one, without the luxury of knowing the best choice beforehand. Why did I choose to address the ethics of end-of-life decision-making in my early career? Partly because it presented itself to me. But also, because the patients I cared for who were living with a terminal illness and impending death, and their families, were at their most vulnerable and lacked advocates—I knew I could help.

Over the years, I've thought a lot about how to teach end-of-life care, ethics, and cultural sensitivity to health care professionals (HCPs) and students. One of the biggest challenges has been addressing the affective component inherent in each. How do we get beyond biases grounded in our own emotional land mines or blind spots, or religious or cultural teachings of which we may not even be aware? The work of Levine (1982, 1984, 1991) and Storti (1999) influenced my work. I was careful to include self-awareness-promoting experiential exercises in a Train-the-Trainer program I created for a local hospital on Communications Competence (i.e., successfully communicating with persons who speak a different language than the health care provider, are from a different culture, and/or who are blind, deaf, hearing-impaired, or speech-impaired). This led to other opportunities to address the topic of diversity in health care. For example, I served as a review panel member in the American Medical Association's Ethical Force Program, "Improving Communication—Improving Care," which focused on a comprehensive approach to improving HCP communication with persons from different cultures and for whom English was not their primary language.

After graduate school, I was fortunate to meet Diane Hoffmann and was able to collaborate with her and others at the Law and Health Care Program at the law school, which gave me a unique perspective about the place of law in ethics, particularly when discussing advocacy, the protection of vulnerable populations, and public policy. I started working with the Maryland Health Care Ethics Committee Network (MHECN), a local ethics network that provides resources to health care ethics committee members. My involvement allowed me to bridge case-based clinical ethics with community and public policy approaches. I am able to interact with HCPs from all areas of both academia and clinical care, and I sense their frustration. They were trained to do more than assembly-line care, but the current trends in health care are pushing in that direction, leading many to question whether they should leave their profession. I see doctors and nurses entering law school to make a change in the health care system to bring about more fair-minded care. Local ethics networks facilitate one way of addressing these concerns through multidisciplinary cross-fertilization, education, and policy initiatives (Tarzian, Hoffman, Volbrecht, & Meyers, 2006).

In 2002–2003 I served on the advisory board of the American Nurses Association's (ANA) Center for Ethics and Human Rights. The ANA's commitment to issues of diversity and addressing disparities impressed me, evident by the many position statements adopted over the past 20 years. As a member of the American Society for Bioethics and Humanities' Board of Directors (ASBH) for the past 4 years, I appreciate the ANA's ability to take stands and participate in lobbying efforts to effect change, promoting better care for patients. In 2001, the ASBH debated whether to take stands or not. The emerging consensus, after heated discussions on the topic, was that a professional bioethics society should be apolitical—because of tax-exempt requirements and ASBH's core of diversity. Given the organization's nature, consensus about substantive moral issues would not be possible or meaningful.

The above examples raise the issues of the relationship between an organization and each individual member and between the organization and the society in which it resides. The ANA, for example, recognizes that nurses are constrained from practicing according to their code of ethics by various societal barriers, including inadequate health care coverage/access for their patients and unsafe workplace environments. Thus, the ANA takes public positions on these issues, which influence ethical practice and individual health. Although, regrettably, relatively few nurses are members, ANA speaks for all nurses, and their example showcases how ethics in nursing is primarily grounded in patient care.

Reflections on My Contributions Thus Far

Commenting on the impact of my work on health care ethics is a daunting task, partly because I feel that I'm only in the late spring or summer of my professional career. How is such impact measured? Nurturing relationships with students or colleagues? Seeds planted for future germination? By peer-reviewed publications? Teaching and lecturing? All of the above, I think. Looking at my scholarly publications, I would categorize them in four domains: pain management (Hoffmann & Tarzian, 2001, 2003a, 2003b; Tarzian, Davidson, & Hoffmann, 2002; Tarzian & Hoffman, 2005), end-of-life care (Cohen, Phillips, & Tarzian, 2001; Hoffmann & Tarzian, 2005; Tarzian, 2005; Tarzian, Neal, & O'Neil, 2005; Tarzian & Schwarz, 2004), health care ethics committees (Hoffmann & Tarzian, 2008; Hoffmann, Tarzian, & O'Neil, 2000; Tarzian, Hoffmann, et al., 2006), and resource allocation (Hoffmann & Tarzian, 2002, 2003c, 2003d; Lisle, Tarzian, Cohen, & Trinkoff, 1999; Tarzian & Silverman, 2002). My publications in end-of-life care represent the domain in which diversity and disparities are most closely addressed. Yet I am left with a dilemma. Persons who are dying deserve to have HCPs address their physical, psychological, and spiritual needs, and the fact that this does not happen for avoidable reasons is unjust. There are many ethical issues that demand attention but go largely unnoticed. Research results have shown that nurses encounter more ethical issues than they identify as such. Why is it that most requests for ethics consultations in health care facilities involve issues related to

EOL care, such as withholding and withdrawing treatment? While clearly "life and death" situations demand prompt attention, what are we to do with the other niggling ethical problems that surface daily?

My own response to the dilemma of focusing my work on end-of-life care when there are so many competing priorities has been to try to incorporate marginalized viewpoints when I can, which might be a rather unorthodox approach. Traditional academic wisdom advocates picking one area to pursue and to continually build on it. Instead, I pursue projects which present themselves to me which have in common the threads of advocacy for vulnerable persons and diversity. In the focus group study I conducted with two colleagues, we addressed an EOL issue within a marginalized population: homeless persons (Tarzian, Neal, & O'Neil, 2005). This provided an opportunity to explore and give voice to individuals typically overlooked when addressing disparities in EOL care. Similarly, I explored perspectives of African-American women regarding breast cancer screening with two colleagues, to see how this culture influences women's views toward cancer and death (Cohen, Phillips, & Tarzian, 2001).

Research findings provide useful tools to advocate for change, but academics often consider their work "finished" when their paper is published in a peer-reviewed journal. While this is important, other venues of dissemination are essential, even critical. As one example, two projects funded by the Mayday Fund received national attention by way of press briefings. In one case, this led to a feature story in the New York Times (Wartik, 2002), which resulted in a contact who had mutual research interests from our very own campus.

What Lies Ahead?

One might ask, what's the value of "professionalizing" ethics in nursing? The nurse who successfully works through an ethical conflict in clinical practice without identifying herself as "doing ethics" likely possesses a similar knowledge and skill set as the nurse ethicist. From my experience, formal education in ethics is beneficial. First, we can help develop a theoretical foundation in ethics that includes a nursing perspective. Ethics promotes thinking more broadly than the individual patient to systems and policies that facilitate "doing the right thing" for groups of patients and society in general. Formally educating nurses will allow them to converse with others in the field and better represent patients and their well-being. The sheer number of nurses in the world provides an opportunity to translate ethical concepts to the lay public, allowing citizens across the globe to make more informed decisions and contribute to public debate about health care priorities in an increasingly complex health care environment. I predict a growing trend toward application of "evidence-based practice" to the field of ethics and related public policy. Yet, there are dangers inherent in equating value with what can be measured as a good "outcome." Nurse ethicists can play a pivotal role in ensuring that patients' rights and best interests are well-represented in clinical care, health care financing, and policy.

In nursing's early years as a professional discipline, members focused internally in an effort to establish credibility. I think the 21st century holds promise for nurses to integrate more fully into all levels of health care, ethics, political life, and professional societies. We must address the inequities in our health care system that prevent us from making fair-minded decisions about the allocation of health care resources. We need a more educated citizenry and basic health care coverage for all citizens that allows limits to be set on high cost-low benefit procedures. Until then, we will continue to practice default rationing, which has resulted in U.S. citizens paying more per capita than any other developed country but showing poorer outcomes (Davis, et al., 2007). In addition to working with other health care professionals, we must also reach out beyond national borders. I would like to think I could have some part in helping make this transition toward a new vision for nurses and bioethics.

Earlier I mentioned my experiences in La Descubierta and how I struggled trying to identify where to start in order to effect needed change. I concluded that sometimes "how" you effect change in an area is just as important (or more so) than what you immediately accomplish, particularly since true change takes time. As Ghandi stated, we must become the change we want to see in the world (cited in Shapiro, 2006). I believe that. And I believe that nurses with solid knowledge and skills in health care ethics are in the best position to promote positive change.

References

Cohen, M. Z., Phillips, J. A., & Tarzian, A. J. (2001). African-American women's experiences with breast cancer screening. *The Journal of Nursing Scholarship, 33*(2), 135–140.

Cortis, J. (2003). Managing society's difference and diversity. *Nursing Standard, 18*, 14–16; 33–39.

Davis, K., Schoen, C., Shih, T., Schoenbaum, C., Weinbaum, I., & Guterman, S. (2007). Slowing the growth of U.S. health care expenditures: What are the options? *The Commonwealth Fund*, January. Retrieved September 23, 2007, from http://www.commonwealthfund.org/publications/publications_show.htm?doc_id=449510

Hoffmann, D., & Tarzian, A. (2001). The girl who cried pain: A bias against women in the treatment of pain. *The Journal of Law, Medicine, & Ethics, 29*(1), 13–27.

Hoffmann, D. E., & Tarzian, A. J. (2002). Third-party reimbursement practices and their influence on pain management in Connecticut, Part 1. *The Pain Clinic, 4*(6), 11–15.

Hoffmann, D. E., & Tarzian, A. J. (2003a). Achieving the right balance in oversight of physician opioid prescribing for pain: The role of state medical boards. *Journal of Law, Medicine & Ethics, 31*(1), 21–40.

Hoffmann, D. E., & Tarzian, A. J. (2003b). Achieving the right balance in oversight of physician opioid prescribing for pain: A survey of state medical boards. *Journal of Medical Licensure and Discipline, 89*(4), 159–170.

Hoffmann, D. E., & Tarzian, A. J. (2003c). Third-party reimbursement practices and their influence on pain management in Connecticut, Part 2. *The Pain Clinic, 5*(1), 38–43.

Hoffmann, D. E., & Tarzian, A. J. (2003d). Third-party reimbursement practices and their influence on pain management in Connecticut, Part 3. *The Pain Clinic, 5*(2), 22–27.

Hoffmann, D. E., & Tarzian, A. J. (2005). Dying in America: An examination of policies that deter adequate end-of-life care in American nursing homes. *Journal of Law, Medicine, & Ethics, 33*(2), 294–309.

Hoffmann, D. E., & Tarzian, A. J. (2008). The role and legal status of health care ethics committees in the U.S. In S. H. Johnson, A. S. Iltis, & B. A. Hinze (Eds.), *Legal perspectives in bioethics: Annals of bioethics series* (pp. 46–67). London: Routledge.

Hoffmann, D., & Tarzian, A., & O'Neil, J. A. (2000). Are ethics committee members competent to consult? *The Journal of Law, Medicine & Ethics, 28*(1), 30–40.

Hunt, L. M. (2001). Beyond cultural competence. *Park Ridge Bulletin, 24,* 3–4. Retrieved February 8, 2008, from www.parkridgecenter.org/Page1882.html

Leininger, M. (1991). *Culture care diversity and universality: A theory of nursing.* New York: National League for Nursing Press.

Leininger, M. (2002). Founder's focus: Cultural diffusion trends, uses, and abuses in transcultural nursing. *Journal of Transcultural Nursing, 13*(1), 70.

Levine, S. (1982). *Who dies? An investigation of conscious living and conscious dying.* Garden City, NY: Anchor.

Levine, S. (1984). *Meetings at the edge: Dialogues with the grieving and the dying, the healing and the healed.* Garden City, NY: Anchor.

Levine, S. (1991). *Guided meditations, explorations, and healings.* New York: Anchor.

Lisle, P. C., Tarzian, A. J., Cohen, M. Z., & Trinkoff, A. M. (1999). Health care reform: Its effects on nurses. *Journal of Nursing Administration, 29*(3), 30–37.

National Academy of Sciences. (2002). *The Institute of Medicine's Report: Unequal treatment: What healthcare providers need to know about racial and ethnic disparities in healthcare.* Washington, DC: National Academy Press.

Shapiro, F. R. (Ed.) (2006). *The Yale book of quotations.* New Haven: Yale University Press.

Storti, C. (1999). *Figuring foreigners out: A practical guide.* Yarmouth, MN: Intercultural Press.

Tarzian, A. J. (2000). Caring for a dying individual who has air hunger. *Journal of Nursing Scholarship, 32*(2), 137–143.

Tarzian, A. J. (2005). Daddy dearest: Influence of culture in end-of-life decision-making. In J. Zimbelman & B. White (Eds.), *Moral dilemmas in community health care: Cases and commentaries* (pp. 289–305). New York: Pearson/Longman.

Tarzian, A. J., Davidson, S. M., & Hoffmann, D. E. (2002). Management of cancer-related and noncancer-related chronic pain in Connecticut: Successes and failures. *Connecticut Medicine, 66*(11), 683–689.

Tarzian, A. J., & Hoffmann, D. E. (2005). Barriers to managing pain in the nursing home: Findings from a statewide survey. *Journal of the American Medical Directors Association, 6*(3 Suppl.), S13–19.

Tarzian, A. J., Hoffmann, D. E., Volbrecht, R. M., & Meyers, J. L. (2006). The role of healthcare ethics committee networks in shaping healthcare policy and practices. *HEC Forum, 18*(1), 85–94.

Tarzian, A. J., Neal, M. T., & O 'Neil, J. A. (2005). Attitudes, experiences, and beliefs affecting end-of-life decision-making among homeless individuals. *Journal of Palliative Medicine, 8*(1), 36–48.

Tarzian, A. J., & Schwarz, J. K. (2004). Ethical and legal aspects of dying and health careresource allocation. In M. Matzo & D. Sherman (Eds.), *Gerontologic palliative care nursing* (pp. 82–104). St. Louis, MO: Mosby.

Tarzian, A. J., & Silverman, H. (2002). Care coordination and utilization review: Clinical case managers' perceptions of dual role obligations. *Journal of Clinical Ethics, 13*(3), 216–229.

U.S. Department of Health and Human Services. (2003). National Healthcare Disparities Report. Rockville, MD: Agency for Healthcare Research and Quality. Retrieved February 21, 2007, from http://www.ahrq.gov/qual/nhdr03/nhdr03.htm

Wartik, N. (June 23, 2002). In search of relief: Hurting more, helping less? *New York Times,* Retrieved September 23, 2007, from http://query,nytimes,com/gst/fullpage.html?sec=health&res=980CE6DD133CF930A15755C0A9649C8B63

Anita J. Tarzian received her PhD in Nursing and Ethics from the University of Maryland School of Nursing in 1998. Prior to that, she earned a Master's degree in Intercultural Nursing from the University of Maryland, a Bachelor of Science in Nursing from Rush University in Chicago, and a Bachelor of Arts from Knox College in Galesburg, IL. Her experiences as a staff nurse in a tertiary care medical center and also during a two-year stint in the Dominican Republic with the United States Peace Corps, deepened her appreciation of both the blessings and burdens of technology, the influence of culture on health care decision-making and behavior, and sources of disparities in health care access. Dr. Tarzian is an independent ethics and research consultant, with affiliations at the Schools of Law and Nursing at the University of Maryland, Baltimore. Her professional energies have been directed toward a diverse range of activities in health care, including ethics consultation, end-of-life care/hospice, palliative care, research ethics, and multiculturalism. She is Program Coordinator of the Maryland Healthcare Ethics Committee Network and Co-Chair of Chesapeake Research Review, Inc.'s Institutional Review Board. Her research and scholarly work has been published in peer-reviewed journals, and she has given professional presentations and invited lectures in the United States and abroad.

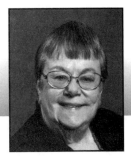

Catherine P. Murphy

CHAPTER 23

Living Out the Mission: Memoirs of a Crusader

My roots and the foundation of my personal development are integral to an understanding of the directions I took in the course of my career. A number of my professional experiences had an impact on the focus of my ultimate career goals in education, research, and public policy, which complete my story.

Enlightenment

When it comes to the source of human values, the nature versus nurture debate has received much attention. I am a believer in the nurture side of the debate. If there is any credence to the nature side of the argument, at least in the case of my ancestry, perhaps it is also true. Going back in Irish history, my ancestors endured 400 years of English domination. My parents were subjected to the tyranny of English rule growing up and their families were very active in the Irish resistance movement leading ultimately to the free state of Ireland. As young adults, my parents immigrated to the land of opportunity at the height of the Great Depression in America, where my father landed a job in the New York City Transit System, helping to found the Transport Workers Union. Moral principles of human dignity, self-determination, justice, and fairness were constantly reinforced in my family. The importance of courage in maintaining values in the face of all odds—even at the cost of life itself—was prominent. Through my family's example, coupled with their unconditional love and support, I grew to have the fortitude to pursue a life based on my own values and beliefs, including the influence of 15 years of Catholic school education.

When I entered the world of clinical nursing in the late 1950s, I was puzzled at the conformity of nursing colleagues to the decisions made by authority figures, even in the face of their own moral conflict. My colleagues stated that they did not think nurses had the authority to make clinical decisions, or when confronted with conflicting loyalties, nurses were obligated to the institution and physicians above patients. As I began postnursing school and graduate studies, I continued to work at bedside nursing. In this era before the establishment of brain death criteria, ethical dilemmas surrounding the use of technology and end-of-life treatment were rapidly escalating in intensity and quantity. My interests led me to pursue doctoral study and research in the area of ethics and nurses' ethical choices in the face of ethical dilemmas. In my research endeavors focusing on nurses' role functioning and role-connected ethical conflict, three models of the nurse-patient relationship emerged from the data—physician advocate, bureaucratic, and patient advocate (Murphy, 1978, 1981, 1983).

During the later 1960s, the American Philosophical Association (APA) had a special section on medicine and philosophy which met to share ideas at their annual convention. The section participants were primarily teaching courses in the emerging medical ethics and philosophy fields in schools of medicine. Through my acquaintance with the Professors Bandman, Bertram Bandman encouraged his wife Elsie Bandman and me to attend these annual sessions. To our dismay, the philosophers' discussions focused solely on the physicians as the decision-makers and moral agents in health care. Elsie and I badgered the members year after year in our quest for them to recognize the possibility that other health care professionals may also face ethical dilemmas, and I now must say they were quite tolerant and accommodating toward us, considering we were not even members of the organization!

Finally in the late 1970s at a Boston meeting of the APA philosophy group, led by Professor Stuart Spicker, a group of us met to begin a dialogue on nursing and ethics to explore the development of a proposal to obtain funding for this uncharted area of study. As a result, a four-state consortium was formed and funded. The first phase was a scholarly exploration of the ethical issues unique to nursing through a series of dialogues between a core group of nurses and humanities scholars. The second phase included a series of forums in each of the four states. In each public community forum, a nurse and a local humanities scholar were paired to present ethical issues, as well as the roles and responsibilities of health care professionals in ethical decision-making. The sessions were well attended and provoked audience participation.

Out of this multiyear project, *Nursing, Images and Ideals: Opening Dialogue with the Humanities* was produced (Spicker & Gadow, 1980). In addition, another book, *Ethical Problems in the Nurse-Patient Relationship,* was published as an outcome (Murphy & Hunter, 1983). These outcomes had great impact on the emerging field of nursing ethics as well as my own professional development.

The project was most likely one of the first interdisciplinary endeavors to comprehensively examine and identify the unique and shared ethical concerns of practicing nurses, as well as the emerging legitimacy of nurses' roles in the centrality of ethical decisions in health care. The probing debates of scholars looking at nursing from the outside challenged us to defend our positions as to why the role of nurses should be central to ethical decision-making. Nurses historically played a role of passive onlooker, dutifully following physician and institutional orders, as employees of hierarchical, bureaucratic practice settings. Noting these constraints, the philosophers questioned if nurses could be considered moral agents able to freely make ethical choices.

Another plus for the profession was that these philosophers and humanities scholars who taught in schools of medicine and health care delivery settings were being educated on the changing role of nurses, and many of them were influential in introducing this perspective in their home institutions. Another important outcome of the project was that the perspective of nursing, as well as the importance of nursing involvement in health care ethical decisions, was very well received and supported by the public.

The impact of the stand taken by the ANA in the Social Policy Statement (1980), which described a much broader role for nurses in making independent judgments, created a rash of new state practice acts reflecting this position. This movement, along with theory development in nursing, helped us to substantiate a philosophical basis which strengthened the argument that nurses were legitimate moral agents because their perspective on the patient as person was unlike the newly developing philosophy of medicine findings whereby medicine's goal focused on disease entities. After all, ethical concerns are about the person—not a disease entity!

Subsequently, I decided on a multifaceted personal mission: educate all nurses in the art of making ethical decisions and the need to create environments that fostered ethically responsible action; educate health care administrators and physicians about the nurse's role to fully participate in the ethical decision-making process; change health care policy to require institutions to support nurses' participation in ethical decision processes at the institutional level; and continue education of the public so it would support the changing role of nurses as advocates in ethical decisions in health care.

Action

The course of my career thereafter took a multifaceted approach in the pursuit of these goals. Activities focused on development of educational programs, publications, research, and health care policy. In 1977, I developed and taught one of the first graduate-level courses in nursing ethics in the country while at Boston University School of Nursing. Later, at Boston College, I developed a concentration in nursing ethics for the PhD program which was one of the first in the country. I developed educational strategies based on cognitive psychology and moral development. I began courses by creating "cognitive disequilibrium" through exposure to moral discussions around the inadequacy of nurses' current ethical reasoning and performance in actual clinical situations. After a period of self-discovery, most students gained insights for the first time that their own practice was at times less than ethically ideal. Students would become highly sensitive to the ethical dimension of practice and would now see ethical questions of patients' rights. A powerful component of these teaching strategies was stimulating the development of political strategies to navigate bureaucratic atmospheres and to create climates that would foster ethically responsible action when the students were in leadership positions. At first nurses saw that the only way to practice the moral ideal was to be a "moral martyr" at great personal cost. I constantly pointed out to them that power is not bestowed; rather it has to be exerted and to come from within. These nurses completely lacked the political skills to navigate and manipulate a climate of advocacy in a bureaucracy. One of the liberating insights I taught was how to educate patients and families to self-advocate in difficult ethical dilemma situations. By bolstering the moral legitimacy of these nurses, their moral confidence and authority flourished.

While at Boston College in the 1980s, I collaborated with Professor Marjory Gordon on a project that produced a continuing education curriculum and educational research tools focusing on teaching clinical judgment skills to practicing nurses. Given our individual areas of expertise, we collaborated in the development of an integrated model of diagnostic, therapeutic, and ethical reasoning (Gordon, Murphy, Candee, & Hiltunen, 1994). The integrated model of judgment proved to be successful, and practicing nurses found it effective in relating the process to diagnostic/therapeutic cognitive reasoning skills with which they were already familiar (Murphy, 1989). Clinical video simulations afforded an opportunity for the application of learning from classroom to practice situations, and through review and feedback and evaluation of the moral action component of their ethical reasoning.

In the 1990s I collaborated with Professor Mary Ann Sweeney when I served as a consultant on a number of her grant-funded projects. My expertise in ethics, coupled with her expertise in technology development, resulted first in an interactive video disc to educate nurses in geriatric settings to make ethical decisions in end-of-life dilemmas. A second project was an interactive CD to teach nurses conflict resolution strategies with families and staff in end-of-life decisions. These interactive media projects received numerous awards.

Another project dealt with teaching elderly in the community about advance directives and how to make end-of-life treatment decisions. The research supported the effectiveness of such an interactive multimedia intervention (Murphy, Sweeney, & Chiriboga, 2000). The educational and research dimensions of my professional goals had come full circle, from focusing on educating nurses to develop skills to be ethical advocates for patients to developing strategies for the public to advocate for themselves.

During the decades of 1970s–1990s, I conducted hundreds of continuing education workshops and guest lectures to various health care professionals on health care ethics and the changing role of the nurse in decision-making. In the early years, I overheard comments as nurses questioned whether they should be adopting my proposed role of more centrality in ethical decision-making because they did not personally want that responsibility. One interesting reaction from some nurses occurred when I promoted this role—my proposal was interpreted as being antiphysician! One time I was invited to the weekly medical grand rounds of a hospital in Massachusetts to talk about ethical problems in the clinical setting. That very day there was a front-page article in the Boston Globe about the start of the nursing shortage and the increasing dissatisfaction of nurses with conditions in the clinical setting and physician relationships. I delivered my message about the emerging nurses' role, and a staff physician became very irate and declared that nursing educators like me were troublemakers, creating all the dissatisfaction in nurses by giving them ideas that could never come about in the practice setting!

As chair of the ANA Committee on Ethics for 5 years, I used the bully pulpit to effect change in the profession and the larger society. As a committee we issued many position statements regarding nurses' roles in decision-making, as well as numerous positions on ethical issues facing nurses and the public. These statements were debated on the floor of the House of Delegates of the ANA conventions, and many positions ended up as press releases.

I served as a member, adviser, and consultant to numerous policy-making bodies, for example, the National Commission Advisory Panel of the U. S. Congress study on Use of Life-Sustaining Technology in the Care of the Elderly, the advisory board of the National Center of the American Society of Law and Medicine, and the President's Commission for the Study of Ethical Problems in Medicine. By the end of the decade of the 1980s, The Joint Commission for the Accreditation of Health Care Institutions in their standards mandated the development of institutional mechanisms for nurses to be involved in ethical decisions and to deal with ethical disagreements. The government health care systems and various other private health care systems followed.

The public recognition of the importance of nurses and their ethical responsibilities created accountability and legal liability. By the mid-1980s, I was being called as a legal expert witness in nursing ethics cases where nurses failed to adhere to the nursing ideals as expressed in the ANA Code for Nurses now being used by attorneys as a standard of practice. The good news was society (and attorneys) now recognized that nurses were responsible for making decisions and they had a code of ethics!

During this increased public awareness of nurses' roles in ethical decisions, I was bombarded by the media as a spokesperson for nursing and ethics. I had the privilege of participating in interviews by numerous newspapers and radio stations throughout the country, and in addition, I appeared on national and local television stations. One appearance was triggered by a nationwide panic caused by an erroneous article reporting on nurses' possible participation in mercy killing. Gauging from the reactions, there was now a great deal of public education and public recognition of the importance of the role of nurses in the ethical decisions of health care.

Reflection

This is my story—a lifelong quest to make a positive difference in my profession and ultimately in the delivery of health care. Caring for patients and teaching generations of nursing students has been my privilege. The journey has never been dull and has always been challenging, resulting in a fulfilling professional career.

In looking toward the future I like to think that some of my professional career goals were achieved in terms of my impact on education, research, and public policy. Like it or not, health care institutions now have to involve nurses in all aspects of ethical decision-making and ensure the creation of mechanisms that foster nursing advocacy. This is not only as a result of mandates by policy-making bodies, but also in the interest of recruitment and retention of nurses—a very scarce resource. Vigilance is needed to ensure that there is no backsliding. The impact of the feminist movement on the predominantly female profession of nursing and the dramatic increase in the female composition of modern medicine have both altered nurse-physician relationships of dominance. This should serve as a further safeguard for the future.

In terms of public perception of nursing, the profession must continue to educate the public on ethical trends affecting them and their relationship with nurses. Members of the profession, as well as the professional organizations, must continue to seek a place at the table of important health policy initiatives. The trend toward nursing militancy in labor disputes must not cause the nursing profession to lose sight of the best ethical interests of the public and the responsibility to advocate for them as a profession.

Ethics courses should be required at all levels of the curriculum in schools of nursing to prepare nurses for the continuing high incidence and emergence of new ethical issues. With the explosion of multimedia technology development and its application, nursing educators must increase its use in education. Traditional teaching methods have to be altered, making them more vibrant and relevant for the young generation of students who have grown up with multimedia. Given the rationing of health care professionals' time spent in patient interaction, use of multimedia patient education tools for making informed decisions will also be a necessity.

In the area of research, many studies need to be conducted in health care ethics. While there are restraints and limitations on the research questions and design in empirical research, creative approaches must be developed. Questions such as whether patients were the victims of ethical violations in institutions will hardly be approved by the institutional review board. In my experience as a member on hospital research review committees, study proposals that posed a threat to the reputation of the institution would be rejected. In terms of ethical questions, a researcher cannot ethically create a design that, for example, randomly assigns patients to just and unjust care, or informed consent/no informed consent.

Descriptive research is needed to identify the type and incidence of nurses' ethical dilemmas in specialized areas of practice in order to discover emerging issues and trends. I previously identified a framework for descriptive research questions regarding the type and incidence of ethical dilemmas that arise out of the multifaceted role of the nurse—as direct care giver, professional colleague, employee, and citizen (Murphy, 1985). Given the aging population and the continuing explosion of biomedical technology developments, the ethical questions of cost, financing, and access to health care will be even more pressing as future ethical dilemmas. Nurses will be involved in designing intervention research to inform patients and the public about the consequences, risks, benefits, costs, and uncertainties in their treatment options offered by biomedical technology. Qualitative research as well as philosophical and historical research approaches will also be needed to further monitor and direct professional ethics in the future.

References

American Nurses Association. (1980). *Nursing: A Social Policy Statement.* Kansas City, MO: Author.

Gordon, M., Murphy, C. P., Candee, D., & Hiltunen, E. (1994). Clinical judgment: An integrated model. *Advances in Nursing Science, 16*(4), 55–70.

Murphy, C. (1978). The moral situation in nursing. In E. L. Bandman & B. Bandman (Eds.), *Bioethics and human rights* (pp. 313–320). Boston: Little, Brown.

Murphy, C. (1981). Moral reasoning in a selected group of nursing practitioners. In S. Ketefian (Ed.), *Perspectives on nursing leadership: Issues and research* (pp. 45–75). New York: Teachers College Press, Columbia University.

Murphy, C. (1983). Models of the nurse-patient relationship. In C. Murphy & H. Hunter (Eds.), *Ethical problems in the nurse-patient relationship* (pp. 8–24). Boston: Allyn and Bacon.

Murphy, C. P. (1985). *Ethical dilemmas in practice. Issues in professional nursing practice, 4,* Kansas City, MO: American Nurses Association.

Murphy, C. (1989). Integration of diagnostic and ethical reasoning in clinical practice: Teaching and evaluation. In R. Carroll-Johnson (Ed.), *Classification of nursing diagnoses: Proceedings of the eighth conference, North American Nursing Diagnosis Association* (pp. 73–76). Philadelphia: J. B. Lippincott.

Murphy, C. P., & Hunter, H. (Eds.). (1983). *Ethical problems in the nurse-patient relationship.* Boston: Allyn and Bacon.

Murphy, C. P., Sweeney, M. A., & Chiriboga, D. (2000). An educational intervention for advance directives. *Journal of Professional Nursing, 16*(1), 21–30.

Spicker, S., & Gadow, S. (Eds.). (1980). *Nursing, images and ideals: Opening dialogue with the humanities.* New York: Springer.

Catherine P. Murphy, RN, EdD was born in New York City. She received her diploma in nursing from St. Clares Hospital School of Nursing in N.Y. and her baccalaureate degree in nursing from Teachers College, Columbia University. She received her MS degree in nursing from Hunter College of the City University of the State of New York and her EdD from Teachers College, Columbia University. During the course of her career she served in the positions of staff nurse, charge nurse, and clinical director in nursing service. In academia she served in the roles of faculty member, department chairperson, director of the graduate program, and dean of the school of nursing. In recognition of her contributions to nursing ethics, she has received numerous awards among them the ANA Honorary Membership Award, the Teachers College Distinguished Achievement Award for Scholarship and Research, Inaugural Inductee to the Teachers College Hall of Fame, and the Massachusetts Nurses Association Award for Excellence in Teaching. She is retired and resides in Rhode Island on Apponaug Cove with a breathtaking view overlooking Narragansett Bay.

⤳ SECTION VIII ⤳
CRITICAL THINKING ACTIVITIES

Diversity and Disparities Issues

◆ During the Legacy Seminar, Tarzian wondered, "Are we nurse ethicists or ethicists who happen to be nurses?" What is your answer to this question and why?

◆ Anne Davis cautions that nurses in other countries and cultures should not adopt the models and approaches in ethics developed in the United States without adaptation to their cultural values. Review the essays in this section and describe a cultural difference in the approach to ethics that would support Davis's argument.

◆ A key point of Murphy's work was to defend the nurse's moral legitimacy in ethical decision-making. Evaluate Murphy's success in mounting this defense.

SECTION IX
Pain and Suffering

Pain can be physical or psychological. As commonly understood among the nursing profession, "pain is whatever the experiencing person says it is and exists whenever he says it does" (M. McCaffery, 1979, [Nursing Management of the Patient with Pain]. *Philadelphia: J. B. Lippincott, p. 11). Suffering is a state of serious distress which can be manifested in physical, mental, or social means. Suffering can result from many factors, or simply result from the threat of those factors materializing.*

Suffering

Cortney Davis

1.
In intensive care,
these sufferings:

a baby whose father had taken him
by both legs, a finger between them,

and hit the baby against the wall
because the baby cried. With the other hand

he held the mother back. A boy
who fell off his bike and was hit by a car.

His mother watched him lying
in the clean sheets, his heart

beating under his chest
as if an animal were trying to escape.

The monitor line straightened;
then she howled for him.

There was a child who drowned
and a crazy woman we tied to the mattress

who rose up
with the mattress still on her back.

Once a man ran naked down the back stairs
into the parking lot

just to feel for the last time
the hard diamonds of snow.

2.
I've seen women
who were beaten

by other women
with a shoe, a stick, a picture frame.

A mother hits
the side of her daughter's face
with a flashlight.

Fathers use their hands,
to women mostly,
to their children
maybe something else.

One woman told me it wasn't the blows
but the love lost,
gone as if they peeled your skin,
sucked all marrow from your bones and now
you walk everywhere hollow.

3.
This is their sound.

It starts as a whine,
like children whine
when they can't have
what they want;

then it becomes
mindless,
a staccato rap
finding your pulse;

then
intermittent,

like the high sound
when intestines churn,
trying to find something left
to pass through;

then it becomes
all there is,
small and pure,
a delicious drop
balanced on the tongue
of the open mouth;

then,
   Silence.

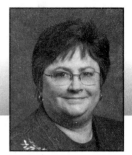

Marsha D. M. Fowler

CHAPTER 24

Come; Give Me a Taste of Shalom

Framing the Theme

There has been many an erudite philosophical discussion of the "hallmarks of the moral," and yet, at the fundamental human level, there is really only one hallmark: tragedy. Moral tragedy gives rise to suffering, both private and social, as patients, families, health care providers, groups within society, and society itself come to grips with the shared human condition, technological advances, constrained resources, social injustice, and global inequities. Some moral quandaries befall us and are the universal and inescapable consequences of human fragility, disease, and trauma. Other moral dilemmas confront us because of human strengths and desires wrongly exercised. Even creation itself suffers and groans under the burden of human decisions. This too is tragic. Whether arising from circumstance or from hubris, moral tragedy requires a response, often an immediate and decisive response, and suffering must be addressed. But, how are we to respond, or more precisely, what are the determinants of our response?

For some, a response proceeds from an analysis of the situation or issue based on moral principles, or an ideal of caring, or a specific end that is sought, or sometimes from a "purely philosophical equation," a professional ideal, a professional standard such as the Code of Ethics for Nurses, or a social norm. For many persons, however, the underlying basis of ethical analysis and moral decision-making remains invisible as it emerges clothed in philosophical or professional terms. Underneath, the basis is often religious in nature. Much of the world is religious (estimated to be 77%), and yet few within nursing consider the influence of specific religious traditions on ethical analysis, deliberation, discourse, and decision-making. Fewer still have examined the perspectives of religious traditions, whether ancient or modern, on discrete moral topics within ethics in nursing and what they might offer to an understanding of, for instance, person, health, society, community, caring, service, hope, suffering, or compassion. The wealth of human understanding contained in the 6,000 years of religious literature, both oral and written, has been sorely neglected by nursing scholars and researchers. This too is a moral tragedy. Until such time as nursing engages in the academic study of religion and the ethical systems religious traditions beget, nursing has no right to lay claim to "holistic care."

The Context

At the age of four, I was shocked to discover that I was a devout left-leaning Christian misplaced in a fundamentalist Christian family. Officially I am a Minister of the Word and Sacrament, Presbyterian Church (USA). Within my family I am still the "leftist-commie-hippie-black-sheep." The working out of these two identities within the context of academic nursing gives rise to my contribution to nursing ethics.

The faithful exercise of one's religious tradition requires of the adherent some discernment in determining what is right or wrong to do. In religious terminology, this is often referred to as what is righteous or what is sinful. At its most primitive, this discernment requires adherence to a shared set of often concrete, invariant, black-and-white norms. While this may reflect an individual's understanding, few religions are actually this morally primitive. In fact, many religioethical systems are complex, nuanced, and even elegant. They contain a view of the consanguinity of the human condition, a vision for the life of faith lived rightly and faithfully, both individually and communally; an understanding of the nature and ordering of the cosmos; and a view of the relationships between God and mortals, humans and humans, and humans and the created world.

As one who has been religious from childhood, my interest in ethics thus predates both learning to ride a bicycle and entry into nursing. While religion has been formative of my thinking and life, I have also been shaped by my social context. My childhood in culturally diverse San Francisco, the loss of friends and classmates to death in Vietnam or flight to Canada, my college education in the Berkeley area in the mid-1960s, the days of folk and protest music and marches, have all had a hand in shaping both me and my specific interests within ethics.

I received a Kennedy Fellowship in Ethics at Harvard in 1978. The Fellowship laid the foundation for the subsequent completion of a doctorate in Social Ethics. My dissertation research focused on the history and development of nursing ethics and the Code of Ethics for nurses, and more specifically on the interaction of nursing's ethics with culture, society, politics, and professions. I utilized Ernst Troeltsch's work of the *Religiongeschichtelische Schule* (a particular German school of thought) as a theoretical base for analysis. He saw the Church as historically conditioned in several respects, but as having its own autonomous and transcendent core meaning and its own independent (that is, socially conditioned but not socially constructed) affect upon society, culture, and history.

It seemed to me that nursing was culturally conditioned, in part by its own aspirations to be regarded as a "profession," but that it too, like the Church, had a distinctive and independent core meaning and its own implications for its unfolding that could neither be collapsed into nor subsumed under "medicine." Through nursing's social ethics and practice, the profession could affect society, culture, and history, though its power to do so was and remains dependent in part upon the social location of women (Fowler, 1984). In following a modified Troeltschian methodology, my analysis of the social conditioning of the Nightingale Pledge, the precursor codes, the Code and its successive iterations, as well as the body of nursing ethics literature from the 1870s to the 1980s led me to conclude that the central moral motif of nursing is "the ideal of service." "Caring," using Troeltsch's framework, could only be regarded as a local metaphor for nursing, "for us, for now," that could not bear the weight of the whole of the profession historically in all its forms and across cultures. "Service," however, seemed to be able to encompass all forms of nursing past and present, whether public health, hospital, retail, or military nursing, and to some degree to transcend culture. It seemed as well to have greater explanatory power and consistency with the plenary body of nursing ethical literature (Fowler, 1984).

My research into the history and development of the Code in 1980 and forward led me into looking at the literature on control of occupational labor and the sociology of professions, about which I have written elsewhere (Fowler, 1990a, 1993, 2000). The sociology of professions was of interest on two counts: (a) nursing's ardent desire to be regarded as a profession, and thus its employment of trait definitions of professions and subsequently setting about "proving" that those traits existed in nursing—while aping the "professional" behaviors of other professions (Bixler & Bixler, 1959), and (b) the effect that various forms of occupational control could exert upon ethics.

From 1976 into the 1990s, I continued to explore and write about ethical issues in long-term ventilatory care and acute respiratory crisis, specifically focusing on withholding and withdrawing life-sustaining treatment, slow codes, and euthanasia. The backdrop to these considerations had been an exploration of the emerging literature on the "technological imperative."

In the early 1990s, I embarked upon a major project in assisting Natalya Mal'tseva, the Deputy Director of the Ministry of Health, Republic of Russia, in creating a new program of education for the 440 *medsistra* schools outside Moscow Oblast. I built a project to convert these schools into baccalaureate programs on a modified Western model that I struggled to have implemented in ways that reflected Russian culture, perspectives, values, and sensibilities. This ended up being a 10-year commitment. My task was largely to work across the 11 time zones of the country with 1,200 leading educators who would then carry out the project within their oblasts and schools.

In the demise of the Soviet system, the 10 percent of all curricula that was given to "ideology" (a.k.a. Marxism) became a void that had to be filled. The Ministry of Health asked me to help fill that void with curricula on duhovnast, that is, spirituality. This necessitated an instant immersion, drowning really, in Russian Orthodox theology, spirituality, praxis, and practice. This required the best of my skills as a theologian, clergywoman, and ecumenist. Quite out of the ordinary, the materials that I prepared for this were published by the ministry as Russian (not foreign) curricular materials (Fowler, 1994). Over the next 10 years I lectured throughout Russia on ethics and spirituality to nursing educators and directors of *medsistra* schools. By the mid-1990s I was working closely with the nursing association to develop a code of ethics which was subsequently published in Saint Petersburg (Association of Medical Sisters of Russia, 1997).

This work in Russia had a significant impact upon me in terms of my own spirituality and enlarged ecumenism, and a return to my "original" interest in the interaction of ethics and spirituality, or more specifically, various traditions of religious spirituality and culture. My interest in suffering, brought over from my days as a pulmonary clinical nurse specialist (CNS), continued but turned more specifically toward religious/spiritual and theological treatments of the topic. I was struck by the wisdom of ancient texts, or sacred writ, that were built upon millennia of observations of the human condition.

In the late 1980s I had providentially done some work in reconsidering health from a theological perspective (Fowler, 1990b). I had come to embrace a concept rooted in ancient Semitic languages as a fuller understanding of health. The concept, shalom or salaam, is often poorly translated as peace in English; it has a far richer and capacious understanding than this. Shalom is one of the most significant theological terms in Scripture, [having] a wide semantic range stressing various nuances of its basic meaning: totality or completeness (Youngblood, 1986, p. 732).

In the Russian context, the World Health Organization (WHO) definition of health (1948), as well as its alternatives in the medical and nursing literature, seemed unserviceable and culturally incompatible with a communally oriented culture. Shalom seemed a far more adequate definition of health. The features of shalom that stood out as more expressive of my understanding of health, as more compatible with the Russian cultural context, and as a corrective to Western nursing approaches were several. Shalom, arising as it did from a communal context, encompasses both the individual and the community. The individual cannot be healthy if the community is sick and the community cannot be healthy without a concern for the health of the individual. In addition shalom as totality or completeness allowed for the realization of health even in the presence of illness or even in one who was dying. A complete understanding of shalom does, however, encompass the absence of disease. There seemed, too, to be more space in shalom to address suffering.

On Suffering

The nursing literature has struggled with suffering, and, like compassion, has paid it disproportionately little attention. What little scientific research exists on suffering in the nursing literature is not without merit; it is simply too thin. In some instances, only one or two studies exist on an entire significant aspect of suffering. Nursing research recognizes that suffering is an intensely personal experience, yet nursing has failed to explore the social nature of suffering. Nursing has to some degree been preoccupied with the physical causes of suffering. The majority of studies involve suffering in instances of breast cancer, HIV/AIDS, or end-of-life situations.

Consistent with the scientific model, nursing has reified the concept of suffering so as to render it measurable, enumerate its causes, and list its pathognomonic "signs and symptoms." Throughout the nursing research literature, there is only thin attention paid to the linkage of suffering and spirituality (despite its inclusion in the North American Nursing Diagnosis Association [NANDA] as the diagnosis of "spiritual distress" [Carpenito-Moyet, 2007]), though that has been changing in recent years. There is still, however, a tendency to collapse the spiritual into the psychological (see Benedict, 1989). A few studies have examined "telling one's story" in the amelioration of suffering. However, these studies completely miss the important distinction between telling one's story as a relational act, and the distinct and crucial act of composing one's story, an aspect that is emphasized in the theological literature.

The Western theological literature, including biblical studies, brings dimensions to the understanding of suffering that are not resident in the nursing or medical literature. However, only broad considerations will be addressed here. Theological literature emphasizes both the inescapability of suffering—that it is a part of the human condition—and that it is universal. In consequence, suffering is seen as a part of life, intrinsically, and to be addressed as such (Brueggermann, 1984, p. 53). In a sense, there is no "why?" to suffering.

The power of suffering to isolate is concurrently the power to cause distortions or disruptions in one's understanding of the world and of God. Fragmentation, even disintegration, may result. For many, this raises the problem of theodicy—a shoal upon which faith may founder.

In the midst of suffering, there is in some cultures a human tendency to seek understanding, self-understanding, and perhaps meaning or simply sense-making of the suffering (Battenfield, 1984; Brallier, 1992, p. 206; Lindholm & Eriksson, 1993). Suffering can make us acutely aware of our mortality and impotence, dashing our illusions of control and power, and yet it can move us to develop in new ways, ways that joy does not.

While in some texts suffering is a consequence of divine and just punishment, these texts do not see suffering as a divine pedagogical instrument, inflicted for the purposes of instruction. I have no use for a God who instructs humankind through human suffering; I have every need of a God who instructs humankind in suffering. These same texts also recognize that some suffering is simply inexplicable (Zuck, 1992; also see Clines, 1989; Habel, 1985; Hartley, 1988). Theology also recognizes that some suffering may have redemptive qualities—not that the person is redeemed by or in suffering, but that the suffering is redeemed; theology also recognizes that some suffering has no redemptive quality whatsoever (Bstan-dzin-rgya-mtsho, Mitchell, & Wiseman, 2003; Pinn, 2002; also see Ayoub, 1978).

More importantly and perhaps more practically for nursing and the patients who suffer, the theological literature emphasizes the necessity of lament and presence with one another in the midst of suffering (Westermann, 1981; also see Brueggermann, 1984). Of course, no one wants a patient who laments. No one wants Job for a patient. Job "did not restrain [his] mouth," spoke "in the anguish of [his] spirit," and "complained in the bitterness of [his] soul." No one wants this kind of patient; they make us feel uncomfortable. This is the patient whose lament we shun; this is the patient who is shunned. There is very little that Job's friends get right, except for this:

> Job's three friends made an appointment together to come and mourn with him, and to comfort him. And when they raised their eyes from afar, and did not recognize him, they lifted their voices and wept. And each one tore his robe and sprinkled dust on his head toward heaven. So they sat down with him on the ground seven days and seven nights, and no one spoke a word to him, for they saw that his grief was great (Job 2:11-13, New Revised Standard Version [NRSV]).

This passage does indicate the importance of presence with the one who suffers, or sharing in the suffering of one who suffers. Yet, we are loath to get that close to suffering. Even those whose calling it is to do so, do not.

Suffering has a cry and that cry is: be. Be with me. Be, not do. Be, even in silence. Just be. Nurses, however, are good at doing, doing, doing, speaking, speaking, speaking. Here, suffering brings us back to the necessity of "shalom," which is rooted and found only in relationship.

In the theological literature, it is in being-with-another and in hearing that person's lament, however Jobian it may be, that the person who suffers comes to "shalom." How that lament is to be expressed is not left to chance. The structure of a psalm of individual lament provides an ancient template for the expression of one's own lament.

There are attributes of a psalm of lament of the individual that are particularly important to note. First, the form demands that the entire, complete, full lament be expressed—that every drop of the lament be squeezed out and nothing be left to sit in the soul. Second, there is no normative judgment in a psalm of lament. Very, very politically incorrect things are said in these psalms. No matter how nonpolitically correct, they must be expressed. Otherwise, it sits within and festers. Though one may hide it from one's self, it is not hidden from God, so one may as well get it all out. Another attribute of a psalm of lament that is important to note is that it always must end on a rising note. While a psalm of lament takes you into the pit and runs you around on the bottom of the pit, and may have you do several extra laps as well, it always helps you begin to climb up and out. You are not simply left in the pit, ever. While most laments are phrased in the language of faith, that is, in "God talk," this need not necessarily be the case. Laments can be created with no religious content and can be used as a template for the expression of suffering, or as a mental template for the nurse working with one who suffers, who needs to express his lament.

Millennia of observation of human suffering are reflected upon in ancient scriptures in many traditions. Western sacred writ reflects theologically upon causes of suffering, suffering of the just and the unjust, and other aspects of suffering. However, in the use of lament, one finds movement beyond the "problem" of suffering to the "experience" of suffering, beyond the "definitional" to the "practical." The emphasis that is placed upon lament and presence, especially in lament, is born of a sizable longitudinal population. As suffering is a part of life, so is lament, whether individual or communal. While we would very much like to do otherwise, we must stick around for those moments when the patient does not restrain his mouth, speaks in the anguish of his spirit, and complains in the bitterness of his soul. In those moments, nurses whose impulse is toward doing, doing, doing, need not scramble to "find the words to say." There are no words to say: just be.

There is, of course, more to this "being" than silence and physical presence. The recognition that suffering is not under our control, however much we might try to control it—through medications, interventions, and more—it remains beyond our control. When I am present for the suffering and lament of a patient, truly present, I am reminded that suffering is also my lot, even if not right here, right now. As I share in the patient's suffering and lament and am present to the patient, I allow the terror and darkness that cannot be controlled to confront me in my own frailty; I too have a lament within. This presence is not the "therapeutic use of self" as nursing discusses. This presence is a presence in vulnerability—the vulnerability of the shared human condition—that, while it still retains identity boundaries, is open to an ontological change in both persons by virtue of human connectedness.

That suffering yearns for and finds comfort in presence is best expressed in the beloved passage from the 23rd Psalm (verse 4): "Even though I walk through the darkest valley, I will fear no evil; for you are with me; your rod and your staff—they comfort me." (King James Version: "Yea, though I walk through the valley of the shadow of death, I will fear no evil: for thou art with me; thy rod and thy staff they comfort me.") This metaphor-laden psalm focuses on God's provision and protection—and presence—even in the צלמות, a compound noun that literally means "very deep shadow" or even "total darkness," but probably implies the threat of death (as in Job 10:21–22). In a measure of linguistic beauty, the term also means the dark circles under one's eyes that result from weeping and grief (Brown, Driver, Briggs, Robinson, & Gesenius, 1952; Gesenius, 1979; Swanson, 1997).

We have all had patients with whom we "fell in love": patients with whom we have had a deep connectedness, often inexplicable. To share in the lament of another is to be open, truly open, to that connection in which one experiences the "donative element" (the gift element) of humanity while being open to a change in the very nature of one's being in response to the immediacy of that sharing and connectedness (May, 1977). Figure 24.1 attempts to capture the most significant factors in a lament welcomed and heard and those that are shunned and silenced.

For the most part, the past 20 years have been devoted at least in part to intersections of spirituality and ethics and religion and ethics. Most, if not all of my career, I have taught spirituality content and developed material around the "spiritual theme" and its interaction with bioethical decision-making by patients and practitioners (Fowler & Peterson, 1997). In my work with my colleague Brenda Simons, we concluded that people tend to have a single, recurrent spiritual theme that surfaces again and again throughout life, not infrequently in moral decisions. We were

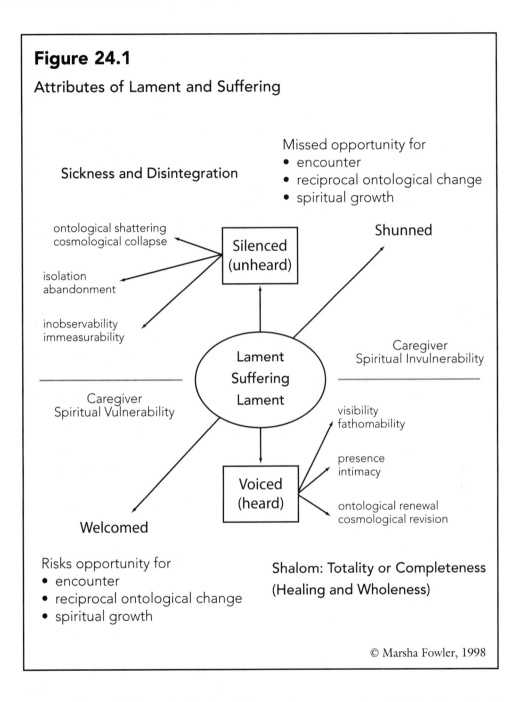

Figure 24.1

Attributes of Lament and Suffering

Sickness and Disintegration

Missed opportunity for
- encounter
- reciprocal ontological change
- spiritual growth

ontological shattering
cosmological collapse

Silenced
(unheard)

Shunned

isolation
abandonment

inobservability
immeasurability

Caregiver
Spiritual Invulnerability

Lament
Suffering
Lament

Caregiver
Spiritual Vulnerability

visibility
fathomability

presence
intimacy

Voiced
(heard)

ontological renewal
cosmological revision

Welcomed

Risks opportunity for
- encounter
- reciprocal ontological change
- spiritual growth

Shalom: Totality or Completeness
(Healing and Wholeness)

© Marsha Fowler, 1998

concerned as well about the limits of the nursing warrant for dabbling in spiritual care. While I believe that there is an important role for nurses to engage in spiritual care, and that all nurses should at least be able to recognize spiritual care needs, I do not believe that the deeper reaches of spiritual care fall within the proper purview of nursing. For the most part, nurses are neither prepared, nor skilled, nor called to dive into the deeper waters of the spirit. Like the person who is not the lifeguard who dives into the water to help the drowning swimmer, more likely both will drown. These deep waters, where silences are named, are not nursing's domain. By silences I do not mean the immediate or underlying causes of grief or suffering, but rather the monsters that live down deep in the human soul—often feeding upon one's spiritual theme—that must be ridden and broken to be tamed. It is the domain of the ineffable, and of the core of the person, and it is dangerous; it does not belong to nursing.

The nursing literature on religion is morbidly anemic, and its attention to the intersections of religion and ethics is nonexistent. For the most part, the nursing literature is attempting to craft a generic spirituality with which it can interact. I have found this vacuous and deeply unsatisfying, and have become more interested in religion per se. I have encountered few patients whose spirituality was not shaped by either a religious faith or by exposure to the "culture of a religion" that has long since ceased to be embraced by the present or preceding generation of his or her family. It is increasingly the case that we will see patients whose genetic memory of a religious tradition will have receded, but that is infrequently the case at present. Religion suffuses culture, even where the religion is no longer embraced. Russia is Eastern Orthodox, even as an atheist state. There are a number of ways in which the academic study of religion is important to nursing, and more specifically to a study of ethics and nursing.

There are at least eight fundamental and separable points at which nursing could begin a fruitful engagement with religion. The first area is that of the formal "theology" of a religious tradition in terms of its view of health, healing, health care, illness, mental illness, personal responsibility for health, serving those who are ill, the role of the community in illness, and so forth. This would also include a study of how ethics is "done" in a given religious tradition. The second is that of the tradition's formal theology as it would undergird, inform, or shape the nursing enterprise—and whether it would view nursing as a morally praiseworthy enterprise. The third area for research is that of the tradition's understanding of concepts important to nursing care such as hope, compassion, service, justice, and caring, and their interaction with ethics. A fourth area is that of the relationship of ethics and faith as it might influence clinical ethical decision-making by nurses. This would also include how the tradition would formulate its social ethics, especially in terms of health policy critique, formulation, and action. A fifth area for scholarship and research is that of a tradition's distinctive influence upon patient/family bioethical decisions. A sixth, very concrete area is that of specific religious proscriptions and prescriptions regarding health and health-related behaviors that might influence nursing practice in individualizing care. A seventh area of research is to explore the historic relationship between nursing and religion, including the religious perspectives of historic nursing figures such as Nightingale, and the ways in which these perspectives might have influenced their leadership and direction in the profession and its ethics. An eighth area of exploration is in postcolonial theology and theory. Postcolonial theory has much to say that is important to nursing, particularly in the domain of social ethics, concern for socially disadvantaged, underserved and vulnerable populations, and health disparities—in hearing voices from the margins (Keller, Nausner, & Rivera, 2004; Sugirtharajah, 2006; also see Smith, 2006).

It is essential that nursing engage in research and scholarship in all eight of these areas if nursing is to understand itself, if nurses are to understand themselves, and if we are to understand our patients and the world in which we live—and presume to declare that we are interested in the whole person, or for our purposes here, whole-person ethics.

References

Association of Medical Sisters of Russia. (1997). *Code of Ethics for Russian Medical Sisters* (pp. 1–28). St. Petersburg, Russia: Author.

Ayoub, M. (1978). *Redemptive suffering in Islam: A study of the devotional aspects of `Ashura in Twelver Shi`Ism*. The Hague, Netherlands: Mouton.

Battenfield, B. L. (1984). Suffering—A conceptual description and content analysis of an operational schema. *Image, 16*(2), 36–41.

Benedict, S. (1989). The suffering associated with lung cancer. *Cancer Nursing, 12*(1), 34–40.

Bixler, G. K., & Bixler, R. W. (1959). The professional status of nursing. *American Journal of Nursing, 59*(8) 1142–1146.

Brallier, L. W. (1992). The suffering of terminal illness: Cancer. In P. Starck & J. McGovern (Eds.), *The hidden dimension of illness: Human suffering* (pp. 203–225). New York: National League for Nursing Press.

Brown, F., Driver, S. R., Briggs, C. A., Robinson, E., & Gesenius, W. (1952). *A Hebrew and English lexicon of the Old Testament* (based on the lexicon of William Gesenius, E. Robinson, Trans.). Oxford, U.K.: Clarendon Press.

Brueggermann, W. (1984). *The message of the Psalms: A theological commentary*. Minneapolis: Augsburg Publishing House.

Bstan-dzin-rgya-mtsho, Dalai Lama XIV, Mitchell, D. W., & Wiseman, J. (2003). *Transforming suffering: Reflections on finding peace in a troubled world*. New York: Image/Doubleday.

Carpenito-Moyet, L. J. (2007). *Nursing diagnosis: Application to clinical practice*. Philadelphia: Lippincott, Williams & Wilkins.

Clines, D. J. A., & Nelson Reference Staff. (1989). *Job 1–20* [Word Biblical Commentary Series]. Dallas, TX: Word Division of Thomas Nelson Incorporated.

Fowler, M. (1984). *Ethics and nursing, 1893–1984: The ideal of service, the reality of history.* Unpublished doctoral dissertation. University of Southern California, Los Angeles.

Fowler, M. D. M. (1990a). Nursing and social ethics. In N. A. Chaska (Ed.), *The nursing profession: Turning points* (pp. 24–30). St. Louis: C.V. Mosby.

Fowler, M. D. M. (1990b). Peace in our time. *Heart & Lung, 19*(3), 315–316.

Fowler, M. D. M. (1993). Professional associations, ethics and society. *Oncology Nursing Forum, 20*(10 suppl.), 13–19.

Fowler, M. (1994). *Spirituality, faith and nursing practice.* Moscow: Ministry of Health (published in Russian).

Fowler, M. D. M. (1998). "The necessity of lament in suffering," presentation to Clark County and Las Vegas Ministerial Association. March 11, 1998.

Fowler, M. (2000). The moral role and responsibility of a professional association. (In Russian). *Сестринское Дело.* St. Petersburg, Russia, 28(8), np.

Fowler, M., & Peterson, B. S. (1997). Spiritual themes in clinical pastoral education. *Journal of Supervision and Training in Ministry, 18,* 46–54.

Gesenius, W. (1979). *Gesenius' Hebrew and Chaldee lexicon to the Old Testament.* (S.P. Tregelles, Trans.). Grand Rapids, MI: Baker Book House.

Habel, N. C. (1985). *The book of Job: A commentary.* Philadelphia: Westminster.

Hartley, J. E. (1988). *The book of Job* [The new international commentary on the Old Testament series]. Grand Rapids, MI: Eerdmans.

Keller, C., Nausner, M., & Rivera, M. (Eds.). (2004). *Postcolonial theologies: Divinity and empire.* St. Louis, MO: Chalice Press.

Lindholm, L., & Eriksson, K. (1993). To understand and alleviate suffering in a caring culture. *Journal of Advanced Nursing, 18*(9), 1354–1361.

May, W. (1977). Code and covenant or philanthropy and contract? In S. J. Reiser, A. J. Dyck, & W. J. Curran (Eds.), *Ethics in medicine: Historical perspectives and contemporary concerns* (pp. 65–76). Boston: MIT Press.

Pinn, A. B. (Ed.). (2002). *Moral evil and redemptive suffering: A history of theodicy in African-American religious thought.* Gainesville, FL: University Press of Florida.

Smith, H. (2006). *A seat at the table: Huston Smith in conversation with Native Americans on religious freedom.* Berkeley: University of California Press.

Sugirtharajah, R. S. (2006). *Voices from the margin: Interpreting the Bible in the third world*. (Rev. & exp. 3rd ed.). Maryknoll, NY: Orbis Books.

Swanson, J. (1997). *Dictionary of Biblical languages with semantic domains: Hebrew (Old Testament)*. Oak Harbor, WA: Logos Research Systems.

Westermann, C. (1981). *Praise and lament in the Psalms* (K. Crim & R. N. Soulen, Trans.). Atlanta, GA: Westminster John Knox.

World Health Organization. (1948). *Constitution of the World Health Organization*. Geneva, Switzerland: Author.

Youngblood, R. F. (1986). Peace. In J. Orr (Ed.), *The international standard Bible encyclopedia* (Rev. ed., vol. 3). Grand Rapids, MI: W. B. Eerdmans.

Zuck, R. B. (Ed.). (1992). *Sitting with Job: Selected studies on the book of Job*. Grand Rapids, MI: Baker Book House.

Marsha D. M. Fowler, Senior Fellow and Professor of Ethics, Spirituality, and Faith Integration, Azusa Pacific University. She is a graduate of Kaiser Foundation School of Nursing (diploma), University of California at San Francisco (BS, MS), Fuller Theological Seminary (MDiv) and the University of Southern California (PhD). She has engaged in teaching and research in bioethics and spirituality since 1974. Her research interests are in the history and development of nursing's ethics and the Code of Ethics for Nurses, social ethics and professions, suffering, the intersections of spirituality and ethics, and religious ethics in nursing.

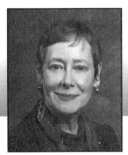

Joy H. Penticuff

CHAPTER 25

Suffering, Compassion, and Ethics: Reflections on Neonatal Nursing

My work in nursing ethics has grown out of my clinical experiences as a neonatal intensive care nurse. Across four decades, my clinical focus has been the well-being of infants and their families in neonatal intensive care. My research and writing have examined how we as professionals can meet our obligation to support families whose infants undergo a technology that has both the beneficial power to cure, and the harmful power to preserve lives filled with suffering. Through my work I have also attempted to analyze some of the challenges neonatal nurses face in maintaining their sense of ethical integrity, and this has led to studies of characteristics of the neonatal intensive care unit (NICU) organizational environments that support or impede open communication and resolution of ethical dilemmas inherent in neonatal intensive care.

I was fortunate to begin my specialization in neonatal intensive care as a master's student in pediatric nursing at the Frances Payne Bolton School of Nursing at Case Western Reserve University (CWRU) in Cleveland, Ohio. The NICU at Rainbow Babies' and Children's Hospital (a part of CWRU's teaching hospitals) specialized in the care of extremely premature newborns under the medical direction of two physicians—Drs. Marshall Klaus and John Kennell—who were as interested in humane care as they were in state-of-the-art, high-tech care. They defined neonatal care in a holistic way, and took into account parents' emotional responses, needs, social support, and the community resources available for families of high-risk infants.

In the NICU of Rainbow Babies' and Children's Hospital, the philosophy of care was based on the recognition that infants in the NICU are first and foremost members of families, and that infants' ultimate flourishing comes about within the nurturing environments of their homes and communities. So I was lucky to have a blend of humane caring and technology modeled from my earliest experiences as a nurse in the NICU (Kennell, 1999). This blend of care and technology, in an interesting way, postponed my entry into ethics, because at that time I did not sense a divergence between what I thought of as "morally right" for infants and families, and what we were carrying out for them in practice.

After I received my master's degree I entered the doctoral program in clinical psychology at CWRU with a specialization in infancy, childhood, and adolescence. I was supervised in therapeutic work with adolescents and, to a more limited extent, their families. My clinical psychology placement was in a residential treatment setting for school-age children with emotional problems. As I experienced the overall culture of what was a state-of-the-art residential treatment facility, I began to question the effectiveness of treatment plans that focused much more on the children than on the families whose interactions with their child or adolescent led to placement in the facility in the first place. But this was a systems problem, and I did not conceptualize it as an ethical dilemma that I had to address, since I knew I did not want to work in residential treatment settings. I knew my real love was work with families of NICU infants. When I graduated with my PhD, I left Cleveland and accepted a tenure-track faculty position in the Family Nursing Division of the School of Nursing, the University of Texas at Austin, where I immediately made contact with the three neonatal intensive care units in the area.

Early on, my clinical focus was on helping parents interact with their infants and make secure affectional ties (Penticuff, 1980). At the same time, I was becoming immersed in the teaching, research, community service, and publishing that are essential faculty activities in a research university. In my academic and community service roles I was able to do a lot of supportive work with families, and I supervised master's nursing students in work with families in crisis—rape crisis, domestic and child abuse, and families with children undergoing pediatric or neonatal intensive care. I worked closely with the staff at the regional NICU, continuing to focus on psychological aspects of the NICU experience. My publications and research from 1976–1982 mirrored my focus at the time (Hawkins, Manosevitz, Sawin, Walker, & Penticuff, 1977–78; Penticuff, 1980; Penticuff & Walker, 1981–1982). But my horizons were broadening, and I was beginning to feel that something was missing as I worked with NICU staff.

Gradually, I realized that what was missing was the humanistic part of neonatal care that had been so important in the NICU at Babies' and Children's Hospital. In Austin, the focus on high-tech care seemed to inhibit staff's recognition that aggressive neonatal therapies carry high risk and burden for infants and families. I became concerned that for some of the sicker, extremely premature infants who had incurred profound neurological impairments, life-prolonging treatment might be more a harm than a benefit. And I was troubled about families' lack of understanding of these complications, as well as the ramifications for their infants' future development. When I brought up my concerns with the medical director of the unit, the response was "The important thing is first to save their lives." No matter where I went in Texas, this mantra seemed to be the official party line, and I felt strongly that this absolutist view was morally wrong.

In 1981 I was fortunate to attend the Intensive Bioethics Course at the Kennedy Institute of Ethics, Georgetown University. I thought that a grounding in bioethics could help me think through my concerns about high-tech neonatal care. Again, my publications were a means for putting forth my evolving interpretation of ethical imperatives in nursing practice. My first ethics publication was in 1982 (Penticuff, 1982a), while on a parallel track the psychology focus continued (Penticuff, 1982b, 1982c; 1984; Walker & Penticuff, 1979–1981).

My ethics focus in the NICU was on parents' moral authority in making decisions about the continuation or withdrawal of burdensome therapies which would merely prolong dying, or would sustain a life overshadowed by devastating impairment and chronic illness (Penticuff, 1988). A central aspect of my focus was the health care professional's obligation (derived from the duty to respect autonomy) to provide clear, understandable information essential to the parents' ability to make informed choices about their infant's treatment (Penticuff, 1988). I reasoned that neonatal intensive care is inherently burdensome for infants, and the only justification for such treatment is that the ultimate benefit to the infant outweighs the harms (Penticuff, 1987).

In 1983, in response to media reports of Down Syndrome and multiply disfigured infants being denied life-sustaining medical treatment, the Reagan administration promulgated its initial "Baby Doe" regulations; the final regulations were enacted after 2 years of public and professional debate (U. S. Department of Health and Human Services [DHHS], 1985). These federal policies prohibited the withholding of life-sustaining therapies from handicapped infants, regardless of an infant's present or predicted quality of life. I felt that I had no choice but to get involved with this issue, since I had seen the havoc and broken lives (Stinson & Stinson, 1983) that could result when quality of life was trumped by what Arthur Caplan termed the "technological imperative" (Caplan & Cohen, 1987).

I decided to do some qualitative research (Penticuff, 1983) in which I interviewed all of the regional NICU neonatologists and a number of the neonatal nurses. In the summer of 1983, as a Hastings Center Visiting Scholar, I worked with Arthur Caplan and Thomas Murray in analyzing the interviews, and subsequently was invited to join the newly formed Hastings Center Research Group on Ethics and the Care of the Newborn. At first I was the only nurse among philosophers and sociologists, and I felt quite nervous and reluctant to express my unschooled ethical views. But I realized that as a clinician I had an important perspective on neonatal intensive care, and I was fortunate to be able to discuss my views with several physicians who shared my concerns. For me, my most important discussion was with Raymond Duff, MD, who put his professional career on the line with his publication of decisions to withdraw life-sustaining treatment in the NICU (Duff & Campbell, 1973). So I "screwed my courage to the sticking point" and spoke up.

The initial premise of the Research Group was that life-sustaining treatments were being withheld (unethically) from some newborns in American NICUs because the newborns had handicaps. My (clearly minority) view was that the much larger problem was a mammoth, unfeeling, unstoppable technology. Early on, no one in the group seemed inclined to look comprehensively at outcomes of high-tech neonatal care. Many believed that it was inherently right to provide neonatal intensive care to save infant lives, and that outcomes were of secondary importance. My concerns were about quality of life, and I believed that allowing some infants to die was morally permissible and sometimes obligatory. My views were based on the idea that in using powerful technology, we are ethically obligated to look at good and harm from the perspectives of the infants and parents who must live with what that technology produces (Penticuff, 1987).

Gradually it became apparent to the group that, in fact, overtreatment and disregard for quality of life were the larger problems in the NICU. The lack of decision authority by caring, informed parents in NICU decision-making also became apparent (Pinch, 2002; Pinch & Spielman, 1989). My 3-year participation (December, 1983–April, 1987) in the discussions of the Hastings Center group, including my contribution to the writing of the *Imperiled Newborns* special issue of the *Hastings Center Report* (Caplan & Cohen, 1987), provided an important foundation for all of my succeeding work in ethics.

I suppose that my contributions in the field of nursing ethics, and bioethics generally, have come out of my deep sense that as nurses, we have a moral obligation to prevent and alleviate unnecessary suffering (Penticuff, 1997, 2006). I have been influenced by the writing of Sally Gadow, who was the first nurse to state that the goal of nursing is to alleviate human vulnerability (Gadow, 1988). When you read the work of Eric Cassell (1991), you see that suffering creates the most profound of all vulnerabilities. My conclusion about neonatal intensive care is that, unless the focus on what technology can achieve is tempered by a humanistic focus on alleviating the suffering and vulnerability of NICU infants and families, there cannot be real involvement of parents in decisions about whether it is morally right to employ aggressive technology for their particular infants.

Neonatal technology is a double-edged sword for infants at the margin of viability, because it holds both promise and peril. The promise is that for some of these infants, outcomes are good. But for others, the burdensome treatments produce suffering without the moral justification of a life experienced as more of a good than a harm for infants and families.

Professionals who care for NICU infants often are reluctant to discuss the burdens of aggressive NICU treatment, during which infants experience pain, air hunger, agitation, and noxious stimulation (Blackburn & Barnard, 1985; Franck, 1987, 1992; Perlman & Volpe, 1989; Walden, et al., 2001). The loving, soothing, nurturing interaction with parents that is so important in calming distressed infants is often precluded by high-tech treatment such as high-frequency ventilation (Penticuff, 1980). For infants whose NICU hospitalization stretches into months, there is deprivation of stimulation appropriate for cognitive and physical development (Aucott, Donohue, Atkins, & Allen, 2002; Gottfried & Gaiter, 1985). If an infant incurs devastating complications (especially large hemorrhages into the brain, resulting in severe neurological impairment), the outcome is likely to be a future of profoundly diminished quality of life (Wilson-Costello, Friedman, Minich, Fanaroff, & Hack, 2005). For some previable infants admitted to the NICU, use of technology merely prolongs dying.

The most high-tech, aggressive therapies required to save the lives of the sickest infants born at the border of viability (i.e., 23–26 weeks' gestation) include multiple invasive procedures, agitation from pain and chronic air hunger, inadequate assessment and management of infant pain, and deprivation of soothing parental interaction (Aucott, et al., 2002; Penticuff, 1989; Walden, et al., 2001). Aggressive neonatal care is, clearly, inherently burdensome to infants and families. The morality of applying aggressive treatment must be judged by the good or harm experienced by infants and families. I also believe that informed, caring parents have the ultimate moral authority to judge when burden to the infant is not offset by benefit. This latter view became the direction that my succeeding research would take (Penticuff, 1995, 1998; Penticuff & Arheart, 2005).

Beginning around 1990, I became interested in how characteristics of practice environments—e.g., staff communication patterns in hospital units—might influence nurses' actions as advocates for infants and families and their involvement in the resolution of ethical dilemmas in clinical practice. I carried out several research studies funded by the National Institute of Nursing Research (NINR), National Institutes of Health (NIH), that focused on these issues (Penticuff, 1989; Penticuff & Walden, 2000).

Perhaps my most outstanding academic achievement was my intervention research funded by NINR from 1997–2001: Parent-Professional Collaboration in NICU Decisions. The study aimed to help families participate collaboratively with NICU professionals in deciding appropriate care when infants sustained severe complications of extreme prematurity. The conceptualization of the study was driven by my view that we (nurses and other health care professionals) are obligated to use our judgment and skill to decrease the vulnerability of parents in the NICU. I was guided by the following premises: For parents to collaborate in decisions, they must have an adequate understanding of their infant's medical condition, treatment options, and associated prognoses, and they must have an opportunity to discuss treatment plans with professionals. Therefore, I wanted to design an intervention that would help parents to accurately understand their infant's medical condition, treatment options, and the probable outcomes of each option. The intervention also had to give parents a venue in which they could sit down with their infant's care providers in a private, quiet place near the NICU and discuss their infant's care and the recommended treatments, and ask questions.

Quantitative findings of this study support the effectiveness of the intervention, especially in increasing collaboration scores for minority mothers (Penticuff & Arheart, 2005). But the qualitative data (analysis of the audiotaped Care Planning Meetings for the intervention group) told a different story about shared decision-making.

We found that in the Care Planning Meetings the neonatologists and nurse practitioners in our study never brought up the topic of withdrawal of life-sustaining treatment, even in infants with chronic lung disease on ventilators who had incurred severe neurological complications. Issues of quality of life were not brought up. Physicians discussed complications in terms of their pathophysiology and avoided discussion of the probable impact of complications on the infant's future health and functional abilities. Parents also avoided stress-producing topics in the discussion of their infant's medical condition and prognosis.

As I reflected upon the qualitative findings of this study, I concluded that it is understandable that professionals in the NICU would avoid emotionally difficult discussions with parents. In the large majority of NICU settings, professionals lack the supervised training, the available time, and the organizational support that such conversations require (Buckman, 1992; Roter & Hall, 2006). For parents, too, the support for such conversations often is lacking, and parents who are emotionally unprepared to hear "bad news" are likely to shun these conversations. My goal in future work is to assist NICU professionals to develop skills in the supportive communication of "bad news," and to assist NICU organizations to develop supportive environments in which such communication can take place. My work to help families understand the information they need to make important health decisions and to facilitate their decision-making process is ongoing.

As I come to the end of this recollection of my work in nursing ethics, I'd like to return to the focus on suffering and compassion. I have wondered about why these two phenomena are so morally intriguing to me. And I think that the intrigue is because it is only within face-to-face encounters that one can understand that another suffers. And the comprehension that another suffers is the moral warrant for compassion. I close with some excerpts from a recent presentation in Hualian, Taiwan:

Nursing ethics—nursing's views of what it means to do good for those who are ill—arise from the interactions that occur within arm's length between patient and nurse. All of the activities of nursing are focused ultimately on the good done within arm's length. ... What do nurses derive from this perspective? All that can be perceived by the senses may be taken in. ... Within arm's length the nurse hears the patient's whisper, sees the small movements of trembling, or tears, or the barely perceptible smile.

Nursing ethics view as relevant the entirety of human experiencing—how it is for the patient who is ill, and how it is for the nurse committed to doing good for that patient. Nursing ethics have evolved from nursing's rich history of collective narratives—stories of compassion, duty, giving, touching, and close contact with an infinite array of human struggles and transcendence. ... Nursing ethics are founded in what it is to be a good nurse: embracing what it feels like, what one must give from within oneself, the disillusionment felt in one's own and others' failures, what one must know, what is learned in encounters with the heroic saving of life, with cures thought impossible, with unexpected deaths, with suffering, and with prolonged dying. The ethical nurse ponders these and brings the sensitivities that are gained in each episode into the next patient encounter. Ethical practice thus evolves as the nurse through experience and reflection comes to understand how to be with patients in ways that allow a valid carrying out of what is good for that patient, what affirms that patient's dignity (Penticuff, 2006).

References

Aucott, S., Donohue, P. K., Atkins, E., & Allen, M. C. (2002). Neurodevelopmental care in the NICU. *Mental Retardation and Developmental Disabilities Research Reviews, 8*(4), 298–308.

Blackburn, S., & Barnard, K. (1985). Analysis of caregiving events in preterm infants in the special care unit. In A. Gottfried & J. Gaiter (Eds.), *Infants under stress: Environmental neonatology* (pp. 113–129). Baltimore: University Park Press.

Buckman, R. (1992). *How to break bad news: A guide for health care professionals.* Baltimore: Johns Hopkins University Press.

Caplan, A., & Cohen, C. B. (Eds.). (1987). Imperiled newborns. *Hastings Center Report, 17*(6), 5–32.

Cassell, E. J. (1991). *The nature of suffering and the goals of medicine.* New York: Oxford University Press.

Duff, R., & Campbell, A.G. M. (1973). Moral and ethical dilemmas in the special-care nursery. *New England Journal of Medicine, 289*(17), 890–894.

Franck, L. S. (1987). A national survey of the assessment and treatment of pain and agitation in the neonatal intensive care unit. *Journal of Obstetric, Gynecologic, and Neonatal Nursing, 16*(6), 387–393.

Franck, L. S. (1992). The influence of sociopolitical, scientific, and technologic forces on the study and treatment of neonatal pain. *Advances in Nursing Science, 15*(1), 11–20.

Gadow, S. (1988). Covenant without cure: Letting go and holding on in chronic illness. In J. Watson & M. Ray (Eds.), *The ethics of care and the ethics of cure: Synthesis in chronicity* (pp. 5–14). New York: National League for Nursing Publication # 15-2237.

Gottfried, A. W., & Gaiter, J. L. (1985). *Infant stress under intensive care: Environmental neonatology.* Baltimore, MD: University Park Press.

Hawkins, R., Manosevitz, M., Sawin, R., Walker, L., & Penticuff, J. Investigators (1977–1988). Psychosocial risks in pregnancy and early infancy. A one-year grant to conduct a symposia series on psychosocial risks in pregnancy and early infancy. Funded by the National Institute of Child Health and Human Development.

Kennell, J. H. (1999). The humane neonatal care initiative. *Acta paediatrica, 88,* 367–70.

Penticuff, J. (1980). Disruption of attachment formation through reproductive casualty and early separation. In D. Sawin, R. Hawkins, L. Walker, & J. Penticuff (Eds.), *Exceptional infant IV: Psychosocial risks in infant-environment transactions* (pp. 161–173). New York: Brunner/Mazel.

Penticuff, J. (1982a). Resolving ethical dilemmas in critical care. *Dimensions of Critical Care Nursing, 1*(1), 22–27.

Penticuff, J. (1982b). Psychologic implications of high-risk pregnancy. *Nursing Clinics of North America, 17*(1), 69–78.

Penticuff, J. (1982c). The strange situation procedure. In S. Humenick (Ed.), *Analysis of current assessment strategies in the health care of young children and childbearing families* (pp. 202–214). New York: Appleton-Century-Crofts.

Penticuff, J. (1983). Nursing assessment and management of the childbearing family in crisis. In K. Vestal & C. McKenzie (Eds.), *Association of critical care nurses' high-risk perinatal nursing* (pp. 80–96). Philadelphia: W. B. Saunders.

Penticuff, J. (PI) (1984). Effects of supportive environment on developmental outcome in neurologically impaired premature infants. Funded by the University Research Institute, The University of Texas at Austin.

Penticuff, J. (1987). Neonatal nursing ethics: Toward a consensus. *Neonatal Network, 5*(6), 7–16.

Penticuff, J. (1988). Neonatal intensive care: Parental prerogatives. *Journal of Perinatal and Neonatal Nursing, 1*(3), 77–86.

Penticuff, J. (1989). Infant suffering and nurse advocacy in Neonatal Intensive Care. *Nursing Clinics of North America, 24*(4), 987–997.

Penticuff, J. (1995). Nursing ethics in perinatal care. In A. Goldworth, W. Silverman, D. Stevenson, & E. Young (Eds.), *Ethics and perinatology: Issues and perspectives* (pp. 405–426). Oxford University Press.

Penticuff, J. (1997). Nursing perspectives in bioethics. In K. Hoshino (Ed.), *Japanese and Western Bioethics: Studies in Moral Diversity* (pp. 49–60). Boston: Kleuwer Academic Publishers.

Penticuff, J. (1998). Defining futility in neonatal intensive care. *Nursing Clinics of North America, 33*(2), 339–352.

Penticuff, J. (2006). Nursing perspectives on ethics: Caring within arm's length. Keynote address, International Conference on Nursing Ethics, Hualian, Taiwan, September, 2006.

Penticuff, J. H., & Arheart, K. (2005). Effectiveness of an intervention to improve parent-professional collaboration in neonatal intensive care. *Journal of Perinatal and Neonatal Nursing, 19*(2), 187–202.

Penticuff, J., & Walden, M. (2000). Influence of practice environment and nurse characteristics on perinatal nurses' responses to ethical dilemmas. *Nursing Research, 49*(2), 64–72.

Penticuff, J., & Walker, L. Co-Investigators. (1981–1982). Antecedents of infant-mother attachment. Funded by the Hogg Foundation for Mental Health.

Perlman, J. M., & Volpe, J. J. (1989). Movement disorder of premature infants with severe bronchopulmonary dysplasia: A new syndrome. *Pediatrics, 84*(2), 215–18.

Pinch, W. J. (2002). *When the bough breaks: Parental perceptions of ethical decision-making in NICU.* Lanham, MD: University Press of America.

Pinch, W. J., & Spielman, M. (1989). Ethical decision-making for high-risk infants: The parents' perspective. *Nursing Clinics of North America, 24*(4), 1017–23.

Roter, D. L., & Hall, J. A. (2006). *Doctors talking with patients/Patients talking with doctors* (2nd ed.). Westport, CN: Praeger.

Stinson, R., & Stinson, P. (1983). *The long dying of baby Andrew.* Boston: Little, Brown & Co.

U.S. Department of Health and Human Services. (April 15, 1985). Child abuse and neglect prevention and treatment program. Final Rule: 45 CFR 1340. *Federal Register: Rules and Regulations, 50*(72), 14878–14892.

Walden, M., Penticuff, J., Stevens, B., Lotas, M., Kozinetz, C., Clark, A., et al. (2001). Maturational changes in physiologic and behavioral responses of preterm neonates to pain. *Advances in Neonatal Care, 1*(2), 94–106.

Walker, L. (PI), & Penticuff, J. Co-Investigator. Toward models of mother-infant dyadic development. A three-year research grant to study the impact of maternal attitudes and infant characteristics on later month-infant interaction. Funded by DHEW, 1979–1981.

Wilson-Costello, D., Friedman, H., Minich, N., Fanaroff, A., & Hack, M. (2005). Improved survival rates with increased neurodevelopmental disability for extremely low birth weight infants in the 1990s. *Pediatrics, 115*(4), 997–1003.

⌒

Joy H. Penticuff is the Lee and Joseph Jamail Professor of Nursing at the University of Texas at Austin School of Nursing. She holds an MSN in Pediatric Nursing and a PhD in Clinical Psychology from Case Western Reserve University and a Bachelor of Science in Nursing from The Medical College of Georgia. Dr. Penticuff's work in bioethics began in 1981 when she attended the Intensive Bioethics Course at the Kennedy Institute of Ethics. In 1983 she was a Visiting Scholar at the Hastings Center in New York and in 1989–90 she was Senior Fellow at the Center for Ethics, Medicine, and Public Issues at Baylor College of Medicine, Houston, Texas. Special interests include empirical ethics research, parent-professional collaboration in treatment decisions for extremely premature infants, and supportive communication of "bad news."

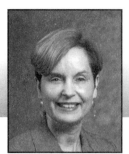

Cynda H. Rushton

CHAPTER 26

Caregiver Suffering: Finding Meaning When Integrity is Threatened

Framing the Issue

Suffering, often unacknowledged, has confronted nurses and other members of the interdisciplinary team for decades. Its incidence and intensity have increased with the growth of technology, complexity of care, and diversity of moral viewpoints.

By definition, to care is to suffer with, to share solidarity. Suffering for and with another person ignites our innate capacities for compassionate action. Caring for others signifies concern for them as persons. It involves creating and sustaining relationships and connotes a strong sense of responsibility to attend to and provide for the holistic needs of another. Caring is demonstrated through the embodiment of healing presence (Koener, 2007). In the context of caregiver suffering, caring can be extended to caring for ourselves and our colleagues.

Suffering can arise intermittently or be sustained over long periods. As Tatelbaum (1989) explained, suffering is the "persistence of painful feelings long after they were provoked." It leaves an indelible imprint. As individuals, we are "hardwired" to remember our suffering, to integrate its details into both conscious and unconscious parts of our psyche. Often caregivers can recount details of a past situation that caused them suffering more vividly than they can describe a recent event. A "moral residue" persists as the aftermath of compromised integrity becomes ingrained in the memory of the person (Webster & Baylis, 2000). When suffering is unresolved and remains in the unconscious, it will likely reappear when similar experiences of suffering occur, or may manifest itself as inappropriate or disproportionate responses to other situations.

The experience of suffering often leaves the person feeling exposed and vulnerable. At its root is the sense of having no control over one's destiny, of submitting to or being forced to endure some particular set of circumstances (Hauerwas, 1986). This view of suffering as a passive process is often reinforced by a view of suffering as an inevitable part of certain experiences, diseases, or roles. Some believe that suffering has redemptive value and "builds character," while others hold that it does not build character, but rather reveals it. Regardless of the meaning assigned to suffering, both positive and negative consequences are possible.

The Context

More than 20 years ago, I began to work as a clinical ethics educator, translating complex ethical concepts into clinical practice within an interdisciplinary model. As a translational ethicist, I taught and mentored nurses to empower them, to give them the knowledge and skills they need to engage in interdisciplinary dialogue and advocate for the patients and families they serve. As a pediatric nurse, I was drawn to difficult cases. Early in my career, when I worked in critical care, I helped care for an infant who had been asphyxiated in a defectively designed crib. Neurologically devastated, she lived in our intensive care unit for almost 2 years in a persistent vegetative state (PVS) with a tracheostomy, a feeding tube, and mechanical ventilation that her parents wanted withdrawn. As we gave her highly specialized nursing care and maintained her personhood by daily bathing and grooming, we witnessed her reflex responses to frequent suctioning and positioning that some interpreted as suffering, despite her impaired brain function. We vacillated between compassion and feelings of disgust, remorse, and objectification. Often outraged by continuing aggressive treatment despite her parents' preferences to allow her to die, we practiced in a climate of ambiguity, uncertain about the ethical boundaries of treatment and fearful of the ramifications of honoring parental requests to limit life-sustaining therapies. For almost 2 years, she was a living reminder of the perils of the unbridled use of our emerging technologies. When she died despite our aggressive efforts to treat an overwhelming sepsis, we were all relieved her journey was finally over. For me, her death marked the beginning of my personal exploration of moral distress and caregiver suffering.

In the mid-1980s, I was a clinical nurse specialist for neonatology and general pediatric surgery at the Henrietta Egleston Hospital for Children in Atlanta, Georgia, where I was often involved in difficult cases involving very premature infants and those born with congenital malformations. During that time, a series of "Baby Doe" cases sparked national debate about the care of and decision-making for imperiled newborns. When the hospital responded to a federal mandate by creating an interdisciplinary infant care review committee, I was invited to serve.

I moved to Washington, DC, and the Children's National Medical Center, where I continued my work in neonatal care and quickly aligned myself with the newly formed Office of Ethics. There, in one of the nation's first institutionally based clinical ethics programs, I worked with Dr. Sanford Leikin and Dr. Jonathan Moreno (Philosopher in Residence). Together we began to create an ethics consultation process, education and support, and interdisciplinary dialogue. As nursing liaison, I learned from other nurses and care team members that their suffering was often a response to their moral distress and threats to their integrity. Their concerns were magnified because of the special moral commitments that arose from caring for critically ill and dying infants and children.

My passion led me to pursue a doctorate focusing on bioethics, and conversations with Dr. Warren T. Reich over several years led me to write one of the first articles about professional caregiver suffering (Rushton, 1992). Reich (1989) defined suffering as "an anguish experienced as a threat to our composure, our integrity, the fulfillment of our intentions, and more deeply as a frustration to the concrete meaning that we have found in our personal experience. It is the anguish over the injury or threat to the injury to the self and thus the meaning of the self that is at the core of suffering." Reich's definition allowed me to define responses to suffering and examine related concepts. Recently, others have expanded the dialogue about the relevance of suffering to professional practice (Browning, 2004; Jesuit, 2000; Sudin-Huard & Fahy, 1999).

For caregivers, the perceived inability to minimize or eliminate tragic outcomes brings on feelings of powerlessness and helplessness (Jellinek, Todres, Catlin, Cassem, & Salzman, 1993). If these concerns are not legitimized by other members of the health care team or by the institution, the caregiver's moral agency is threatened (Hamric, Davis, & Childress, 2006). Enforcing rules and policies that discount the role of nurses or other health care professionals in decision-making processes renders them powerless, suppresses their values, and undermines their capacity for compassion (Halifax, Dossey, & Rushton, 2006; Hamric, et al., 2006; Rushton, 1995).

In my explorations, I examined claims of conscience as expressions of the moral conflict nurses experience as they struggle to balance competing professional and ethical obligations and preserve a sense of wholeness (Oberle & Hughes, 2001; Rushton, 1992, 2004; Rushton, Williams, & Sabatier, 2002). I found conflicts of conscience were not limited to nurses. A national, multisite survey found that almost half (47%) of the health care professionals caring for the terminally ill reported they had acted against their consciences in doing so; 7 out of 10 house officers reported distress, and 5 out of 10 nurses (Solomon, et al., 1993). Similar findings were later validated in a pediatric population (Solomon, et al., 2005).

I also explored the meaning of integrity. Whatever their source, threats to the integrity of health care professionals involve arbitrary decisions and actions that alienate them from their convictions and morality, threaten their authenticity, and cause them to neglect what matters most personally and professionally (Gutierrez, 2005; Meltzner & Huckaby, 2004). When caregivers act in a way they believe to be wrong or harmful, their loss of integrity results in suffering (Hardingham, 2004; Rushton, 1995). The provision of care deemed "futile" is a prominent source of moral distress (Ferrell, 2006; Taylor, 1995) and by extension a source of profound suffering.

According to Reich (1989), the threat to one's wholeness is a particular kind of suffering. Caregivers struggle to maintain their integrity so that they do not suffer for and with others to the point of their own demise. Because suffering and loss are inevitable dimensions of caring for patients and their families, health care professionals may feel their integrity is threatened if they "get too close" (Barnard, 1995) and allow themselves to experience grief or love (Peter & Liaschenko, 2004). Intimacy with patients and families requires a balance between empathizing with and sharing their suffering while cultivating equanimity and embodying a healing presence (Halifax, et al., 2006; Peter & Liaschenko, 2004; Rushton, Halifax, & Dossey, 2007).

Understanding these threats is the key to understanding suffering. Underlying them all is a threat to the individual's integrity, that internal state of wholeness in all dimensions of a person's being—physical, emotional, and spiritual. Integrity relies on the balance and harmony of the various dimensions of human existence. Because we are whole beings, suffering occurs at the level of the whole being (Singh, 1998). Threats to bodily integrity can become evident as disease, injury, or illness. For caregivers, physical symptoms may be manifestations of their own conscious and unconscious suffering within their professional roles. Their psychological integrity may be undermined by a disintegration of the self by psychopathology or threats to personhood. Their self-image may be undermined by unrealistic expectations, suppressed feelings, maladaptive coping, dysfunctional relationships, and flawed communication. Because spiritual integrity involves an integration of moral character, adherence to moral norms, and coherent and consistent behavior within a set of principles, it too is vulnerable to disruptions.

At the core of each threat is the sense of loss—of integrity, self-image, relationships, and hopes for the future—and of grief in the face of loss. For health care professionals, this includes threats to their integrity when they cannot resolve core issues. They may feel incapable of honoring their core commitments to their patients, or of seeing a dignified death as a healing act. For caregivers, suffering can be more personal as they become disconnected from their own needs and desires, personal or professional relationships, and the deepest meaning of their lives.

Another concept related to caregiver suffering is moral distress. Jameton (1984) described moral distress as a phenomenon that occurs when individuals are unable to translate their moral choices into action (Jameton, 1984, 1987, 1993). Jameton's definition was later expanded to include the distress that occurs when individuals "attempt" to implement actions they perceive to be correct, but their effort fails to resolve the underlying conflict (Gutierrez, 2005). When health care professionals cannot live up to their personal values by acting in an ethical manner, they experience moral distress in response to their own suffering.

According to Jameton, individuals may initially experience frustration, anger, and anxiety in response to the obstacles and conflicts with others about important values. Their real or perceived inability to act upon their initial moral distress involves an appraisal of how the situation and the actions taken or not taken promote or undermine integrity, and/or result in participation in actions that are viewed as wrong (Jameton, 1993).

For some time, I vacillated in my thinking. Did moral distress cause suffering, or was suffering a type of moral distress? I have come to believe that moral distress is a special form of suffering and that the concepts are inextricably linked. There is an expanding literature on moral distress in nursing (Austin, Lemermeyer, Goldberg, Bergum, & Johnson, 2005; Corley, 1995, 1998; Gutierrez, 2005; Hanna, 2004), and now extending to other disciplines (Austin, Rankel, Kagan, Bergum, & Lemermeyer, 2005; Kälvemark, Höglund, Hansson, Westerholm, & Atnetz, 2004).

The sense of being disconnected from oneself characterizes caregiver suffering. Burnout is "a state of gradual physical, emotional, mental exhaustion caused by long-term involvement in emotionally demanding situations" (Malakin-Pines & Aronson, 1988). In contrast, compassion fatigue is characterized by a sense of helplessness and confusion, isolation from supporters, and can have a more rapid onset and resolution (Figley, 1995). I began to see both as outcomes when individuals were unable to make sense of their suffering, or when their capacity to maintain wholeness and integrity was exceeded. More recently, these consequences have led me to explore the concepts of resilience and renewal and their relationship to suffering (see Figure 26.1).

Over the last 10 years, my work in ethics has focused on palliative and end-of-life care. As an ethics consultant since the late 1980s and cochair of the Johns Hopkins Hospital Ethics Committee and Consultation Service since 1999, I found that most ethics consults focused on some aspect of end-of-life care and involved moral distress and caregiver suffering. When I began to examine the nature of suffering related to end-of-life care, I began to appreciate different worldviews. I was deeply influenced by my training in the program "Being With Dying: Compassionate End of Life Care" (Halifax, et al., 2006; Rushton, et al., 2007). The Buddhist notions of suffering and compassion resonated with my clinical experiences and intuitions about how to begin to create a more holistic and healing environment for practice. The program also led me to consider the broader context of organizational ethics and their implications for integrity (Rushton & Brooks-Brunn, 1997; Rushton & Scanlon, 1995; Rushton, et al., 2002), and to explore the interconnections among suffering, moral distress, trust, betrayal, respect, and integrity (Reina, Reina, & Rushton, 2007; Rushton, 1992, 2006, 2007; Rushton, Reina, & Reina, 2007).

Impact on Health Care Ethics

Although I initially framed the issue of caregiver suffering broadly, for many years others and I have focused on nurses and the practice of nursing. During my chairmanship, the American Association of Critical-Care Nurses (AACN) Ethics Workgroup developed a position statement on moral distress, along with a model, curriculum, and process for clinical settings (AACN, 2005, 2006). Based on my prior work, it is the first of its kind and includes a "tool kit" that has been widely adopted and applied to clinical cases (Rushton, 2006).

Building on this work, I collaborated with Dr. Gail Geller to lead an interdisciplinary team funded by the National Institutes of Health's Ethical, Legal, and Social Implications of the Human Genome Project, to study moral distress and suffering among genetics service providers. Preliminary work suggests that the definition of moral distress must be broadened to capture the range of threats to the integrity of these professionals. The final outcome will be recommendations for a national agenda to address moral distress in clinical genetics practice.

Figure 26.1

Provisional Relationships Among Concepts

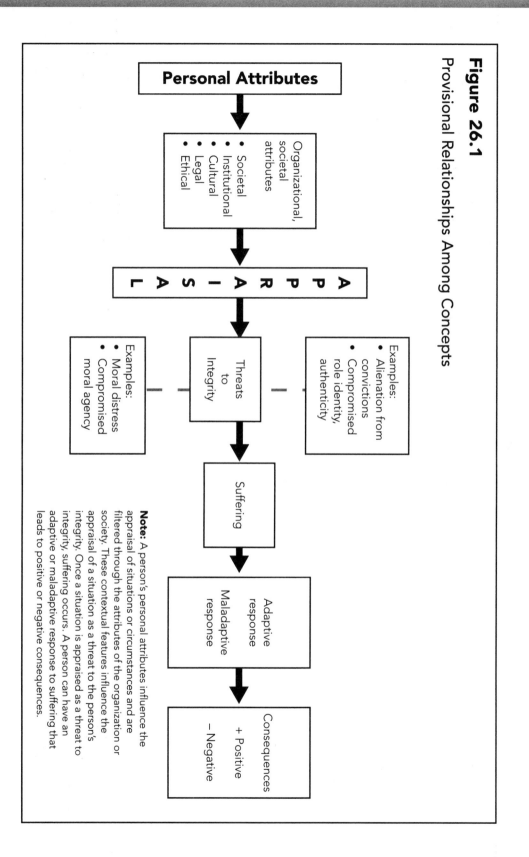

Personal Attributes

Organizational, societal attributes

- Societal
- Institutional
- Cultural
- Legal
- Ethical

A P P R A I S A L

Examples:
- Alienation from convictions
- Compromised role identity, authenticity

Threats to Integrity

Examples:
- Moral distress
- Compromised moral agency

Suffering

Adaptive response

Maladaptive response

Consequences
+ Positive
– Negative

Note: A person's personal attributes influence the appraisal of situations or circumstances and are filtered through the attributes of the organization or society. These contextual features influence the appraisal of a situation as a threat to the person's integrity. Once a situation is appraised as a threat to integrity, suffering occurs. A person can have an adaptive or maladaptive response to suffering that leads to positive or negative consequences.

Meaning of This Work for the Future

Caregiver suffering is real and has profound implications for individuals, their professions, and the people they serve. My explorations underscore its universality and significance; its meaning and consequences highlight the moral responsibility of health care professionals and institutions to address it compassionately. Thoughts of totally eliminating it are unrealistic and undesirable. Contrary to contemporary Western views of suffering as negative and without value, befriending our suffering and ourselves has the potential to transform medical and nursing practice. It can take nurses back to the holistic vision of nursing described by Florence Nightingale as a calling to service, rather than rote technicians who are solely focused on statistics and tasks (Dossey, 2000; Dossey, Selanders, Beck, & Attewell, 2005).

The way health care professionals respond to their own suffering is mirrored in their responses to the suffering of patients and families. If we can respond to our own suffering with compassion and nonjudgment, we can respond similarly to the sufferings of patients and families (Rushton, Reder, et al., 2006). Still, health care professionals, including nurses, are sorely lacking skills in self-compassion, renewal, and the cultivation of resilience.

Creating an environment that allows caregivers to practice with integrity is no simple task. Strategies to promote the integrity of the person being cared for, their family, the health care professional, the institution, and the community require multipronged efforts. Only through a commitment to a shared vision can health care professionals and the institutions successfully impact the experience of suffering and its effect on the quality of patient care. Addressing this important issue involves more than individual interventions. To evolve to a place where interdisciplinary sharing and problem solving are possible, the entire care team needs to engage in interdisciplinary forums where they can discuss suffering and define coping strategies.

Acknowledging and bearing witness to suffering are important steps toward creating an environment of integrity. Educational sessions that include experiential exercises can sensitize professionals to the issues. Forums such as ethics rounds, patient care conferences, and debriefings following patient deaths can help interdisciplinary teams address their own suffering and moral distress and create a supportive space for sharing, reflection, and resolution (Rushton, Reder, et al., 2006). Suffering for and with our patients will always be a dimension of nursing practice. Our challenge is to care for ourselves so we can continue to care for others.

To this end, the profession has asserted that nurses can no longer disregard their deepest needs; they must address their own suffering. The latest revision of the ANA

Code of Ethics mandates that nurses transform their professional norms to honor values of wholeness, appropriate boundaries, self-respect, and integrity (ANA, 2001). Nurses themselves must develop new professional accountabilities and reward them visibly and often.

Nurses must also partner with the institutions where they practice to create environments grounded in integrity. As the nursing shortage escalates, institutions must acknowledge and respond to the impact of caregiver suffering on the workforce, or risk further erosion of the profession. Nursing must unite, as a profession, to advocate for practice models that respect the contributions of nurses and nurture their physical, emotional, and spiritual well-being.

Broader Significance (Beyond the Discipline of Nursing)

Recognizing moral distress as a special form of suffering allows nurses to enter into interdisciplinary dialogue with other health care professionals about its incidence and intensity (Kälvemark, et al., 2004; Rushton, 2006; Rushton, Reder, et al., 2006). Today, programs and textbooks focused on pediatric palliative and end-of-life care acknowledge the suffering of the entire interdisciplinary team (Carter & Levetown, 2004; The Initiative for Pediatric Palliative Care, 2003). Today, more interdisciplinary dialogue is occurring within hospitals and other settings about these issues (Kane, 2006; Rushton, Reder, et al., 2006).

I believe that recognizing and understanding caregiver suffering can transform clinical practice. If health care professionals, administrators, organizations, and institutions join forces, they can create a more compassionate practice environment (Barden, 2005; Ulrich, et al., 2007) for caregivers and for patients and their families alike.

References

American Association of Critical-Care Nurses. (2005). *4 A's to rise above moral distress toolkit.* Aliso Viejo, CA: Author.

American Association of Critical-Care Nurses. (2006). *Moral distress position statement.* Aliso Viejo, CA: Author.

American Nurses Association. (2001). *Code of ethics for nurses with interpretive statements.* Washington, DC: Author.

Austin, W., Lemermeyer, G., Goldberg, L., Bergum, V., & Johnson, M. (2005). Moral distress in healthcare practice: The situation of nurses. *HEC Forum, 17*(1), 33–48.

Austin, W., Rankel, M., Kagan, L., Bergum, V., & Lemermeyer, G. (2005). To stay or to go, to speak or stay silent, to act or not to act: Moral distress as experienced by psychologists. *Ethics & Behavior, 15*(3), 197–212.

Barden, C. (Ed.). (2005). *AACN standards for establishing and sustaining healthy work environments: A journey to excellence.* Aliso Viejo, CA: American Association of Critical-Care Nurses.

Barnard, D. (1995). The promise of intimacy and the fear of our own undoing. *Journal of Palliative Care, 11*(4), 22–26.

Browning, D. M. (2004). Fragments of love: Explorations in the ethnography of suffering and professional caregiving. In J. Berzoff & P. Silverman (Eds.), *Living with dying: A handbook for end-of-life healthcare practitioners* (pp. 21–42). New York: Columbia University Press.

Carter, B. S., & Levetown, M. (2004). *Palliative care for infants, children, and adolescents: A practical handbook.* Baltimore: Johns Hopkins University Press.

Corley, M. (1995). Moral distress of critical care nurses. *American Journal of Critical Care, 4*(4), 280–285.

Corley, M. C. (1998). Ethical dimensions of nurse-physician relations in intensive care. *Nursing Clinics of North America, 33*(2), 325–337.

Dossey, B. M. (2000). *Florence Nightingale: Mystic, visionary, healer.* Springhouse, PA: Springhouse Corp.

Dossey, B. M., Selanders, L. C., Beck, D. M., & Attewell, A. (2005). *Florence Nightingale today: Healing, leadership, global action.* Silver Spring, MD: American Nurses Association.

Ferrell, B. R. (2006). Understanding moral distress of nurses witnessing medically futile care. *Oncology Nursing Forum, 33*(5), 992–930.

Figley, C. R. (1995). *Compassion fatigue: Coping with secondary traumatic stress disorder in those who treat the traumatized.* New York: Brunner/Mazel.

Gutierrez, K. M. (2005). Critical care nurses' perceptions of and responses to moral distress. *Dimensions in Critical Care Nursing, 24*(5), 229–241.

Halifax, J., Dossey, B., & Rushton, C. (2006). *Compassionate care of the dying: An integral approach.* Santa Fe, NM: Prajna Mountain Publishers.

Hamric, A. B., Davis, W. A., & Childress, M. D. (2006). Moral distress in health care professionals. *The Pharos of Alpha Omega Alpha-Honor Medical Society, 69*(1), 16–23.

Hanna, D. R. (2004). Moral distress: The state of the science. *Research & Theory for Nursing Practice, 18*(1), 73–93.

Hardingham, L. B. (2004). Integrity and moral residue: Nurses as participants in a moral community. *Nursing Philosophy, 5*(2), 127–134.

Hauerwas, S. (1986). *Suffering presence: Theological reflections on medicine, the mentally handicapped and the church.* Notre Dame, IN: University of Notre Dame Press.

The Initiative for Pediatric Palliative Care. (2003). [Online]. Available from http://www.ippcweb.org/

Jameton, A. (1984). *Nursing practice, the ethical issues.* Englewood Cliffs, NJ: Prentice-Hall.

Jameton, A. (1987). Duties to self: Professional nursing in the critical care unit. In M. D. M. Fowler & J. Levine-Ariff (Eds.), *Ethics at the bedside: A source book for the critical care nurse* (pp. 115–135). Philadelphia: Lippincott.

Jameton, A. (1993). Dilemmas of moral distress: Moral responsibility and nursing practice. *AWHONN'S Clinical Issues in Perinatal & Women's Health Nursing, 4*(4), 542–551.

Jellinek, M. S., Todres, I. D., Catlin, E. A., Cassem, E. H., & Salzman, A. (1993). Pediatric intensive care training: Confronting the dark side. *Critical Care Medicine, 21*(5), 775–779.

Jesuit, D. (2000). Suffering of critical care nurses with end-of-life decisions. *MEDSURG Nursing, 9*(3), 145–152.

Kälvemark, S., Höglund, A. T., Hansson, M. G., Westerholm, P., & Arnetz, B. (2004). Living with conflicts—ethical dilemmas and moral distress in the health care system. *Social Science & Medicine, 58*(6), 1075–1084.

Kane, J. R. (2006). Pediatric palliative care moving forward: Empathy, competence, quality, and the need for systematic change. *Journal of Palliative Medicine, 9*(4), 847–849.

Koerner, J. G. (2007). *Healing presence: The essence of nursing.* New York: Springer Publishing.

Malakin-Pines, A. M., & Aronson, E. (1988). *Career burnout: Causes and cures.* New York: Free Press.

Meltzner, L. S., & Huckaby, L. M. (2004). Critical care nurses' perceptions of futile care and its effect on burnout. *American Journal of Critical Care, 13*(3), 202–208.

Oberle, K., & Hughes, D. (2001). Doctors' and nurses' perceptions of ethical problems in end-of-life decisions. *Journal of Advanced Nursing, 33*(6), 707–715.

Peter, E., & Liaschenko, J. (2004). Perils of proximity: A spatiotemporal analysis of moral distress and ambiguity. *Nursing Inquiry, 11*(4), 218–225.

Reich, W. T. (1989). Speaking of suffering: A moral account of compassion. *Soundings, 72*(1), 83–108.

Reina, D., Reina, M., & Rushton, C. (2007). Trust: The foundation for team collaboration and healthy work environments. *AACN Advanced Critical Care, 18*(2), 103–108.

Rushton, C. H. (1992). Caregiver suffering in critical care nursing. *Heart Lung, 21*(3), 303–306.

Rushton, C. H. (1995). The baby K case: Ethical challenges of preserving professional integrity. *Pediatric Nursing, 21*(4), 367–372.

Rushton, C. H. (2004). The other side of caring: Caregiver suffering. In B. S. Carter & M. Levetown (Eds.), *Palliative care for infants, children, and adolescents. A practical handbook* (pp. 220–243). Baltimore: Johns Hopkins University Press.

Rushton, C. H. (2006). Defining and addressing moral distress. *AACN Advanced Critical Care, 17*(2), 161–168.

Rushton, C. H. (2007). Respect in critical care: A foundational ethical principle. *AACN Advanced Critical Care, 18*(2), 149–156.

Rushton, C. H., & Brooks-Brunn, J. A. (1997). Environments that support ethical practice. *New Horizons, 5*(1), 20–29.

Rushton, C. H., Halifax, J., & Dossey, B. (2007). Being with dying: Contemplative practices for compassionate end of life care. *American Nurse Today, 2*(a), 16–19.

Rushton, C. H., Reder, E., Hall, B., Comello, K., Sellers, D. E., & Hutton, N. (2006). Interdisciplinary interventions to improve pediatric palliative care and reduce health care professional suffering. *Journal of Palliative Medicine, 9*(4), 922–933.

Rushton, C. H., Reina, M. L., & Reina, D. S. (2007). Building trustworthy relationships with critically ill patients and families. *AACN Advanced Critical Care, 18*(1) 19–30.

Rushton, C. H., & Scanlon, C. (1995). When values conflict with obligations: Safeguards for nurses. *Pediatric Nursing, 21*(3), 260–261, 268.

Rushton, C. H., Williams, M. A., & Sabatier, K. H. (2002). The integration of palliative care and critical care: One vision, one voice. *Critical Care Nursing Clinics of North America, 14*(2), 133–140.

Singh, K. D. (1998). *The grace in dying: How we are transformed spiritually as we die.* San Francisco: Harper San Francisco.

Solomon, M. Z., O'Donnell, L., Jennings, B., Guilfoy, V., Wolf, S. M., Nolan, K., et al. (1993). Decisions near the end of life: Professional views on life-sustaining treatments. *American Journal of Public Health, 83,* 14–23.

Solomon, M. Z., Sellers, D. E., Heller, K. S., Dokken, D. L., Levetown, M., Rushton, C., et al. (2005). New and lingering controversies in pediatric end-of-life care. *Pediatrics, 116*(4), 872–883.

Sudin-Huard, D., & Fahy, K. (1999). Moral distress, advocacy and burnout: Theorizing the relationships. *International Journal of Nursing Practice, 5*(1), 8–13.

Tatelbaum, J. (1989). *You don't have to suffer: A handbook for moving beyond life's crises.* New York: Harper & Row.

Taylor, C. (1995). *Medical futility and nursing. Image—The Journal of Nursing Scholarship, 27*(4), 301–306.

Ulrich, C., O'Donnell, P., Taylor, C., Farrar, A., Danis, M., & Grady, C. (2007). Ethical climate, ethics stress, and job satisfaction of nurses and social workers in the United States. *Social Science & Medicine, 65*(8), 1708–1719.

Webster, G. C., & Baylis, F. (2000). Moral residue. In S. B. Rubin & L. Zoloth (Eds.), *Margin of error: The ethics of mistakes in practice of medicine* (pp. 217–230). Hagerstown, MD: University Publishing Corp.

Cynda H. Rushton, PhD, RN, FAAN is an associate professor at the Johns Hopkins University School of Nursing (JHUSON) and program director of Johns Hopkins Harriet Lane Compassionate Care Program. She is a graduate of Catholic University of America (PhD), Medical University of South Carolina (MSN), and University of Kentucky (BSN). Throughout her career, Rushton has participated in national initiatives, delivered testimony to Congress, and collaborated with professional organizations to create better systems of pediatric palliative care and to see her vision for improving care at the end of life become a reality. Rushton was instrumental in creating the Harriet Lane Compassionate Care Program, the first pediatric palliative care program in Maryland. She has served as Program Director since 2000, working closely with other team members to create a 70-member interdisciplinary palliative care network, establish innovative educational programs, create a comprehensive bereavement program for families and health care professionals, and develop support systems for health care professionals who care for these children. Dr. Rushton is a frequent national and international speaker and has provided leadership and service to a variety of professional associations and societies, health care institutions, and policy agencies. In 2001 she received the American Association of Critical-Care Nurses Pioneering Spirit Award for her work in advancing palliative care across the life-span. She was selected as one of 20 Robert Wood Johnson Nurse Executive Fellows in 2006.

⤳ SECTION IX ⤳
CRITICAL THINKING ACTIVITIES

Pain and Suffering

✦ Merely being present to someone who is suffering is extremely difficult for many nurses. Why do you think this is so? What types of educational programs or support could be offered to help nurses learn how to be present and still in the face of suffering?

✦ Religious beliefs and their influence on the moral life are often ignored. Can you identify a particular religious belief that clearly influences how you approach patient care? Can you recall a patient's religious belief that had a clear impact on how a decision was made?

✦ Fowler claims, "That which heals suffering is intimacy." Think of an experience from clinical practice with a patient or family in which suffering was healed by intimacy. Explain or discuss.

✦ Penticuff asserts "Nursing ethics ... arise from the interactions that occur within arm's length between nurses and patient." Why does this have moral significance? How does nursing differ from other health professionals who are also just arm's length away from patients?

✦ Caregivers suffer as well as patients and families. Name some of the suffering that "fractures the identity of nurses," as Rushton noted in her presentation at the Legacy Seminar, from your clinical practice. What strategies work to relieve the suffering of nurses?

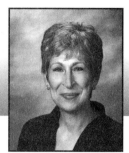

Amy M. Haddad

Endnotes:
A Mix of Metaphors

The task of summarizing what the Legacy project means is a daunting task for many reasons, not the least of which is the caliber of the contributors and the measure of their years of experience in nursing and ethics that their lives collectively represent. Since Dr. Pinch and I have had the opportunity to read the contributors' papers numerous times and listen to their comments during the Legacy seminar in April 2007, we have a good sense of the overall project and whether we attained the goals we established for the project. I believe we have met out goals and in some ways surpassed them in ways we are only beginning to understand. As Dr. Pinch notes in the introduction, we set out to gather a group of outstanding scholars in nursing ethics, many of them esteemed colleagues, some of them dear friends, in order to discuss and exchange ideas about the contributions of nurses to ethics in health care and the profession of nursing. I think that the time we spent together at the Legacy seminar and the discourse that ensued was invaluable as it informed and enriched all of the contributions and our collective understanding of what has been accomplished in nursing ethics over the past three plus decades and what challenges lie ahead.

When I think about the Legacy project from the broader perspective of summarizing the entire book rather than each individual contribution, I am struck by the mix of metaphors that come to mind. By examining the major metaphors the contributors used to talk about their work in ethics and the impact of their work in nursing and health care, I believe that it will provide some insights into the Legacy project that otherwise would be overlooked. I begin with a brief description of what a metaphor is and then turn to an exploration of the various metaphors that appear most often in the contributors' papers, what they show, what they hide, and what questions they raise.

Metaphors

A metaphor is a form of imagery. In a true metaphor we say, "A = B." A metaphor fuses together two separate things. It offers no comfortable distance between two objects as compared to a simile that allows some space. For example, "War is hell" is a strong metaphor that is immediately understandable. A simile version would be "War is like hell," which loses the impact of the metaphor and opens up the option that war could also be like many other things such as a game. Metaphors are more than words and figures of speech. In their landmark book, *Metaphors We Live By*, Lakoff and Johnson (1980) argued that metaphors are not mere poetical or rhetorical embellishments to language, but are a part of everyday speech that affects the ways in which we perceive, think, and act. Metaphors define and shape realities. It is worthwhile to quote Lakoff and Johnson in full to set the stage for the focus on the metaphors in the Legacy contributors' work.

> The concepts that govern our thought are not just matters of the intellect. They also govern our everyday functioning, down to the most mundane details. Our concepts structure what we perceive, how we get around in the world, and how we relate to people. Our conceptual system thus plays a central role in defining everyday realities. If we are right in suggesting that our conceptual system is largely metaphorical, then the way we think, what we experience, and what we do every day is very much a matter of metaphors (p.3).

But, we are largely unaware of our conceptual system. We function on a sort of "auto-pilot," thinking and acting automatically along certain lines. By purposefully looking at language, we can see that our ordinary conceptual system is metaphorical in nature. The language of the Legacy contributors is in many ways remarkably similar as they describe what they have been through in their personal and professional lives as well as the kind of scholarly work that has attracted their interest and passion. I will identify and briefly discuss the major metaphors that I noticed through these many readings of the contributors' work.

The Journey Metaphor

The first metaphor that shapes each of the contributors' papers is the "life is a journey" metaphor. To be fair, the journey metaphor was imposed on the contributors from the beginning of the project by Dr. Ellenchild Pinch and me. We wanted each contributor to critically reflect on her body of work in nursing ethics within the context of her experience as a nurse. Furthermore, we wanted the contributors to evaluate the impact their work has had in nursing, ethics, and health care and indicate future directions for scholarship in nursing ethics. The fact that we asked the nurse ethicists themselves to reflect on their body of work and what it means rather than enlisting objective others to do so is what makes this book and the perspectives therein unique. As Jonsen (1998) explains in the preface of *The Birth of Bioethics,* "The biographies of the pioneer bioethicists and the birth of bioethics are entwined. Turns in personal careers move with events in the surrounding world of medicine and science and morality; the events are analyzed through the eyes of persons whose academic careers educated them to see those events in a certain way (p.viii)." So, not only is the journey of these nurse ethicists described, the tale is told through the eyes of those who traveled it. Furthermore, the personal careers of the nurses in this book moved not only with events in the wider world but those closer to home such as interactions with the patients and families for whom they cared.

We chose the general term "legacy" to describe the project and the image of the Roman god Janus to depict what we asked the contributors to do, i.e., look backward and forward at their life's work. Of course, since all of the contributors were women, we found a more androgynous version of Janus to use as our logo rather than the traditional bearded representations. Janus is the Roman god of all beginnings, gates and doors, endings and transitions (Johnson, 2004). Statues and drawings of Janus show the god double-faced with each face looking in opposite directions, a rare and difficult skill. The contributors were asked to apply this forward and backward view to their own work. Thus, as editors we set the contributors off on a journey to explore their pasts and see where the road took them.

One aspect of the journey metaphor that was particularly interesting was what the contributors took with them or carried on their journeys and what they discarded along the way. Many of them acknowledged specific people, mentors or experiences that inculcated values early in their work as nurses that they held throughout their careers. Several took a turn in their professional development to seek further education from another discipline outside of nursing in order to accomplish the tasks they felt were important or to answer the questions that puzzled or intrigued them. Speaking of questions, many of the contributors carried the same question forward through much of their work even though they might have asked the question of different populations or in different practice settings.

The journey metaphor also refers to a direction or path in life toward deeper understanding. Lorde (1997) uses the journey metaphor repeatedly in her work describing her struggle with breast cancer. Although certainly not the life-threatening experience that Lorde wrote about, the contributors were asked to complete the difficult task of life review, which is a sort of journey. As Lorde challenges,

> I am talking about the need for every woman to live a considered life. The necessity for that consideration grows and deepens as one faces directly one's own mortality and death. Self scrutiny and an evaluation of our lives, while painful, can be rewarding and strengthening journeys toward a deeper self (p. 59).

Although none of the contributors described the writing and reflection that it took as "painful," I think they all expressed how hard this task was to accomplish, i.e., to make meaning out of the various twists and turns of their lives. Many of the contributors began the account of their journey by describing why they became nurses in the first place although they were not specifically asked to start at that place. Some went back even further in their lives to describe a childhood experience that was significant to their path to nursing. The journey metaphor gives permission to figure out what is important on the trip. In the contributions, we have evidence of the intersections of many of the contributors' life paths, detours, and roads not taken. Many of the contributors expressed surprise and pleasure at seeing how everything fit together in a pattern that was not evident before writing these papers. Thus, the journey was not only personally worthwhile but provides readers with critical self-reflection on personal and professional development rarely found in the nursing literature on this scale.

The "Finding My Place" Metaphor

The "finding my place" metaphor is the second major metaphor that runs through all of the contributors' essays. During their journeys, the contributors frequently mentioned that they struggled to find their place in the broader world of ethics in health care. Many expressed frustration at the lack of a place for nurses at the table, another metaphor, where the real decisions are made. There was also considerable discussion about the place of ethics in the work of nurses and the meaning to the nursing profession. What does this say about contemporary nursing ethics and these nurse ethicists? The kinds of issues and ethical concerns the contributors wrote about are those experienced from their place within health care and society. From this place, whether it is "in the middle" or "at the margins" or mediating between conflicting obligations, it is always one where issues of power and powerlessness, voice and interconnectedness are central and reflect the major themes of feminist perspectives in ethics.

There is more than one use of the finding my place metaphor in the essays as prior to asking the contributors to join the Legacy project, Dr. Pinch and I chose to organize the large volume of past scholarly publications by the contributors into eight themes and placed each contribution into one of the themes. Several of the contributors did not agree with their place in a particular theme. Some persisted to the end that their work certainly belonged in more than one category. We agree. The designation of various contributors to the eight themes was not arbitrary, but we did realize the contextual nature of all of the pieces and recognized the interrelationships of the themes and the contributors' work. The eight themes are evident, to one degree or another, in all of the contributions, often overlapping with no one piece fitting neatly into only one theme.

The Planting for the Future Metaphor

The last metaphor I will mention, although there are certainly others to be found in the contributors' essays, is one of planting the seeds for the future of the profession and work in ethics. For example, the Legacy participants nurtured a veritable legion of undergraduate and graduate nursing students, established guidelines, position statements, and contributed to the development of the Code of Ethics, all of which contributes to the care of the field now and for future generations of nurses, the profession, and the public. Many contributors expressed the hope that others will take on research questions they dealt with and build on the findings or insights from their work to deal with developing issues in health care. All of the contributors were modest about what their work has meant or might mean yet there was a sense of hopefulness in their essays that the work will be cultivated and nurtured by others. The Legacy project is clearly fertile ground for growing novel ideas, branching off into new directions of scholarship and sustaining projects with deep roots. All the contributors share a passion for their profession. Readers are invited into the ongoing discussion and are encouraged to take a look backward and forward in their own professional lives.

References

Johnson, Sarah Isles (Ed.) (2004). *Religions of the ancient world: A guide.* Harvard University Press Reference Library. Cambridge, MA: Belknap Press.

Jonsen, A.R. (1998). *The birth of bioethics.* New York: Oxford University Press.

Lakoff, G. & Johnson, M. (1980). *Metaphors we live by.* Chicago: University of Chicago Press.

Lorde, A. (1997). *The cancer journals.* San Francisco: Aunt Lute Books.

Amy M. Haddad, BSN, MSN, PhD, is Director of the Center for Health Policy and Ethics and Dr. C.C. and Mabel L. Criss Endowed Chair in Health Sciences at Creighton University, Omaha, Nebraska. Dr. Haddad is a nationally known expert in ethics education, providing leadership in the development of novel methods to shape ethically competent and committed health professionals. She has been teaching ethics in Creighton University's Schools of Pharmacy and Health Professions, Nursing and Medicine since 1984. Dr. Haddad's recent honors include being named a Carnegie Scholar by the Carnegie Center for the Advancement of the Scholarship of Teaching in 2001. Dr. Haddad was the recipient of the 2003 Robert K. Chalmers Distinguished Pharmacy Educator Award from the American Association of Colleges of Pharmacy (AACP). She received the Pellegrino Medal from the Healthcare Ethics and Law Institute of Samford University in 2007.

Contributor Biographies

Mila Ann Aroskar, retired Associate Professor, School of Public Health Adjunct Associate Professor, School of Nursing, is an emeritus Faculty Associate, Center for Bioethics, University of Minnesota, Minneapolis, MN. She is a graduate of the College of Wooster (BA); Columbia University School of Nursing (BS); Teachers College, Columbia University (MEd); State University of New York at Buffalo (EdD), and has an honorary DSc from Creighton University. Her career in bioethics and professional ethics spanned three decades in nursing, patient care, healthcare administration, public health, and health policy.

Laurie Badzek, RN, MS, JD, LLM, is currently Director for the American Nurses Association Center of Ethics and Human Rights, a role in which she previously served from 1998–1999. During that time, Badzek was instrumental in developing a plan that ultimately resulted in the approval of a new Code of Ethics for Nurses by the 2001 House of Delegates. Currently a tenured, full professor at the West Virginia University School of Nursing, Badzek, a nurse attorney, teaches nursing, ethics, law and health policy. Having practiced in a variety of nursing and law positions, she is an active researcher, investigating ethical and legal health care issues. Her current research interests include patient and family decision making, nutraceutical use, mature minors and professional healthcare ethics. Her research has been published in nursing, medical and communication studies journals including the *Journal of Nursing Law, Nephrology Nursing Journal,* the *Annals of Internal Medicine, Journal of Palliative Care,* and *Health Communication.*

Anne H. Bishop is Professor of Nursing Emerita, Lynchburg College in Virginia. She is a graduate of the University of Virginia (BSN, MSN, EdD). She has been writing on nursing as practice and nursing ethics since the early 1980s. She has co-authored books, articles, and presentations with John R. Scudder, Jr., Emeritus Professor of Philosophy, Lynchburg College in Virginia.

Leah L. Curtin, Clinical Professor of Nursing at the University of Cincinnati College of Nursing and Health, is a managing partner in Metier Consultants. A graduate of the University of Cincinnati (BS and MS), and the Athenaeum of Ohio (MA), she was awarded two honorary doctorates: one from the State University of New York at Utica for her work in ethics and one from the Medical College of Ohio for humanitarian services following the publication of her work on the impact of war on children. A Fellow of the American Academy of Nursing since 1982, Curtin's interest in ethics arose out of her experiences in clinical practice and its intersections with social justice, workplace environment—particularly autonomous decision-making for nurses—and the impact of laws and social and/or institutional policies on patients and nursing practice.

Patricia D'Antonio, RN, PhD, FAAN is an Associate Professor of Nursing, the Associate Director of the Barbara Bates Center for the Study of the History of Nursing, University of Pennsylvania, and a Fellow of the American Academy of Nursing. She is also the editor of the *Nursing History Review,* the official journal of the American Association for the History of Nursing. She received her BS from Boston College, her MSN from the Catholic University of America, and her PhD from the University of Pennsylvania. Her clinical background includes specialization in psychiatric nursing; her research focuses on the history of psychiatry and psychiatric nursing, and 19th and early 20th century nursing and health care.

Anne J. Davis is a Professor Emerita, retired, from the University of California, San Francisco. Her career at UCSF spanned 34 years. Beginning in 1962, Dr. Davis's teaching experience took on an international component with appointments in Israel, Japan, Korea, and Taiwan. These rich experiences led to the development of her overriding interest in cultural diversity and nursing ethics. She is a graduate of Emory University, Atlanta (BS, Nursing), Boston University (MS, Psychiatry), and University of California, Berkeley (PhD, Higher Education). Dr. Davis has been the recipient of numerous awards including an honorary Doctor of Science from Emory University and election as a Fellow in the American Academy of Nursing.

Cortney Davis, an Adult Nurse Practitioner currently working in Sacred Heart University in Fairfield, CT., is the author of three poetry collections, most recently *Leopold's Maneuvers* (University of Nebraska Press, 2004), winner of the Prairie Schooner Poetry Prize and of the *American Journal of Nursing* Book of the Year

Award. Her memoir, *The Experience of the Female Body,* was published by Random House in 2001 and won the Center for the Book Nonfiction Award. She is coeditor of two anthologies of poetry and prose by nurses, *Between the Heartbeats* and *Intensive Care* (University of Iowa Press, 1994 and 2003). Her essay collection, *The Heart's Truth: Essays about the Art of Nursing,* is forthcoming in 2009 from Kent State University Press. Recipient of an NEA Poetry Fellowship and three Connecticut Commission on the Arts Poetry Grants, She lives in Redding, CT and holds a BA and MA in English Literature in addition to her nursing credentials.

Judith A. Erlen, Professor and PhD Program Coordinator, School of Nursing, also holds a secondary appointment in the Center for Bioethics and Health Law at the University of Pittsburgh, Pittsburgh, PA. She is the Associate Director of the Center for Research in Chronic Disorders in the School of Nursing, as well as the Director of the Center's Research Development Core. She received a Bachelor of Science in Nursing from the University of Pittsburgh, a Master of Science in Nursing from Wayne State University, and a PhD in Nursing from the Texas Women's University. Ethics in nursing and healthcare has been a focus of her research and teaching since the late 1970s. Her work centers on powerlessness in relation to the nurse's role in affecting ethical decisions, respect for persons and its relationship to vulnerable populations, and quality of life.

Marsha D. M. Fowler, Senior Fellow and Professor of Ethics, Spirituality, and Faith Integration, Azusa Pacific University. She is a graduate of Kaiser Foundation School of Nursing (diploma), University of California at San Francisco (BS, MS), Fuller Theological Seminary (MDiv) and the University of Southern California (PhD). She has engaged in teaching and research in bioethics and spirituality since 1974. Her research interests are in the history and development of nursing's ethics and the Code of Ethics for Nurses, social ethics and professions, suffering, the intersections of spirituality and ethics, and religious ethics in nursing.

Sara T. Fry, BS, MS, MA, PhD, RN, is former Henry R. Luce Professor of Nursing Ethics at the Boston College School of Nursing, Chestnut Hill, MA. Her education includes degrees at Georgetown University (MA and PhD in philosophy), University of North Carolina, Chapel Hill (MS), University of South Carolina, Columbia (BS) and The Johns Hopkins Hospital School of Nursing. She is co-author with Dr. Robert Veatch of *Case Studies in Nursing Ethics.* Dr. Fry's role in nursing ethics covers a broad spectrum of experiences and contributions to the field including but not limited to funded and unfunded research projects, consultations and other professional services, editorial and scholarly review functions, positions in various professional organizations and committees, presentations and publications (books, book chapters, journal articles, reviews, and letters).

Amy M. Haddad, BSN, MSN, PhD, is Director of the Center for Health Policy and Ethics and Dr. C.C. and Mabel L. Criss Endowed Chair in Health Sciences at Creighton University, Omaha, Nebraska. Dr. Haddad is a nationally known expert in ethics education, providing leadership in the development of novel methods to shape ethically competent and committed health professionals. She has been teaching ethics in Creighton University's Schools of Pharmacy and Health Professions, Nursing and Medicine since 1984. Dr. Haddad's recent honors include being named a Carnegie Scholar by the Carnegie Center for the Advancement of the Scholarship of Teaching in 2001. Dr. Haddad was the recipient of the 2003 Robert K. Chalmers Distinguished Pharmacy Educator Award from the American Association of Colleges of Pharmacy (AACP). She received the Pellegrino Medal from the Healthcare Ethics and Law Institute of Samford University in 2007.

Shaké Ketefian is Professor of Nursing at the University of Michigan School of Nursing. She is a graduate of the American University of Beirut (BS), and Teachers College, Columbia University (MEd, EdD). Her areas of teaching have been research in nursing ethics, research methods, and scientific integrity. Her scholarship has dealt with international doctoral education, international nursing, ethical decision-making, and scientific integrity. She has conducted several meta-analytic studies of research within nursing ethics.

Joan Liaschenko, MA, MS, RN, PhD, FAAN, is originally from Philadelphia where she completed basic nursing studies and obtained a BS from Hahnemann University and an MA from Bryn Mawr College. She migrated west where she obtained an MS, PhD, and completed a postdoctoral fellowship at the University of California, San Francisco. She joined the University of Minnesota Faculty in January of 2001 where she is jointly appointed in the Center for Bioethics and the School of Nursing. Both her research and teaching are largely informed by feminist scholarship. She teaches masters and doctoral students in the School of Nursing, which is noteworthy for their commitment to ethics education, requiring ethics at all educational levels: baccalaureate, masters, and doctoral. Through the Center for Bioethics, she has taught courses on 'The Social Construction of Health and Illness' and 'Stories of Illness,' a course that relies primarily on the writings of ill people. Her major research interest is the morality of nursing work, specifically, the ways in which the context of the work shapes nurses' moral concerns, the language they use to articulate them, and how they seek to resolve them. She has studied home care, intensive care units, and psychiatric nurses as well as nurses who run biomedical clinical trials. She has published widely and has been a visiting scholar in Australia, Canada, Germany, Japan, Turkey, and upcoming, New Zealand. She holds adjunct faculty appointments at the Universities of Toronto and Calgary.

Beverly J. McElmurry is Professor, Public Health Nursing, and Associate Dean, Global Leadership, University of Illinois at Chicago. She is a graduate of the University of Minnesota at Minneapolis (BS, MEd) and Northern Illinois University (EdD). Women's health, nursing ethics, and community-based primary health care have been enduring areas of interest throughout her academic career. As a long term Director of the UIC WHO Collaborating Center for International Nursing Development of Primary Health Care, she has had extensive opportunities to work with international colleagues and students to strengthen nursing's contribution to global health and development.

Pamela A. Miya is Director, Program Services, March of Dimes, Nebraska Chapter. She recently accepted this position after 30 years as a faculty member in the College of Nursing, University of Nebraska Medical Center, where she served as an Associate Professor. Teaching responsibilities included both undergraduate and graduate courses centering on maternal-newborn nursing and women's health. Research interests focused on ethical issues confronting nurses in a variety of clinical settings. She is a graduate of Purdue University (AAS and BSN), Indiana University (MSN), and the University of Nebraska (PhD). She is serving as Chair of the ANA's Advisory Board, Center for Ethics and Human Rights (2006–2008).

Catherine P. Murphy, RN, EdD, was born in New York City. She received her diploma in nursing from St. Clares Hospital School of Nursing in N.Y. and her baccalaureate degree in nursing from Teachers College, Columbia University. She received her MS degree in nursing from Hunter College of the City University of the State of New York and her EdD from Teachers College, Columbia University. During the course of her career she served in the positions of staff nurse, charge nurse, and clinical director in nursing service. In academia she served in the roles of faculty member, department chairperson, director of the graduate program, and dean of the school of nursing. In recognition of her contributions to nursing ethics, she has received numerous awards among them the ANA Honorary Membership Award, the Teachers College Distinguished Achievement Award for Scholarship and Research, Inaugural Inductee to the Teachers College Hall of Fame, and the Massachusetts Nurses Association Award for Excellence in Teaching. She is retired and resides in Rhode Island on Apponaug Cove with a breathtaking view overlooking Narragansett Bay.

Joy H. Penticuff is the Lee and Joseph Jamail Professor of Nursing at the University of Texas at Austin School of Nursing. She holds an MSN in Pediatric Nursing and a PhD in Clinical Psychology from Case Western Reserve University and a Bachelor of Science in Nursing from The Medical College of Georgia. Dr. Penticuff's work in bioethics began in 1981 when she attended the Intensive Bioethics Course at the Kennedy Institute of Ethics. In 1983 she was a Visiting Scholar at the Hastings Center in New York and in 1989–90 she was Senior Fellow at the Center for Ethics, Medicine, and Public Issues at Baylor College of Medicine, Houston, Texas. Special interests include empirical ethics research, parent-professional collaboration in treatment decisions for extremely premature infants, and supportive communication of "bad news."

Winifred J. Ellenchild Pinch, Professor Emerita School of Nursing, is a faculty member at the Center for Health Policy and Ethics, Creighton University. She is a graduate of Temple University (BS), State University of New York at Buffalo (MEd), Creighton University (MS), and Boston University (EdD). Bioethics has been a focus of her teaching and research since 1976, beginning with her doctoral program. Special interests include ethical decision making by parents in the neonatal intensive care unit, feminist perspectives in bioethics, and reproductive issues.

Shireen S. Rajaram is a Professor of Sociology at the University of Nebraska at Omaha (UNO). She is the chair of the Department of Sociology and Anthropology at UNO. She has a courtesy joint-appointment with the College of Public Health at the University of Nebraska Medical Center. She is a member of the Women's Studies, Latino and Latin American Studies, and Environmental Studies programs at UNO. She received her PhD in Medical Sociology from the University of Kentucky and has a Certificate in Medical Behavioral Science from the Department of Behavioral Sciences at the University of Kentucky. Her main areas of interest are women's health, minority health, and environmental health. She has done research in breast and cervical cancer, diabetes, and childhood lead poisoning. She has published extensively in journals such as *Women and Health, Health Care for Women International, Preventive Medicine,* and *Sociology of Health and Illness.* She teaches graduate and undergraduate classes on Women's Health, Ethnicity and Health, and Society and Health.

Warren T. Reich, regarded throughout the world as a founding figure in the field of Bioethics, is Distinguished Research Professor of Religion and Ethics in the Theology Department of Georgetown University, and Professor Emeritus of Bioethics in the Department of Family Medicine at Georgetown. He is currently Director of the Project for the History of Care. Funded by the Lilly Endowment, this Project is examining the history of a full range of ideas and practices of care in the Western world. Dr. Reich was a founding member of Georgetown's Kennedy Institute of Ethics and originated and edited the first two editions of the *Encyclopedia of Bioethics.* He was also the founder and, for twenty years, director of the clinical bioethics and medical humanities program in the Georgetown University Medical Center, one of the world's first comprehensive programs of this kind in an academic medical center. Dr. Reich is the recipient of numerous national and international awards for his contributions to bioethics, especially the ethics of care. Although he taught moral theology principally at the Catholic University of America, he has been a Fellow or Visiting Professor both in the U.S. and abroad. Dr. Reich is currently writing a book on *The Idea of Care: A History and Analysis* and is editing (with Jonathan Riley-Smith as co-editor) a book on *Chivalry and Care.*

Marie Simone Roach, CSM, PhD was born in Scotchtown, on the outskirts of New Waterford, Cape Breton, Nova Scotia. She did primary education there before entering a diploma program in Nursing at St. Joseph's Hospital, Glace Bay, NS, graduating in 1944. She entered the Sisters of St. Martha, Antigonish, NS in 1945. Engaged in health care ministry, she obtained a BSc in Nursing at St. Francis Xavier University, Antigonish; a Masters in Nursing Education Administration at Boston University, and a PhD in Education from The Catholic University of America with a major in Philosophical Foundations. She did further study in ethics in a post-doctoral fellowship at Harvard Divinity School, and a year as Reader at Regis College, Toronto School of Theology for further research and writing on the Ontology of Human Caring, a focus of her professional research and writing. Her studies in ethics were grounded in this research. She is presently engaged in study and writing in the area of Transformative Suffering using the spiritual journey of her own biography as context.

Cynda H. Rushton, PhD, RN, FAAN is an associate professor at the Johns Hopkins University School of Nursing (JHUSON) and program director of Johns Hopkins Harriet Lane Compassionate Care Program. She is a graduate of Catholic University of America (PhD), Medical University of South Carolina (MSN), and University of Kentucky (BSN). Throughout her career, Rushton has participated in national initiatives, delivered testimony to Congress, and collaborated with professional organizations to create better systems of pediatric palliative care and to see her vision for improving care at the end of life become a reality. Rushton was instrumental in creating the Harriet Lane Compassionate Care Program, the first pediatric palliative care program in Maryland. She has served as Program Director since 2000, working closely with other team members to create a 70-member interdisciplinary palliative care network, establish innovative educational programs, create a comprehensive bereavement program for families and health care professionals, and develop support systems for health care professionals who care for these children. Dr. Rushton is a frequent national and international speaker and has provided leadership and service to a variety of professional associations and societies, health care institutions, and policy agencies. In 2001 she received the American Association of Critical-Care Nurses Pioneering Spirit Award for her work in advancing palliative care across the life-span. She was selected as one of 20 Robert Wood Johnson Nurse Executive Fellows in 2006.

M. Colleen Scanlon, RN, JD is Senior Vice President, Advocacy at Catholic Health Initiatives in Denver, Colorado. In this role, she has the responsibility for directing the development and integration of a comprehensive advocacy program within one of the largest Catholic health care systems in the country. Prior to this, she was the Director of the American Nurses Association Center for Ethics and Human Rights in Washington, DC and served as a Clinical Scholar in the Center for Clinical Bioethics at Georgetown University Medical Center. Colleen received her BSN from Georgetown University, an MS in Gerontology from the College of New Rochelle and a JD with a health law and policy certificate from Pace University School of Law. Special interests include palliative care ethics, advocacy on behalf of vulnerable persons, and professional and organizational integrity.

John (Jack) R. Scudder, Jr. is Professor of Philosophy Emeritus, Lynchburg College in Virginia. He is a graduate of Vanderbilt University (BA), University of Alabama (MA), and Duke University (EdD). At the time he began working with Anne Bishop, he had been interpreting philosophy of education from a phenomenological perspective. Anne recognized possibilities for interpreting nursing phenomenologically. They have been thinking and writing together since the early 1980s.

Sarah E. Shannon is an Associate Professor in the Department of Biobehavioral Nursing and Health Systems, School of Nursing, and Adjunct in Department of Medical History and Ethics, School of Medicine, at the University of Washington in Seattle. She is a graduate of the University of Arizona (BSN) and University of Washington (PhD and MS). Her research focus has been primarily in improving the care of dying ICU patients through improving team communication around end-of-life decision-making with patients and their families. More recently she has collaborated on looking at team disclosure of medical errors to patients. Dr. Shannon's teaching and service has also been focused in bioethics.

Mary Cipriano Silva received her BSN and MS from Ohio State University and her PhD from the University of Maryland. Her interest in bioethics spans several decades, and her scholarship on ethics focuses on informed consent, administrative ethics, and ethical guidelines. She is a Professor Emerita in nursing from George Mason University, Fairfax, Virginia.

Anita J. Tarzian received her PhD in Nursing and Ethics from the University of Maryland School of Nursing in 1998. Prior to that, she earned a Master's degree in Intercultural Nursing from the University of Maryland, a Bachelor of Science in Nursing from Rush University in Chicago, and a Bachelor of Arts from Knox College in Galesburg, IL. Her experiences as a staff nurse in a tertiary care medical center and also during a two-year stint in the Dominican Republic with the United States Peace Corps, deepened her appreciation of both the blessings and burdens of technology, the influence of culture on health care decision-making and behavior, and sources of disparities in health care access. Dr. Tarzian is an independent ethics and research consultant, with affiliations at the Schools of Law and Nursing at the University of Maryland, Baltimore. Her professional energies have been directed toward a diverse range of activities in health care, including ethics consultation, end-of-life care/hospice, palliative care, research ethics, and multiculturalism. She is Program Coordinator of the Maryland Healthcare Ethics Committee Network and Co-Chair of Chesapeake Research Review, Inc.'s Institutional Review Board. Her research and scholarly work has been published in peer-reviewed journals, and she has given professional presentations and invited lectures in the United States and abroad.

Carol Rae Taylor is a faculty member of the Georgetown University School of Nursing and Health Studies and Director of the Georgetown University Center for Clinical Bioethics. She is a graduate of Holy Family University (BSN), the Catholic University of America (MSN), and Georgetown University (PhD in Philosophy with a concentration in bioethics). Bioethics has been a focus of her teaching and research since 1980 linked to her passion to "make health care work" for those who need it. Special interests include health care decision-making and professional ethics.

Joyce E. Beebe Thompson, RN, CNM, DrPH, FAAN, FACNM is currently the Lacey Professor of Community Health Nursing at the Bronson School of Nursing, Western Michigan University, and Professor Emerita of Nursing at the University of Pennsylvania. She is a graduate of the University of Michigan (BSN, MPH), Maternity Center Association (CNM) and Columbia University (DrPH). In 1983 she completed the Intensive Bioethics Course at the Kennedy Institute of Ethics, Georgetown University. She has taught health care ethics since 1975 at Columbia, Penn, and in Japan, sub-Saharan Africa, and Latin America. Most of her ethics teaching and writing was with Rev. Dr. Henry O. Thompson until his death in 1997. She continues to write and teach ethics in the relatively new PhD program in Interdisciplinary Health Studies at WMU and within the community-based BSN and MSN programs. Her particular interest in health care ethics is helping professionals make ethical decisions in practice, informed by understanding the importance of values and moral development on decision-making. She has also contributed to the revision of the ANA code and development of the first codes of ethics for the American College of Nurse-Midwives and the International Confederation of Midwives. Her life passion is helping girls and women of the world be viewed as fully human, as persons, with full human rights.

Gladys B. White is an adjunct faculty member at Georgetown University, University of Maryland University College, and Montgomery College. She teaches bioethics, workplace ethics and philosophy at these three institutions. She is a graduate of Duke University (BSN), Catholic University of America (MSN), and Georgetown University (PhD in philosophy). Bioethics has been the focus of her work since 1985. Special interests include reprogenetics, access to health care, and ethical issues in the professions.

Mary Ellen Wurzbach is a Professor of Nursing at the University of Wisconsin-Oshkosh, where she was recently named a Triss Endowed Professor. She is a graduate of the University of Wisconsin-Oshkosh (BSN), University of Wisconsin-Oshkosh (MSN), and the University of Minnesota (PhD). Bioethics has been the focus of her teaching and research since 1980, beginning with her graduation from the Primary Health Care Nursing Masters Program at UW-Oshkosh. Special interests include the role moral conviction plays in nurses' ethical decision-making, comfort as an ethical principle utilized by nurses to make ethical decisions, and moral theory and philosophy.

APPENDIX A

American Nurses Association Code of Ethics for Nurses

1. The nurse, in all professional relationships, practices with compassion and respect for inherent dignity, worth, and uniqueness of every individual, unrestricted by considerations of social or economic status, personal attributes, or the nature of health problems.

2. The nurse's primary commitment is to the patient, whether an individual, family group, or community.

3. The nurse promotes, advocates for, and strives to protect the health, safety, and rights of the patient.

4. The nurse is responsible and accountable for individual nursing practice and determines the appropriate delegation of tasks consistent with the nurse's obligation to provide optimum patient care.

5. The nurse owes the same duties to self as to others, including the responsibility to preserve integrity and safety, to maintain competence, and to continue personal and professional growth.

6. The nurse participates in establishing, maintaining, and improving health care environments and conditions of employment conducive to the provision of quality health care and consistent with the values of the profession through individual and collective action.

7. The nurse participates in the advancement of the profession through contributions to practice, education, administration, and knowledge development.

8. The nurse collaborates with other health professionals and the public in promoting community, national, and international efforts to meet health needs.

9. The profession of nursing, as represented by associations and their members, is responsible for articulating nursing values, for maintaining the integrity of the profession and its practice, and for shaping social policy.

From: American Nurses Association. (2001). *Code of ethics for nurses with interpretive statements.* Silver Spring, MD: Nursesbooks.org, p. 2. Used with permission.

(For online access: Go to http://www.nursingworld.org for ANA home page. Click on "Professional Nursing Practice," next on "Ethics and Standards," and then on "Code of Ethics for Nurses." *Code of Ethics for Nurses with Interpretive Statements* is available as a view-only file.)

APPENDIX B

The Evolution of Nursing's Code of Ethics

Whatever the version of the Code, it has always been fundamentally concerned with the principles of doing no harm, of benefiting others, of loyalty, and of truthfulness. As well, the Code has been concerned with social justice and, in later versions, with the changing context of health care as well as the autonomy of the patient and the nurse.

1893   The "Nightingale Pledge," patterned after medicine's Hippocratic Oath, is understood as the first nursing code of ethics.

1896   The Nurses' Associated Alumnae of the United States and Canada (later to become the American Nurses Association), whose first purpose was to establish and maintain a code of ethics.

1926   "A Suggested Code" is provisionally adopted and published in the *American Journal of Nursing (AJN)* but is never formally adopted.

1940   "A Tentative Code" is published in the *American Journal of Nursing*, but also is never formally adopted.

1950   The Code for Professional Nurses, in the form of 17 provisions that are a substantive revision of the "Tentative Code" of 1940, is unanimously accepted by the ANA House of Delegates.

1956   The Code for Professional Nurses is amended.

1960   The Code for Professional Nurses is revised.

1968   The Code for Professional Nurses is substantively revised, condensing the 17 provisions of the 1960 Code into 10 provisions.

1976   The *Code for Nurses with Interpretive Statements,* a modification of the provisions and interpretive statements, is published as 11 provisions.

1985   The *Code for Nurses with Interpretive Statements* retains the provisions of the 1976 version and includes revised interpretive statements.

2001   The *Code of Ethics for Nurses with Interpretive Statements* is accepted by the ANA House of Delegates.

From: American Nurses Association. (2001). *Code of ethics for nurses with interpretive statements.* Silver Spring, MD: Nursesbooks.org, p. 27. Used with permission.

APPENDIX C

ANA Center for Ethics and Human Rights Mission Statement

The Center is committed to addressing the complex ethical and human rights issues confronting nurses, and designing activities and programs to increase the ethical competence and human rights sensitivity of nurses. Through the Center, ANA's abiding commitment to the human rights dimensions of health care is demonstrated.

Background

In September 1990, the Center for Ethics and Human Rights was established with the following guiding objectives:

- *Promulgate* in collaboration with ANA constituents, a body of knowledge, both theoretical and practical, designed to address issues in ethics and human rights at the state, national, and international level;

- *Develop and disseminate* information about and advocate for public policy to assure that ethics and human rights are addressed in health care; and

- *Assure* that short- and long-range objectives regarding ethics and human rights will be addressed within the Association, and expressed to appropriate bodies external to the Association.

The Center continues to advance these originating goals and has become respected as an authority within the nursing community. The Center remains responsive to the changing realities within health care and the nursing profession, and is committed to addressing professional, ethical, and human rights challenges and ultimately to improving the quality of care rendered to patients and their families.

To access this site, go to www.http://nursingworld.org for ANA home page. Click on "Professional Nursing Practice" and select "Ethics and Standards." In left column, click on "Center for Ethics and Human Rights." Used with permission.

APPENDIX D

Selected Bioethics Resources on the Web

American Journal of Bioethics
http://www.bioethics.net/

American Nurses Association Center for Ethics and Human Rights
http://nursingworld.org/ (Follow path: Professional Nursing Practice > Ethics and Standards > Center for Ethics and Human Rights)

American Society for Bioethics and Humanities
http://www.asbh.org/

Barbara Bates Center for the Study of Nursing History
http://www.nursing.upenn.edu/history/

Center for Health Policy and Ethics, Creighton University
http://chpe.creighton.edu/

The Hastings Center
http://www.thehastingscenter.org/

International Centre for Nursing Ethics
http://www.nursing-ethics.org/

The Journal of Clinical Ethics
http://www.clinicalethics.com/

National Human Genome Research Institute, National Institutes of Health
http://www.genome.gov/

National Institutes of Health, Clinical Center, Department of Bioethics
http://www.bioethics.nih.gov/

National Reference Center for Bioethics Literature, Kennedy Institute
http://bioethics.georgetown.edu/

Nursing Ethics: An International Journal for Health Care Professionals
http://www.nursing-ethics.com/

Index